Fluids&Electrolytes

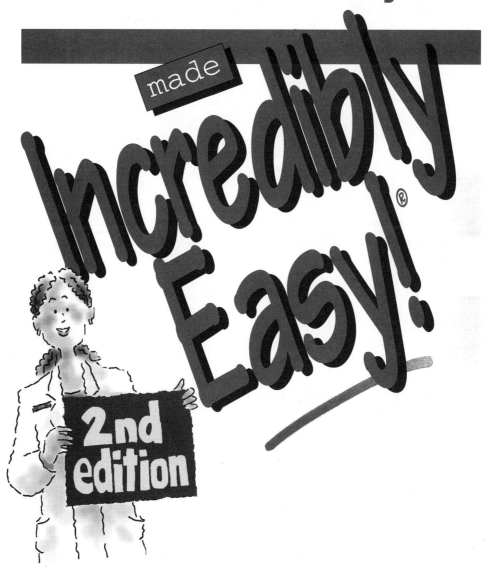

made

Incredibly

Easy!®

2nd edition

Springhouse
Springhouse, Pennsylvania

Staff

Publisher
Judith A. Schilling McCann, RN, MSN

Executive Editor
Kate Jackson

Clinical Manager
Joan M. Robinson, RN, MSN, CCRN

Clinical Editors
Collette Bishop Hendler, RN, CCRN,
(clinical project manager),
Beverly Ann Tscheschlog, RN

Editors
Brenna H. Mayer (senior associate editor),
Ty Eggenberger, Stacey Ann Follin,
Kirk Robinson

Copy Editors
Jaime L. Stockslager (supervisor),
Virginia Baskerville, Kimberly Bilotta,
Tom DeZego, Heather Ditch,
Amy Furman, Fruma Klass, Marcia Ryan,
Pamela Wingrod, Helen Winton

Designers
Arlene Putterman (associate design
director), Mary Ludwicki (art director),
Lynn Foulk

Illustrators
Scott Thorn Barrows, Barbara Cousins,
John Cymerman, Mark Lefkowitz,
Judy Newhouse, Bot Roda, Mary Stangl,
Nina Wallace, Larry Ward

Electronic Production Services
Diane Paluba (manager), Joyce Rossi Biletz

Manufacturing
Patricia K. Dorshaw (manager), Otto Mezei
(book production manager)

Projects Coordinator
Liz Schaeffer

Editorial Assistants
Beverly Lane, Beth Janae Orr,
Elfriede Young

Indexer
Barbara Hodgson

Printed in the United States of America.

IEF&E2 – D N O S A J J M A M
03   10 9 8 7 6 5 4

Library of Congress Cataloging-in-Publication Data

Fluids & electrolytes made incredibly easy.—
2nd ed.
    p. ; cm.
    Includes index.
    1. Water-electrolyte imbalances. 2. Body fluid
    disorders. I. Titles: Fluids and
    electrolytes made incredibly easy. II.
    Springhouse Corporation.
    [DNLM: 1. Water-Electrolyte Imbalance—
    Nurses' Instruction. 2. Water-Electrolyte
    Balance—Nurses' Instruction. WD 220 F6462
    2001]
RC630 .F596 2001
616.3'99s—dc21   2001020925
ISBN 1-58255-136-7 (alk. paper)

Contents

Contributors and consultants

Cheryl A. Westlake Canary, RN, PhD, CS
Assistant Professor
California State University
Fullerton

Peggi Guenter, RN, PhD, CNSN
Editor-in-Chief
Nutrition in Clinical Practice
American Society for Parenteral and
  Enteral Nutrition
Silver Spring, Md.

Gayla H. Love, RN, BSN, CCM
Case Manager
Blue Cross-Blue Shield of Georgia
Atlanta

Georgia McCoy O'Neal, RN, MSN
Nursing Instructor
Jefferson State Community College
Birmingham, Ala.

Anne Marie Palatnik, RN, MSN, CS
Clinical Nurse Specialist—Adult Services
Our Lady of Lourdes Medical Center
Camden, N.J.

Janet L. Parker, RN,CS, MSN, CCP, FNP
Clinical Perfusionist
Deborah Heart and Lung Center
Browns Mills, N.J.

Janet A. Rudolph, RN, MSN
Nursing Instructor
Brandywine School of Nursing
Coatesville, Pa.

Bruce Austin Scott, RN, MSN, CS
Nursing Instructor
San Joaquin Delta College
Stockton, Calif.

Allison Squires, RN,C, MSN
Clinical Development Specialist
Lewistown (Pa.) Hospital

Billie Ward, RN, MSN
Nursing Instructor
Bishop State Community College
Mobile, Ala.

Pat Weiskittel, RN, MSN, CNN, CS
Renal Clinical Nurse Specialist
University Hospital
Cincinnati

Dianne Weyer, RN, MS, CFNP
Assistant Professor
Georgia State University
School of Nursing
Atlanta

*We extend special thanks to the
following people who contributed
to the previous edition:*

Deborah Becker, RN, MSN, CCRN
Kathleen Ellstrom, RN, MS, CS
Theresa P. Fulginiti, RN, BSN, CEN
Joyce Lyne Heise, RN, MSN
Luana Martindale, RN, MSN
Karen E. Michael, RN, MSN
Barbara A. Moyer, RN, EdD
Carol Muha-Ronneau, RN, MSN
Denise Netz, CRNP, MSN
Margaret R. Rateau, RN, MSN
Lucille A. Rosso, RN, MSN
Carla Roy, RN, BSN
Mary Ellen Santucci, RN, MSN, CRRN
Patricia P. Shoemaker, RN, MSN
Dawn M. Specht, RN, MSN, CEN, CCRN, PHRN
Alice Vrsan, RN, MSN, CCRN

Foreword

The first time I was exposed to fluids, electrolytes, and acid-base balance, I was so intimidated that I *actually calculated* how many questions on those subjects I could miss and still pass the examination! In the long run, that approach failed because almost every major health care problem has the potential to cause fluid, electrolyte, and acid-base imbalances.

Many nurses feel overwhelmed when it comes to evaluating the patient's signs and symptoms and interpreting diagnostic findings for imbalances. If you want to be confident about fluid, electrolyte, and acid-base imbalances, *Fluids & Electrolytes Made Incredibly Easy*, Second Edition, is for you!

If you're a nursing student, this book will make your life much easier as you strive to learn about fluids and electrolytes — the most important concepts you'll have to learn. This fun, interesting, and concise text will help you understand the significance of abnormal test results in acutely and chronically ill patients. What's more, you'll be able to anticipate which abnormalities might accompany major health problems.

Numerous charts, illustrations, and other graphics present difficult concepts in an incredibly clear manner. This book will guide you through the maze of "hypo's" and "hyper's," so you'll be able to assess your patients in a focused, systematic manner — and quickly recognize clinical changes related to fluid, electrolyte, and acid-base imbalances.

Fluids & Electrolytes Made Incredibly Easy, Second Edition, provides several organizational tools to help you learn quickly, such as memory joggers (for example, *SUCTION*, which can help you assess a patient for hypokalemia), bulleted "cheat sheets" to highlight key points, a glossary, and quick quizzes with each chapter to evaluate your knowledge.

The text is organized into four parts, beginning with "Balancing basics," which reviews fundamental information about fluids, electrolytes, and acid-base balance. Part II, "Fluid and electrolyte imbalances," discusses abnormal findings related to fluids, sodium, potassium, magnesium, calcium, phosphorus, chloride, acids, and bases. This section explores the major causes of fluid and electrolyte imbalances along with the diagnostic tests and nursing interventions for each. Part III, "Disorders that cause imbalances," discusses five major health problems — heart failure, respiratory failure, excessive GI fluid loss, renal failure, and burns — and the fluid, electrolyte, and acid-base imbalances associated with each. Finally, Part IV, "Treating imbalances," provides useful information about nursing and medical interventions for these problems.

Of particular interest throughout the text are graphic logos that alert you to critical information. These include:

"Uh-oh," which lists dangerous signs and symptoms and enables you to quickly recognize trouble

"It's not working," which helps you find alternative interventions and prioritize

"Chart smart," which features critical documentation elements that help you avoid legal problems

 "Teaching points," which provides clear patient-teaching tips that you can use to help your patients prevent recurrence of the problem

 "Ages and stages," which identifies issues to watch for in your pediatric and geriatric patients.

Fluids & Electrolytes Made Incredibly Easy, Second Edition, will be an important part of your clinical library. It will help you become comfortable with these concepts so you can evaluate your patient's progress and begin formulating nursing interventions of your own with ease. If you've been feeling insecure about your knowledge of fluids, electrolytes, and acid-base balance, this book is for you!

Sheri Innerarity, RN, PhD, CNS, FNP
Assistant Professor of Clinical Nursing
The University of Texas at Austin
Clinical Nurse Specialist
Adult Health & Family Nurse Practitioner
Smithville (Tex.) Medical Clinic

Part I

Balancing basics

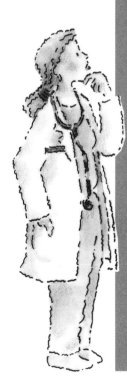

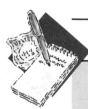

Balancing fluids

Just the facts

This chapter lays the groundwork for understanding fluids and the way the body balances them. In this chapter, you'll learn:

♦ how fluids are distributed throughout the body

♦ what certain fluid-related terms mean

♦ how fluid moves through the body

♦ what roles hormones and the kidneys play in fluid balance.

A look at fluids

Where would we be without body fluids? Nowhere. Fluids are vital to all forms of life: They help maintain body temperature and cell shape, and they help transport nutrients, gases, and wastes. Let's take a close look at fluids and the way the body balances them.

Making gains = losses

The skin, the lungs, the kidneys—just about all major organs—work together to maintain the proper balance of fluid. To maintain that balance, the amount of fluid gained throughout the day must equal the amount lost. Some of those losses can be measured; others can't.

It's insensible

Fluid losses from the skin and lungs are referred to as *insensible losses* because they can't be measured or seen. Losses from the evaporation of fluid through the skin are fairly constant but depend on a person's body surface area. For example, the body surface area of an infant is greater than that of an adult relative to

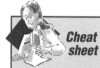

Cheat sheet

Fluid losses

• *Insensible losses*— immeasurable; evaporation through skin (affected by humidity) and lungs (affected by respiratory rate and depth); fever causes loss through the skin and lungs

• *Sensible losses*— measurable; from urination, defecation, and wounds

Now I get it!

Sites involved in fluid loss

Each day the body gains and loses fluid through several different processes. This illustration shows the primary sites involved and the normal daily fluid losses. Gastric, intestinal, pancreatic, and biliary secretions are almost completely reabsorbed and aren't usually counted in daily fluid gains and losses.

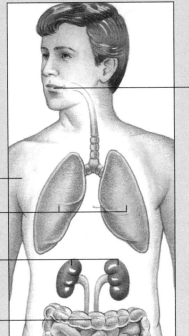

Daily total intake   2,600 ml

Liquids	1,500 ml
Solid foods	800 ml
Water of oxidation	300 ml

Daily total output   2,600 ml

Skin	600 ml
Lungs	400 ml
Kidneys (urine)	1,500 ml
Intestines (feces)	100 ml

their respective weights. As a result, infants typically lose more water from their skin than do adults.

Changes in humidity levels affect the amount of fluid lost through the skin. Likewise, respiratory rate and depth affect the amount of fluid lost through the lungs. Tachypnea, for example, causes more water to be lost; bradypnea, less. Fever increases insensible losses of fluid from both the skin and lungs.

Now that's sensible

Fluid losses from urination, defecation, wounds, and other means are referred to as *sensible losses* because they can be measured.

A typical adult loses 100 to 200 ml/day of fluid through defecation. In cases of severe diarrhea, losses may exceed 5,000 ml/day. (For more information about insensible and sensible losses, see *Sites involved in fluid loss.*)

Memory jogger

To help you remember which fluid belongs to which compartment, keep in mind that INTER means between (as in interval — between two events) and INTRA means within or inside (as in intravenous — inside a vein).

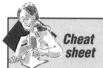

Fluid compartments

This illustration shows the primary fluid compartments in the body: intracellular and extracellular, the latter of which is further divided into interstitial and intravascular. Capillary walls and cell membranes separate intracellular fluids from extracellular fluids.

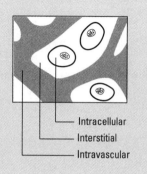

└── Intracellular
└── Interstitial
└── Intravascular

Cheat sheet

Fluid distribution

• *Intracellular*—inside the cells; must be balanced with extracellular
• *Extracellular*—outside the cells; must be balanced with intracellular
• *Transcellular*—in the cerebrospinal column, pleural cavity, lymph system, joints, and eyes

Following the fluid

The body holds fluid in two basic areas, or compartments—inside the cells and outside the cells. Fluid found inside the cells is called intracellular fluid; fluid found outside the cells, extracellular fluid. Capillary walls and cell membranes separate the intracellular and extracellular compartments. (See *Fluid compartments*.)

To maintain proper fluid balance, the distribution of fluid between the two compartments must remain relatively constant. In an adult, the total amount of intracellular fluid averages 40% of the person's body weight, or about 28 L. The total amount of extracellular fluid averages 20% of the person's body weight, or about 14 L.

Extracellular fluid can be broken down further into interstitial fluid, which surrounds the cells, and intravascular fluid or plasma, which is the liquid portion of blood. In an adult, interstitial fluid accounts for about 75% of the extracellular fluid. Plasma accounts for the remaining 25%.

The body contains other fluids, called transcellular fluids, in the cerebrospinal column, pleural cavity, lymph system, joints, and eyes. Transcellular fluids generally aren't subject to significant gains and losses throughout the day, however, so they aren't discussed in detail here.

Water here, water there

The distribution of fluid within the body's compartments varies with age. Compared with adults, infants have a greater percentage of body water stored inside interstitial spaces. About 80% of the body weight of a full-term neonate is water. About 90% of the body weight of a premature infant is water. The amount of water as a percentage of body weight decreases with age until puberty. In a

Ages and stages

The evaporation of time

The risk of suffering a fluid imbalance increases with age. Why? Skeletal muscle mass declines, and the proportion of fat within the body increases. After age 60, water content drops to about 45%.

Likewise, the distribution of fluid within the body changes with age. For instance, about 15% of a typical young adult's total body weight is made up of interstitial fluid. That percentage progressively decreases with age.

About 5% of the body's total fluid volume is made up of plasma. Plasma volume remains stable throughout life.

typical 154-lb (70-kg), lean adult male, about 60% (93 lb [42 kg]) of body weight is water. (See *The evaporation of time*.)

Skeletal muscle cells hold much of that water; fat cells contain little of it. Women, who normally have a higher ratio of fat to skeletal muscle than men, typically have a somewhat lower relative water content. Likewise, an obese person may have a relative water content level as low as 45%. Accumulated body fat in these individuals increases weight without boosting the body's water content.

Fluid types

Fluids in the body generally aren't found in pure forms. They're usually found in three types of solutions: isotonic, hypotonic, and hypertonic.

Meet iso "the match" tonic

An isotonic solution has the same solute concentration as another solution. For instance, if two fluids in adjacent compartments are equally concentrated, they're already in balance, so the fluid inside each compartment stays put. No imbalance means no net fluid shift.

For example, normal saline solution is considered isotonic because the concentration of sodium in the solution nearly equals the concentration of sodium in the blood. (See *Isotonic fluids*.)

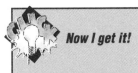

Now I get it!

Isotonic fluids

No net fluid shifts occur between isotonic solutions, because the solutions are equally concentrated.

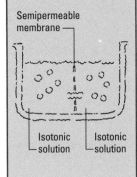

Semipermeable membrane

Isotonic solution   Isotonic solution

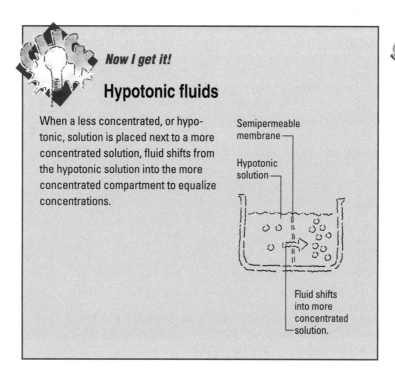

Now I get it!

Hypotonic fluids

When a less concentrated, or hypotonic, solution is placed next to a more concentrated solution, fluid shifts from the hypotonic solution into the more concentrated compartment to equalize concentrations.

Semipermeable membrane

Hypotonic solution

Fluid shifts into more concentrated solution.

Now I get it!

Hypertonic fluids

If one solution has more solutes than an adjacent solution, it has less fluid relative to the adjacent solution. Fluid will move out of the less concentrated solution into the more concentrated, or hypertonic, solution until both solutions have the same amount of solutes and fluid.

Semipermeable membrane

Hypertonic solution

Fluid shifts into more concentrated solution.

Meet hypo "low-low" tonic

A hypotonic solution has a lower solute concentration than another solution. For instance, say one solution contains only a little sodium and another solution contains more. The first solution is hypotonic compared with the second solution. As a result, fluid from the hypotonic solution would shift into the second solution until the two solutions had equal concentrations. Remember that the body constantly strives to maintain a state of balance, or equilibrium.

Half-normal saline solution is considered hypotonic because the concentration of sodium in the solution is lower than the concentration of sodium in the patient's blood. (See *Hypotonic fluids.*)

Meet hyper "over-the-top" tonic

A hypertonic solution has a higher solute concentration than another solution. For instance, say one solution contains a large amount of sodium and a second solution contains hardly any. The first solution is hypertonic compared with the second solution. As a result, fluid from the sec-

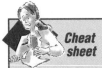
ond solution would shift into the hypertonic solution until the two solutions had equal concentrations. Again, the body constantly strives to maintain a state of equilibrium.

For instance, a solution of dextrose 5% in normal saline solution is considered hypertonic because the concentration of solutes in the solution is greater than the concentration of solutes in the patient's blood. (See *Hypertonic fluids*, page 7.)

Fluid movement

Just as the heart beats constantly, fluids and solutes move constantly within the body. That movement allows the body to maintain homeostasis, the constant state of balance the body seeks. (See *Fluid tips*.)

Within the cells

Solutes within the intracellular, interstitial, and intravascular compartments of the body move through the membranes, separating those compartments in different ways. The membranes are semipermeable, meaning that they allow some solutes to pass through but not others. Following are the different ways fluids and solutes move through membranes at the cellular level.

Diffusion goes with the flow

In diffusion, solutes move from an area of higher concentration to an area of lower concentration, which eventually results in an

Cheat sheet

Three types of body fluids

- *Isotonic* — equally concentrated with other solutions
- *Hypotonic* — less concentrated than other solutions
- *Hypertonic* — more concentrated than other solutions

Now I get it!

Fluid tips

Fluids, nutrients, and waste products constantly shift within the body's compartments—from the cells to the interstitial spaces, to the blood vessels, and back again. A change in one compartment can affect all of the others.

Keeping track of the shifts
That continuous fluid shifting can have important implications for your nursing care. For instance, if you give a hypotonic fluid to a patient, it may cause too much fluid to move from the veins into the cells, and the cells can swell.

Conversely, if you give a hypertonic solution to a patient, it may cause too much fluid to be pulled from cells into the bloodstream, and the cells can shrink.

For more information about I.V. solutions, see chapter 18, Total parenteral nutrition.

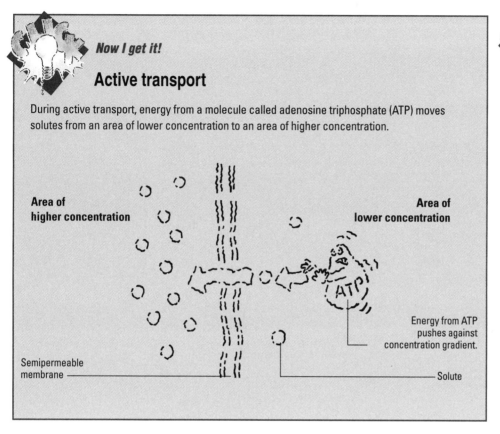

Now I get it!

Active transport

During active transport, energy from a molecule called adenosine triphosphate (ATP) moves solutes from an area of lower concentration to an area of higher concentration.

Area of higher concentration

Area of lower concentration

Energy from ATP pushes against concentration gradient.

Semipermeable membrane

Solute

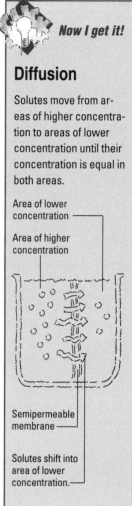

Now I get it!

Diffusion

Solutes move from areas of higher concentration to areas of lower concentration until their concentration is equal in both areas.

Area of lower concentration

Area of higher concentration

Semipermeable membrane

Solutes shift into area of lower concentration.

equal distribution of solutes within the two areas. Diffusion is a form of passive transport because no energy is required to make it happen; it just happens. Like fish traveling downstream, the solutes simply go with the flow. (See *Diffusion*.)

Actively transporting

In active transport, solutes move from an area of lower concentration to an area of higher concentration. Like swimming upstream, active transport requires energy to make it happen.

The energy required for a solute to move against a concentration gradient comes from a substance called adenosine triphosphate, or ATP. Stored in all cells, ATP supplies energy for solute movement in and out of cells. (See *Active transport*.)

Some solutes, such as sodium and potassium, use ATP to move in and out of cells in a

Osmosis

In osmosis, fluid moves passively from areas with more fluid (and fewer solutes) to areas with less fluid (and more solutes). Remember that in osmosis fluid moves, whereas in diffusion solutes move.

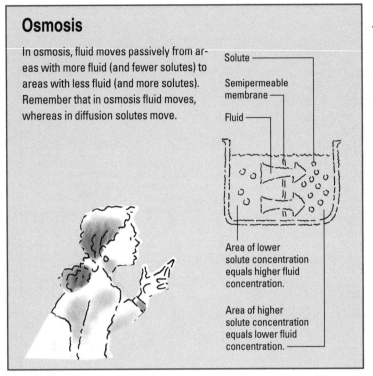

Solute

Semipermeable membrane

Fluid

Area of lower solute concentration equals higher fluid concentration.

Area of higher solute concentration equals lower fluid concentration.

Cheat sheet

ATP

- Also known as *adenosine triphosphate*
- Gives solutes energy to move against concentration gradient
- Used by sodium and potassium to move in and out of cells

form of active transport called the sodium-potassium pump. (For more information on this physiologic pump, see chapter 5, When sodium tips the balance.) Other solutes that require active transport to cross cell membranes include calcium ions, hydrogen ions, amino acids, and certain sugars.

Osmosis lets fluids through

Osmosis refers to the passive movement of fluid across a membrane from an area of lower solute concentration and comparatively more fluid into an area of higher solute concentration and comparatively less fluid. Osmosis stops when enough fluid has moved through the membrane to equalize the solute concentration on both sides of the membrane. (See *Osmosis.*)

Within the vascular system

Within the vascular system, only capillaries have walls thin enough to let solutes pass through. The movement of fluids and solutes through the walls of the body's capillaries plays a critical role in fluid balance.

Fluid movement through capillaries

When fluid-pushing, or hydrostatic, pressure builds inside a capillary, it forces fluids and solutes out through the capillary walls into the interstitial fluid.

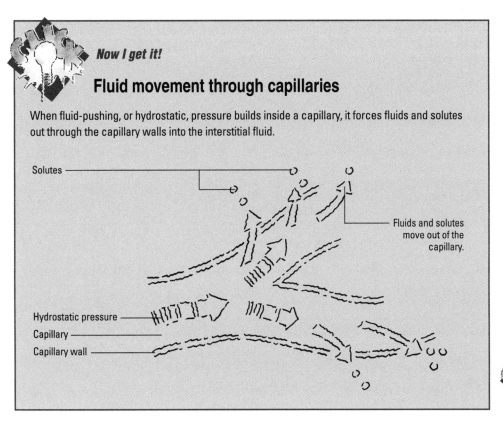

Solutes

Fluids and solutes move out of the capillary.

Hydrostatic pressure

Capillary

Capillary wall

The pressure is on

The movement of fluids through capillaries—a process called capillary filtration—results from blood pushing against the walls of the capillary. That pressure, called hydrostatic (or fluid-pushing) pressure, forces fluids and solutes through the capillary wall.

When the hydrostatic pressure inside a capillary is greater than the pressure in the surrounding interstitial space, fluids and solutes inside the capillary are forced out into the interstitial space. When the pressure inside the capillary is less than the pressure outside of it, fluids and solutes move back into the capillary. (See *Fluid movement through capillaries.*)

Keeping the fluid in

A process called reabsorption prevents too much fluid from leaving the capillaries no matter how much hydrostatic pressure exists within the capillaries. When fluid filters through a capillary, the protein albumin remains behind in the diminishing volume of water. Albumin is a large molecule that normally can't pass

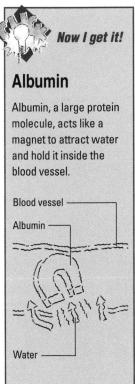

Albumin

Albumin, a large protein molecule, acts like a magnet to attract water and hold it inside the blood vessel.

Blood vessel

Albumin

Water

through capillary membranes. As the concentration of albumin inside a capillary increases, fluid begins to move back into the capillaries through osmosis.

Think of albumin as a water magnet. The osmotic, or pulling, force of albumin in the intravascular space is referred to as the plasma colloid osmotic pressure. The plasma colloid osmotic pressure in capillaries averages about 25 mm Hg. (See *Albumin*, page 11.)

As long as capillary blood pressure (the hydrostatic pressure) exceeds plasma colloid osmotic pressure, water and solutes can leave the capillaries and enter the interstitial fluid. When capillary blood pressure falls below plasma colloid osmotic pressure, water and diffusible solutes return to the capillaries.

Normally, blood pressure in a capillary exceeds plasma colloid osmotic pressure in the arteriole end and falls below it in the venule end. As a result, capillary filtration occurs along the first half of the vessel; reabsorption, along the second half. As long as capillary blood pressure and plasma albumin levels remain nor-

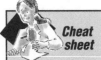

Cheat sheet

Capillary blood pressure

• If pressure exceeds plasma colloid osmotic pressure (COP), then water and solutes move to interstitial fluid.
• If pressure falls below plasma COP, water and diffusible solutes return to capillaries.

Now I get it!

Typical nephron

The nephron (shown below) filters blood, produces urine, and excretes excess solutes, electrolytes, fluids, and metabolic waste products while keeping blood composition and volume constant.

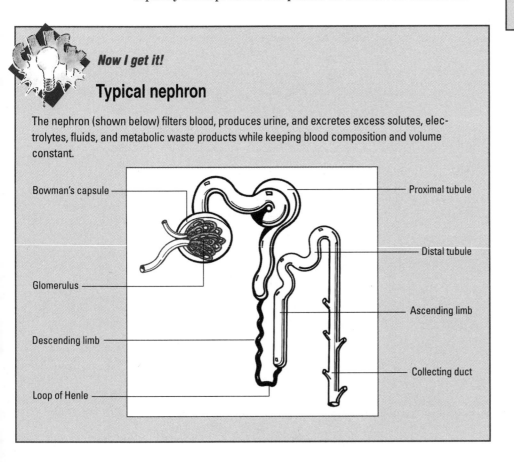

Bowman's capsule
Proximal tubule
Distal tubule
Glomerulus
Ascending limb
Descending limb
Collecting duct
Loop of Henle

mal, the amount of water that moves into the vessel equals the amount that moves out.

Occasionally, extra fluid filters out of the capillary. When that happens, the excess fluid shifts into the lymphatic vessels located just outside the capillaries and eventually returns to the heart for recirculation.

Maintaining the balance

Various things in the body work together to maintain fluid balance. Because one problem can affect the entire fluid-maintenance system, it's important to keep all things in check. Here's a closer look at the things that make this balancing act possible.

The kidneys

The kidneys play a vital role in fluid balance. If the kidneys don't work properly, the body has great difficulty controlling fluid balance. The workhorse of the kidney is the nephron, which forms urine. The body puts the nephrons through their paces every day. (See *Typical nephron*.)

A nephron consists of a glomerulus and a tubule. The tubule, sometimes convoluted, ends in a collecting duct. The glomerulus is a cluster of capillaries that filters blood. Like a vascular cradle, Bowman's capsule surrounds the glomerulus.

Capillary blood pressure forces fluid through the capillary walls and into Bowman's capsule at the proximal end of the tubule. Along the length of the tubule, water and electrolytes are either excreted or retained according to the body's needs. If the body needs more fluid, for instance, it retains more. If it needs less fluid, less is reabsorbed and more is excreted. Electrolytes, such as sodium and potassium, are either filtered or reabsorbed throughout the same area. The resulting filtrate, which eventually becomes urine, flows through the tubule into the collecting ducts and eventually into the bladder as urine.

Superabsorbent

Nephrons filter about 125 ml of blood every minute, or about 180 L/day. That rate, called the glomerular filtration rate, leads to the production of 1 to 2 L of urine per day. The nephrons reabsorb the remaining 178 L or more of fluid, an amount equivalent to more than 30 oil changes for the family car!

Ages and stages

The higher the rate, the greater the waste

Infants and young children excrete urine at a higher rate than adults because their higher metabolic rates produce more waste. Also, an infant's kidneys can't concentrate urine until about age 3 months, and they remain less efficient than an adult's kidneys until about age 2 years.

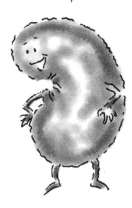

Do I look like I'm retaining water?

A strict conservationist

If the body loses even 1% to 2% of its fluid, the kidneys take steps to conserve water. Perhaps the most important step involves reabsorbing more water from the filtrate, which produces a more concentrated urine.

The kidneys must continue to excrete at least 20 ml of urine every hour (500 ml/day) to eliminate body wastes. A urine excretion rate that's less than 20 ml/hour usually indicates renal pathology. The minimum excretion rate varies with age. (See *The higher the rate, the greater the waste*, page 13.)

The kidneys respond to fluid excesses by excreting a more dilute urine, which rids the body of fluid and conserves electrolytes.

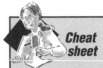

Cheat sheet

ADH

- Also known as *antidiuretic hormone* or *vasopressin*
- Reduces diuresis
- Increases urine retention
- Restores blood volume

Antidiuretic hormone

Several hormones affect fluid balance, among them a water retainer called antidiuretic hormone (ADH). (You may also hear the hormone called vasopressin.) The hypothalamus produces ADH, but the posterior pituitary gland stores and releases it. If you can remember what ADH stands for, you can remember its job: to re-

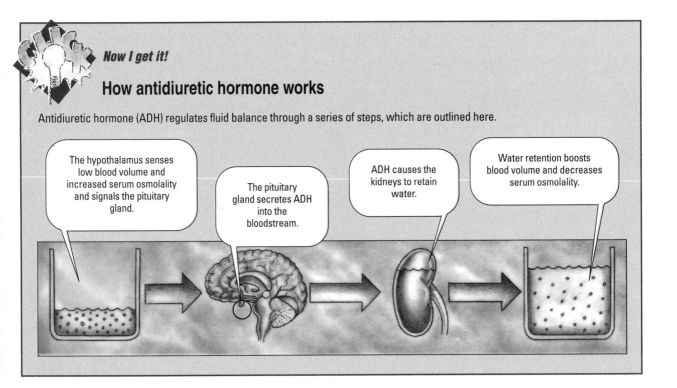

Now I get it!

How antidiuretic hormone works

Antidiuretic hormone (ADH) regulates fluid balance through a series of steps, which are outlined here.

The hypothalamus senses low blood volume and increased serum osmolality and signals the pituitary gland.

The pituitary gland secretes ADH into the bloodstream.

ADH causes the kidneys to retain water.

Water retention boosts blood volume and decreases serum osmolality.

store blood volume by reducing diuresis and increasing water retention. (See *How antidiuretic hormone works.*)

Sensitive to changes

Increased serum osmolality or decreased blood volume can stimulate the release of ADH, which in turn increases the kidneys' reabsorption of water. The increased reabsorption of water results in more concentrated urine.

Likewise, decreased serum osmolality or increased blood volume inhibits the release of ADH and causes less water to be reabsorbed, making the urine less concentrated. The amount of ADH released varies throughout the day, depending on the body's needs.

This up-and-down cycle of ADH release keeps fluid levels in balance all day long. Like a dam on a river, the body holds water when fluid levels drop and releases it when fluid levels rise.

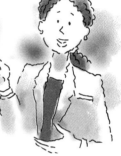

Juxtaglomerular: that's easy for you to say.

Now I get it!

Aldosterone production

The illustration shows the steps involved in the production of aldosterone (a hormone that helps to regulate fluid balance) through the renin-angiotensin-aldosterone system.

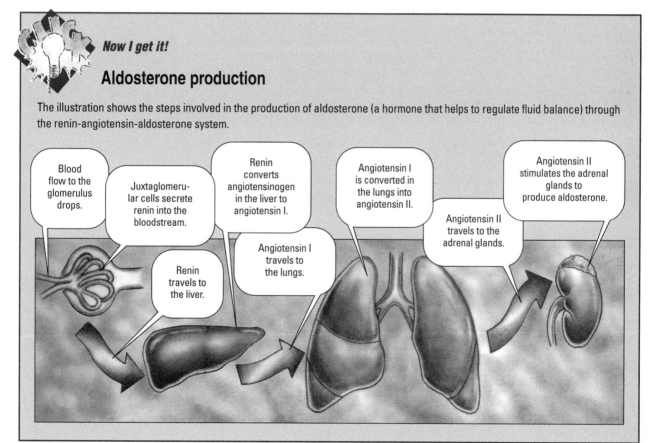

Blood flow to the glomerulus drops.

Juxtaglomerular cells secrete renin into the bloodstream.

Renin travels to the liver.

Renin converts angiotensinogen in the liver to angiotensin I.

Angiotensin I travels to the lungs.

Angiotensin I is converted in the lungs into angiotensin II.

Angiotensin II travels to the adrenal glands.

Angiotensin II stimulates the adrenal glands to produce aldosterone.

Renin-angiotensin-aldosterone system

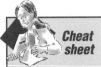

To help maintain a balance of sodium and water in the body as well as to maintain a healthy blood volume and blood pressure, special cells (juxtaglomerular cells) near each glomerulus secrete an enzyme called renin. Through a complex series of steps, renin leads to the production of angiotensin II, a powerful vasoconstrictor.

Angiotensin II causes peripheral vasoconstriction and stimulates the production of aldosterone. Both actions raise blood pressure. (See *Aldosterone production*, page 15.)

As soon as the blood pressure reaches a normal level, the body stops releasing renin, and this feedback cycle of renin to angiotensin to aldosterone stops.

The ups and downs of renin

The amount of renin secreted depends on blood flow and the level of sodium in the bloodstream. If blood flow to the kidneys diminishes, as happens in a patient who is hemorrhaging, or if the amount of sodium reaching the glomerulus drops, the juxtaglomerular cells secrete more renin. The renin causes vasoconstriction and a subsequent increase in blood pressure.

Conversely, if blood flow to the kidneys increases, or if the amount of sodium reaching the glomerulus increases, juxtaglomerular cells secrete less renin. A drop-off in renin secretion reduces vasoconstriction and helps to normalize blood pressure.

Sodium and water regulator

The hormone aldosterone also plays a role in maintaining blood pressure and fluid balance. Secreted by the adrenal cortex, aldosterone regulates the reabsorption of sodium and water within the nephron. (See *How aldosterone works*.)

Triggering active transport

When blood volume drops, aldosterone initiates the active transport of sodium from the distal tubules and the collecting ducts into the bloodstream. That active transport forces sodium back into the bloodstream. When sodium is forced into the bloodstream, more water is reabsorbed and blood volume expands.

Atrial natriuretic peptide

The renin-angiotensin-aldosterone system isn't the only factor at work balancing fluids in the body. A cardiac hormone called atrial natriuretic peptide (ANP) also helps keep that balance. Stored in the cells of the atria, ANP is released when atrial pressure increases. The hormone opposes the renin-angiotensin-aldosterone system by decreasing blood pressure and reducing intravascular blood volume. (See *How atrial natriuretic peptide works*, page 18.)

This powerful hormone:
- suppresses serum renin levels
- decreases aldosterone release from the adrenal glands
- increases glomerular filtration, which increases urine excretion of sodium and water
- decreases ADH release from the posterior pituitary gland
- reduces vascular resistance by causing vasodilation.

Maintaining body fluid levels is a real balancing act.

Stretch that atrium.

The amount of ANP that atria release rises in response to a number of conditions, including chronic renal failure and heart failure.

Anything that causes atrial stretching can also lead to increases in the amount of ANP released, including ortho-static changes, atrial tachycardia, high sodium intake,

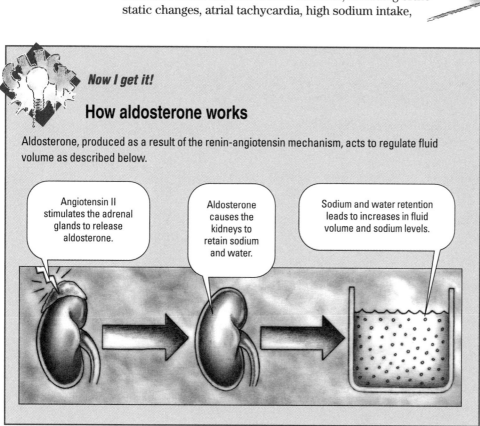

Now I get it!

How aldosterone works

Aldosterone, produced as a result of the renin-angiotensin mechanism, acts to regulate fluid volume as described below.

Angiotensin II stimulates the adrenal glands to release aldosterone.

Aldosterone causes the kidneys to retain sodium and water.

Sodium and water retention leads to increases in fluid volume and sodium levels.

sodium chloride infusions, and use of drugs that cause vasoconstriction.

Thirst

Perhaps the simplest mechanism for maintaining fluid balance is
the thirst mechanism. Thirst occurs as a result of even small losses of fluid. Losing body fluids or eating highly salty foods leads to
an increase in extracellular fluid osmolality. This increase leads to
the drying of mucus membranes in the mouth, which in turn stimulates the thirst center in the hypothalamus.

In an elderly person, the thirst mechanism is less effective than
it is in a younger person, leaving the older person more prone to
dehydration. (See *Signs and symptoms of dehydration in the
elderly.*)

Quenching that thirst

Normally, when a person is thirsty, he drinks fluid. The ingested
fluid is absorbed from the intestine into the bloodstream, where it

**Ages
and stages**

Signs and symptoms of dehydration in the elderly

- Confusion
- Subnormal tempera-
ture
- Tachycardia
- Pinched facial expres-
sion

Now I get it!

How atrial natriuretic peptide works

When blood volume and blood pressure rise and begin to stretch the atria, the heart's atrial natriuretic peptide (ANP) shuts off the renin-angiotensin-aldosterone system, which stabilizes blood
volume and blood pressure.

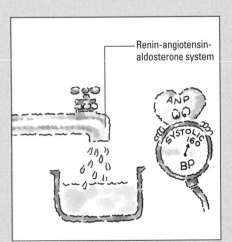

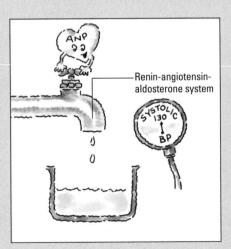

moves freely between fluid compartments. This movement leads to an increase in the amount of fluid in the body and a decrease in the concentration of solutes, thus balancing fluid levels throughout the body.

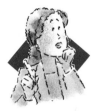

Quick quiz

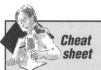

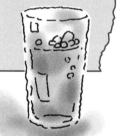

1. If you were walking across the Sahara Desert with an empty canteen, the amount of antidiuretic hormone (ADH) secreted would most likely:
    A.   increase.
    B.   decrease.
    C.   stay the same.

Answer: A. Because your body would probably be dehydrated, it would try to retain as much fluid as possible. To retain fluid, ADH secretion increases.

2. If you placed two containers next to each other, separated only by a semipermeable membrane, and the solution in one container was hypotonic relative to the other, fluid in the hypotonic container would:
    A.   move out of the hypotonic container into the other.
    B.   pull fluid from the other container into the hypotonic container.
    C.   stay unchanged within the hypotonic container.

Answer: A. Fluid would move out of the hypotonic container into the other container to equalize the concentration of fluid within the two containers.

3. Hydrostatic pressure, which pushes fluid out of the capillaries, is opposed by colloid osmotic pressure, which involves:
    A.   reduced renin secretion.
    B.   the pulling power of albumin to reabsorb water.
    C.   an increase in ADH secretion.

Answer: B. Albumin in capillaries draws water toward it, a process called reabsorption.

4. When a person's blood pressure drops, the kidneys respond by:
    A.   secreting renin.
    B.   producing aldosterone.
    C.   slowing the release of ADH.

Answer: A. Juxtaglomerular cells in the kidneys secrete renin in response to low blood flow or a low sodium level. The eventual effect of renin secretion is an increase in blood pressure.

5.   Giving a hypertonic I.V. solution to a patient may cause too much fluid to be:

    A.   pulled from the cells into the bloodstream.
    B.   pulled out of the bloodstream into the cells.
    C.   pushed out of the bloodstream into the extravascular spaces.

Answer: A. Because the concentration of solutes in the I.V. solution is greater than the concentration of solutes in the patient's blood, a hypertonic solution may cause fluid to be pulled from the cells into the bloodstream.

Scoring

☆☆☆   If you answered all five questions correctly, congratulations! You're a fluid whiz.

☆☆   If you answered three or four correctly, take a swig of water; you're just a little dry.

☆   If you answered fewer than three correctly, pour yourself a glass of sports drink and enjoy an invigorating burst of fluid refreshment!

2

Balancing electrolytes

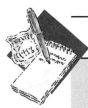

Just the facts

This chapter discusses electrolytes and how the body balances them. In this chapter, you'll learn:

♦ the difference between cations and anions

♦ which serum electrolyte results are normal and which are abnormal

♦ the role nephrons play in electrolyte balance

♦ how and where diuretics affect electrolytes in the kidney

♦ about the electrolyte concentration of selected I.V. fluids.

A look at electrolytes

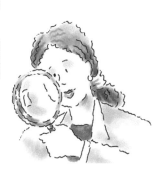

Electrolytes work with fluids to maintain health and well-being. They're found in various concentrations, depending on whether they're inside or outside the cells. Electrolytes are crucial for nearly all cellular reactions and functions. Let's take a look at what electrolytes are, how they function, and what upsets their balance.

Ions

Electrolytes are substances that, when in solution, separate (or dissociate) into electrically charged particles called ions. Some ions are positively charged; others, negatively charged. Several pairs of opposite-charged ions are so closely linked that a problem with one ion causes a problem with the other. Sodium and chloride are linked that way, as are calcium and phosphorus.

A wide variety of diseases can offset the normal balance of electrolytes in the body. Understanding electrolytes and recognizing imbalances will make your patient assessment more accurate.

Anions and cations

Anions are electrolytes that generate a negative charge; cations are electrolytes that produce a positive charge. An electrical charge makes cells function normally. Chloride, phosphorus, and bicarbonate are anions; sodium, potassium, calcium, and magnesium are cations. (See *Looking on the plus and minus sides.*)

The anion gap is a useful test for distinguishing types and causes of acid-base imbalances because it reflects serum anion-cation balance. (The anion gap is discussed in chapter 3, Balancing acids and bases.)

Balancing the pluses and minuses

Electrolytes operate outside the cell in extracellular fluid compartments and inside the cell in intracellular fluid compartments. Individual electrolytes differ in concentration, but electrolyte totals balance to achieve a neutral electrical charge (positives and negatives balance each other). This balance is called electroneutrality.

Interacting electrolytes

Most electrolytes interact with hydrogen ions to maintain acid-base balance. The major electrolytes have specialized functions that contribute to metabolism and fluid and electrolyte balance.

> **Memory jogger**
>
> To remind yourself about the difference between anions and cations, remember that the *T* in "cation" looks like the positive symbol, "+."

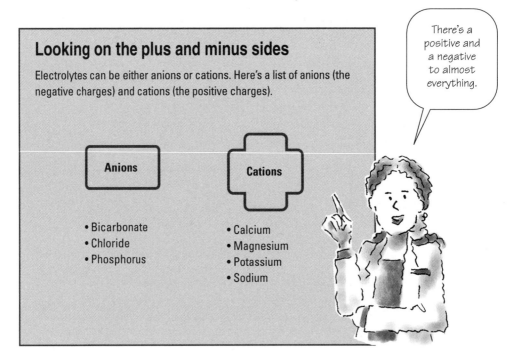

Looking on the plus and minus sides

Electrolytes can be either anions or cations. Here's a list of anions (the negative charges) and cations (the positive charges).

Anions

- Bicarbonate
- Chloride
- Phosphorus

Cations

- Calcium
- Magnesium
- Potassium
- Sodium

> There's a positive and a negative to almost everything.

Major electrolytes outside the cell

Sodium and chloride, the major electrolytes in extracellular fluid, exert most of their effects outside the cell. Sodium concentration affects serum osmolality (solute concentration in 1 L of water) and extracellular fluid volume. Sodium also helps nerve and muscle cells interact. Chloride helps maintain osmotic pressure (water-pulling pressure). Gastric mucosal cells need chloride to produce hydrochloric acid, which breaks down food into absorbable components.

Calcium and bicarbonate are two other electrolytes found in extracellular fluid. Calcium is the major cation involved in the structure and function of bones and teeth and is needed to:
• stabilize the cell membrane and reduce its permeability to sodium
• transmit nerve impulses
• contract muscles
• coagulate blood
• form bone and teeth.

Bicarbonate plays a vital role in acid-base balance.

Major electrolytes inside the cell

Potassium, phosphate, and magnesium are among the most abundant electrolytes inside the cell.

Potassium plays an important role in:
• cell excitability regulation
• nerve impulse conduction
• resting membrane potential
• muscle contraction and myocardial membrane responsiveness
• intracellular osmolality control.

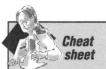

Cheat sheet

Extracellular electrolytes

• *Sodium*—helps nerve cells and muscle cells interact
• *Chloride*—maintains osmotic pressure and helps gastric mucosal cells produce hydrochloric acid
• *Calcium*—stabilizes cell membrane and reduces permeability, transmits nerve impulses, contracts muscles, coagulates blood, and forms bones and teeth
• *Bicarbonate*—plays a role in acid-base balance

Cheat sheet

Intracellular electrolytes

• *Potassium*—responsible for cell excitability, nerve impulse conduction, resting membrane potential, muscle contraction, myocardial membrane responsiveness, and intracellular osmolality
• *Phosphate*—responsible for energy metabolism
• *Magnesium*—responsible for enzyme reactions, neuromuscular contractions, normal functioning of nervous and cardiovascular systems, protein synthesis, and sodium and potassium ion transportation

The body contains phosphorus in the form of phosphate salts. Sometimes the words *phosphorus* and *phosphate* are used interchangeably. Phosphate is essential for energy metabolism. Combined with calcium, phosphate plays a key role in bone and tooth mineralization. It also helps maintain acid-base balance.

Magnesium acts as a catalyst for enzyme reactions. It regulates neuromuscular contraction, promotes normal functioning of the nervous system and the cardiovascular system, and aids in protein synthesis and sodium and potassium ion transportation.

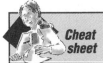

Cheat sheet

Factors affecting electrolyte balance

- Fluid intake and output
- Acid-base balance
- Hormone secretion
- Normal cell functioning

Electrolyte movement

When cells die (for example, from trauma or chemotherapy), their contents spill into the extracellular area and upset the balance. In this case, elevated levels of intracellular electrolytes, such as phosphorus and potassium, are found in plasma.

Although electrolytes are concentrated in one compartment or another, they aren't locked or frozen in these areas. Like fluids, electrolytes move about trying to maintain balance and electroneutrality.

Electrolyte balance

Fluid intake and output, acid-base balance, hormone secretion, and normal cell functioning all influence electrolyte balance. Because electrolytes function both collaboratively with other electrolytes and individually, imbalances in one electrolyte can affect balance in others. (See *Understanding electrolytes.*)

You need phosphate to convert energy.

Electrolyte levels

Even though electrolytes exist inside and outside the cell, only the levels outside the cell in the bloodstream are measured. Although serum levels remain fairly stable throughout a person's life span, understanding which levels are normal and which are abnormal is critical to reacting quickly and appropriately to a patient's electrolyte imbalance.

The patient's condition determines how often electrolyte levels are checked. Results for many laboratory tests are reported in milliequivalents per liter (mEq/L), which is a measure of the ion's chemical activity or its power. (See *Interpreting serum electrolyte test results*, page 26, for a look at normal and abnormal electrolyte levels in the blood.)

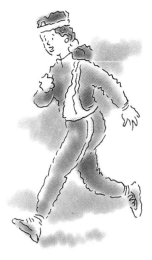

Now I get it!

Understanding electrolytes

Electrolytes help regulate water distribution, govern acid-base balance, and transmit nerve impulses. They also contribute to energy generation and blood clotting. This table summarizes what the body's major electrolytes do. Check the illustration below to see how electrolytes are distributed in and around the cell.

Potassium (K)
• Main intracellular fluid (ICF) cation
• Regulates cell excitability
• Permeates cell membranes, thereby affecting the cell's electrical status
• Helps to control ICF osmolality and, consequently, ICF osmotic pressure

Magnesium (Mg)
• A leading ICF cation
• Contributes to many enzymatic and metabolic processes, particularly protein synthesis
• Modifies nerve impulse transmission and skeletal muscle response (unbalanced Mg concentrations dramatically affect neuromuscular processes)

Phosphorus (P)
• Main ICF anion
• Promotes energy storage and carbohydrate, protein, and fat metabolism
• Acts as a hydrogen buffer

Sodium (Na)
• Main extracellular fluid (ECF) cation
• Helps govern normal ECF osmolality (A shift in Na concentrations triggers a fluid volume change to restore normal solute and water ratios.)
• Helps maintain acid-base balance
• Activates nerve and muscle cells
• Influences water distribution (with chloride)

Chloride (Cl)
• Main ECF anion
• Helps maintain normal ECF osmolality
• Affects body pH
• Plays a vital role in maintaining acid-base balance; combines with hydrogen ions to produce hydrochloric acid

Calcium (Ca)
• A major cation in teeth and bones; found in fairly equal concentrations in ICF and ECF
• Also found in cell membranes, where it helps cells adhere to one another and maintain their shape
• Acts as an enzyme activator within cells (muscles must have Ca to contract)
• Aids coagulation
• Affects cell membrane permeability and firing level

Bicarbonate (HCO_3^-)
• Present in ECF
• Primary function is regulating acid-base balance

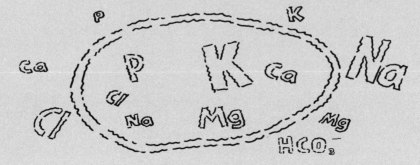

Interpreting serum electrolyte test results

Use the quick-reference chart below to interpret serum electrolyte test results in adult patients. This chart also lists disorders that can cause imbalances.

Electrolyte	Results	Implications	Common causes
Serum sodium	135 to 145 mEq/L	Normal	
	<135 mEq/L	Hyponatremia	Syndrome of inappropriate antidiuretic hormone secretion
	>145 mEq/L	Hypernatremia	Diabetes insipidus
Serum potassium	3.5 to 5 mEq/L	Normal	
	<3.5 mEq/L	Hypokalemia	Diarrhea
	>5 mEq/L	Hyperkalemia	Burns and renal failure
Total serum calcium	8.9 to 10.1 mg/dL	Normal	
	<8.9 mg/dL	Hypocalcemia	Acute pancreatitis
	>10.1 mg/dL	Hypercalcemia	Hyperparathyroidism
Ionized calcium	4.5 to 5.1 mg/dL	Normal	
	<4.5 mg/dL	Hypocalcemia	Massive transfusion
	>5.1 mg/dL	Hypercalcemia	Acidosis
Serum phosphates	2.5 to 4.5 mg/dL or 1.8 to 2.6 mEq/L	Normal	
	<2.5 mg/dL or 1.8 mEq/L	Hypophosphatemia	Diabetic ketoacidosis
	>4.5 mg/dL or 2.6 mEq/L	Hyperphosphatemia	Renal insufficiency
Serum magnesium	1.5 to 2.5 mEq/L	Normal	
	<1.5 mEq/L	Hypomagnesemia	Malnutrition
	>2.5 mEq/L	Hypermagnesemia	Renal failure
Serum chloride	96 to 106 mEq/L	Normal	
	<96 mEq/L	Hypochloremia	Prolonged vomiting
	>106 mEq/L	Hyperchloremia	Hypernatremia

See the whole picture

When you see an abnormal laboratory test result, consider it in the context of what you know about the patient. For instance, a serum potassium level of 7 mEq/L for a patient with previously normal serum potassium levels and no apparent reason for the increase may be an inaccurate result. Perhaps the patient's blood sample was hemolyzed from trauma to the cells.

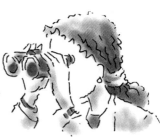

With that said, look at the whole picture before you act, including what you know about the patient, his symptoms, and his electrolyte levels. (See *Documenting electrolyte imbalances.*)

Fluid regulation

Many activities and factors are involved in regulating fluid and electrolyte balance. A quick review of some of the basics will help you understand this regulation better.

Fluid and solute movement

Active transport moves solutes upstream and requires pumps within the body to move the substances from areas of lower concentration to areas of higher concentration—against a concentration gradient. Adenosine triphosphate (ATP) is the energy that moves solutes upstream.

Pushing fluids

The sodium-potassium pump, an example of active transport, moves sodium ions from intracellular fluid (an area of lower concentration) to extracellular fluid (an area of higher concentration). With potassium, the reverse happens: A large amount of potassium in intracellular fluid causes an electrical potential at the cell membrane. As ions rapidly shift in and out of the cell, electrical impulses are conducted. These impulses are essential for maintaining life.

Organ and gland involvement

Most major organs and glands in the body—the lungs, liver, adrenal glands, kidneys, heart, hypothalamus, pituitary gland, skin, GI tract, and parathyroid glands—help to regulate fluid and electrolyte balance.

As part of the renin-angiotensin-aldosterone system, the lungs and liver help regulate sodium and water balance as well as blood pressure. The adrenal glands secrete aldosterone, which influences sodium and potassium balance in the kidneys. These levels are affected because the kidneys excrete potassium, or hydrogen ions, in exchange for retained sodium.

The heart says no

The heart opposes the renin-angiotensin-aldosterone system when it secretes atrial natriuretic peptide (ANP), causing sodium excre-

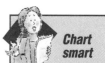

Documenting electrolyte imbalances

Document the patient's electrolyte imbalance by noting:
• assessment findings
• laboratory results pertaining to the imbalance
• related nursing diagnoses
• notification of the doctor
• interventions and treatment for the electrolyte imbalance, including safety measures
• patient teaching
• patient's response to interventions.

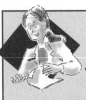

tion. The hypothalamus and posterior pituitary gland produce and secrete an antidiuretic hormone that causes the body to retain water which, in turn, affects solute concentration in the blood.

Where electrolytes are lost

Sodium, potassium, chloride, and water are lost in sweat and from the GI tract; however, electrolytes are also absorbed from the GI tract. Discussion of individual electrolytes in upcoming chapters explains how GI absorption of foods and fluids affects their balances.

The glands play on

The parathyroid glands also play a role in electrolyte balance, specifically the balance of calcium and phosphorus. The parathyroid glands (usually two pairs) are located behind and to the side of the thyroid gland. They secrete parathyroid hormone, which draws calcium into the blood from the bones, intestines, and kidneys and helps move phosphorus from the blood to the kidneys, where it's excreted in urine.

The thyroid gland is also involved in electrolyte balance by secreting calcitonin. This hormone lowers an elevated calcium level by preventing calcium release from bone. Calcitonin also decreases intestinal absorption and kidney reabsorption of calcium.

Kidney involvement

Remember filtration? It's the process of removing particles from a solution by allowing the liquid portion to pass through a membrane. Filtration occurs in the nephron (the anatomic and functional unit of the kidneys). As blood circulates through the glo-

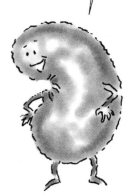

Filtration occurs in my nephron.

Now I get it!

How the nephron regulates balance

In the illustration below, the nephron is stretched to show where and how fluids and electrolytes are regulated.

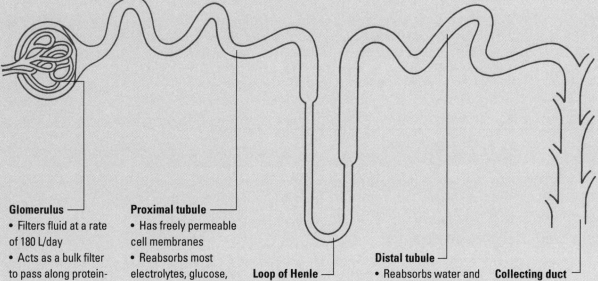

Glomerulus
• Filters fluid at a rate of 180 L/day
• Acts as a bulk filter to pass along protein-free and red blood cell–free filtrate (liquid that has been filtered)

Proximal tubule
• Has freely permeable cell membranes
• Reabsorbs most electrolytes, glucose, urea, and amino acids
• Carries large amounts of water with electrolytes back to circulation
• Reduces water content of filtrate by 70%

Loop of Henle
• Contains a high concentration of salts, mostly sodium
• Further concentrates filtrate because of water lost by osmosis
• Pulls chloride and sodium out of filtrate without water and reabsorbs them in ascending limb
• Causes filtrate to become more dilute as it moves into distal tubule

Distal tubule
• Reabsorbs water and concentrates urine as a result of antidiuretic hormone (ADH) action
• Reabsorbs sodium and water; secretes potassium as a result of aldosterone action

Collecting duct
• Has ADH, which acts to reabsorb water
• Absorbs or secretes potassium, sodium, urea, hydrogen ions, and ammonia, according to the body's needs

merulus (a tuft of capillaries), fluids and electrolytes are filtered and collected in the nephron's tubule.

Some fluids and electrolytes are reabsorbed through capillaries at various points along the nephron; others are secreted. Age can play an important role in the way kidneys function—or malfunction. (See *Who is at risk?*)

Keeping electrolyte levels in check

A vital part of the kidneys' job is to regulate electrolyte levels in the body. Normally functioning kidneys maintain the correct fluid level in the body. Sodium and fluid balance are closely related. When too much sodium is released, the body's fluid level drops.

The kidneys also rid the body of excess potassium. When the kidneys fail, potassium builds up in the body. High levels of potassium in the blood can be fatal. (For more information about which areas of the nephron control fluid and electrolyte balance, see *How the nephron regulates balance*, page 29.)

How diuretics affect balance

Many patients—whether hospitalized or at home—take a diuretic to increase urine production. Diuretics are used to treat many disorders, such as hypertension, heart failure, electrolyte imbalances, and kidney disease.

Monitoring a diuretic's effects

The health care team monitors the effects of a diuretic, including its effect on electrolyte balance. A diuretic causes electrolyte loss, whereas an I.V. fluid causes electrolyte gain.

Older adults, who are at risk for fluid and electrolyte imbalances, need careful monitoring because a diuretic can worsen an existing imbalance. When you know how the nephron functions

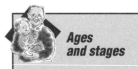

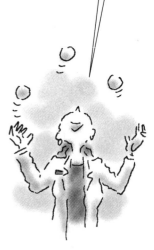

The kidney is a master juggler.

Cheat sheet

Diuretics upset the balance

- Increase urine production
- Treat hypertension, heart failure, electrolyte imbalances, and kidney disease
- Cause electrolyte loss
- Require careful monitoring of electrolytes

Now I get it!

Where diuretics work

Here's a look at the effects of diuretics and other drugs along the nephron.

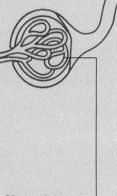

Glomerulus
Dopamine. Not generally classified as a diuretic, dopamine is included here because it may increase urine output. Dopaminergic receptor sites exist along the afferent arterioles (tiny vessels that bring blood to the glomerulus). In low doses (0.5 to 3 mcg/kg/minute), dopamine acts here to dilate the vessels to increase blood flow to the glomerulus. This, in turn, increases filtration in the nephron.

Proximal tubule
Osmotic diuretics (mannitol and glucose). Mannitol isn't reabsorbed in the tubule; it remains in high concentrations throughout its journey, increasing filtrate osmolality and hindering water, sodium, and chloride reabsorption, thereby increasing their excretion.

High blood glucose levels cause excess glucose to spill over into the tubules. The osmotic effect of glucose also results in increased urine output.

Carbonic anhydrase inhibitors (acetazolamide [Diamox]). These drugs reduce hydrogen ion (acid) concentration in the tubule, which causes increased excretion of bicarbonate, water, sodium, and potassium.

Loop of Henle
Loop diuretics (furosemide [Lasix], bumetanide [Bumex], and ethacrynic acid [Edecrin]). These diuretics act on the ascending loop of Henle to prevent water and sodium reabsorption. As a result, volume in the tubules is increased and blood volume is decreased. Potassium and chloride are also excreted here.

Distal tubule
Thiazide diuretics (hydrochlorothiazide [HydroDIURIL] and metolazone [Zaroxolyn]). Thiazide diuretics act high in the distal tubule to prevent sodium reabsorption, which increases the amount of tubular fluid and electrolytes farther down the nephron. Blood volume decreases, aldosterone increases sodium reabsorption and, in exchange, potassium is lost from the body.

Potassium-sparing diuretics (spironolactone [Aldactone]). These diuretics interfere with sodium and chloride reabsorption in the tubule. Potassium is spared, and sodium, chloride, and water are excreted. Urine output increases, and the body retains potassium.

What I.V. fluids contain

This table lists the electrolyte content of some commonly used I.V. fluids.

I.V. solution	Electrolyte	Amount
Dextrose	None	——
Sodium chloride		
5%	Sodium chloride	855 mEq/L
3%	Sodium chloride	513 mEq/L
0.9%	Sodium chloride	154 mEq/L
0.45%	Sodium chloride	77 mEq/L
Dextrose and sodium chloride		
5% dextrose and 0.9% sodium chloride	Sodium chloride	154 mEq/L
5% dextrose and 0.45% sodium chloride	Sodium chloride	77 mEq/L
Ringer's solution (plain)		
	Chloride	156 mEq/L
	Sodium	147 mEq/L
	Calcium	4.5 mEq/L
	Potassium	4 mEq/L
Lactated Ringer's solution		
	Sodium	130 mEq/L
	Chloride	109 mEq/L
	Lactate	28 mEq/L
	Potassium	4 mEq/L
	Calcium	3 mEq/L

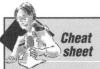

Cheat sheet

Key issues in I.V. fluid treatment

- Patient's normal electrolyte requirements
- Correct amount of electrolytes prescribed and given
- Length of treatment
- Concomitant oral electrolyte supplementation

normally, you can predict a diuretic's effects on your patient by knowing where along the nephron the drug acts.

This knowledge and understanding can help you provide optimal care for a patient taking a diuretic. (See *Where diuretics work*, page 31.)

I.V. fluids

Like diuretics, I.V. fluids affect electrolyte balance in the body. When providing I.V. fluid, keep in mind the patient's normal electrolyte requirements. For instance, the patient may require:
- 1 to 2 mEq/kg/day of sodium
- 0.5 to 1 mEq/kg/day of potassium
- 1 to 2 mEq/kg/day of chloride.

Improving your I.V. IQ

To evaluate I.V. fluid treatment, ask:
- Is the I.V. fluid providing the correct amount of electrolytes?
- How long has the patient been receiving I.V. fluids?
- Is the patient receiving oral supplementation of electrolytes?
 For more about I.V. fluids, see chapter 17, I.V. fluid replacement. (For the electrolyte content of some commonly used I.V. fluids, see *What I.V. fluids contain.*)

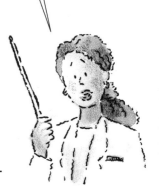

Keep in mind the patient's normal electrolyte needs.

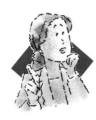

Quick quiz

1. When a burn damages cells, you would expect the cells to release the major electrolyte:
    A. calcium.
    B. chloride.
    C. potassium.

Answer: C. Potassium is one of the major electrolytes inside the cell that leaks out into the extracellular fluid after a major trauma such as a burn. This puts the patient at risk for hyperkalemia.

2. Diuretics affect the kidneys by altering the reabsorption and excretion of:
    A. water only.
    B. electrolytes only.
    C. water and electrolytes.

Answer: C. Diuretics generally affect how much water and sodium the body excretes. At the same time, other electrolytes such as potassium can also be excreted in urine.

3. The main extracellular cation is:
    A. calcium.
    B. potassium.
    C. sodium.

Answer: C. Sodium is the main extracellular cation. Among other things, it helps regulate fluid balance in the body.

4. In the nephron, most electrolytes are reabsorbed in the:
   A.   proximal tubule.
   B.   glomerulus.
   C.   loop of Henle.

Answer: A. The proximal tubule reabsorbs most of the electrolytes from the filtrate. It also reabsorbs glucose, urea, amino acids, and water.

5. Potassium is essential for conducting electrical impulses because it causes ions to:
   A.   clump together to generate a current.
   B.   shift in and out of the cell to conduct a current.
   C.   trap sodium inside the cell to maintain a current.

Answer: B. Potassium in the intracellular fluid causes ions to shift in and out of the cell, which allows electrical impulses to be conducted from cell to cell.

Scoring

☆☆☆ If you answered all five questions correctly, congratulations! You understand balance so well, you're ready to walk the high wire.

☆☆ If you answered four correctly, great! You still have all the qualities of a well-balanced individual!

☆ If you answered fewer than three correctly, no need to feel too unbalanced! Just review the chapter and you'll be fine.

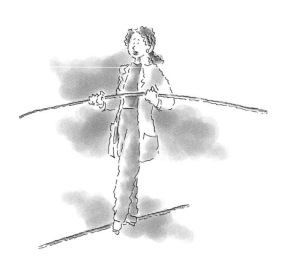

Balancing acids and bases

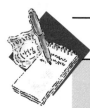

Just the facts

This chapter discusses acids and bases and the way the body balances them. In this chapter, you'll learn:

♦ what acids and bases are

♦ what pH is and what role it plays in metabolism

♦ how the body regulates its acid-base balance

♦ what diagnostic tests are used to assess acid-base balance.

A look at acids and bases

The chemical reactions that sustain life depend on a delicate balance — or homeostasis — between acids and bases in the body. Even a slight imbalance can profoundly affect metabolism and essential body functions. Several conditions, such as infection and trauma, and medications can affect acid-base balance. However, to understand this balance, you need to understand some basic chemistry.

Understanding pH

Understanding acids and bases requires an understanding of pH, a calculation based on the percentage of hydrogen ions in a solution and the amount of acids and bases in the solution.

Acids consist of molecules that can give up, or donate, hydrogen ions to other molecules. Carbonic acid is an acid that occurs naturally in the body. Bases consist of molecules that can accept hydrogen ions; bicarbonate is one example of a base.

A solution that contains more base than acid has fewer hydrogen ions, so it has a higher pH. A solution with a pH above 7 is a base. A solution that contains more acid than base has more hy-

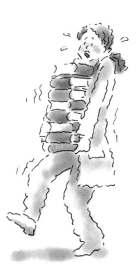

Balancing acids and bases must be easier than balancing these books!

Now I get it!

Normal pH

The illustration shows that the blood pH normally stays slightly alkaline, between 7.35 to 7.45. At that point, the amount of acid (H) is balanced with the amount of base (bicarbonate). A pH below 7.35 is abnormally acidic; a pH above 7.45, abnormally alkaline.

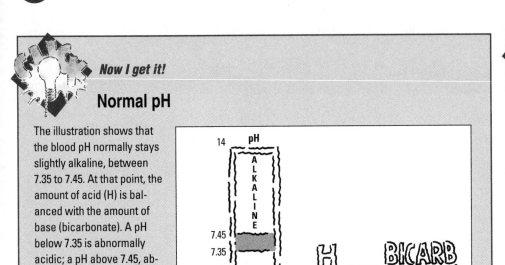

Cheat sheet

Acids and bases

• *Acids*—consist of molecules that can give up hydrogen molecules to other molecules; solutions with a pH below 7
• *Bases*—consist of molecules that can accept hydrogen molecules; solutions with a pH above 7

drogen ions, so it has a lower pH. A solution with a pH below 7 is an acid.

Getting your PhD in pH

You can assess a patient's acid-base balance if you know the pH of his blood. Because arterial blood is usually used to measure pH, this discussion focuses on arterial samples.

Arterial blood is normally slightly alkaline, ranging from 7.35 to 7.45. That pH represents a balance between the percentage of hydrogen ions and bicarbonate ions.

Generally, pH is maintained in a ratio of 20 parts bicarbonate to 1 part carbonic acid. A pH below 6.8 or above 7.8 is usually fatal. (See *Normal pH*.)

Low pH

Under certain conditions, the pH of arterial blood may deviate significantly from its normal narrow range. If the hydrogen ion concentration of the blood increases or the bicarbonate level decreases, pH may decrease. In either case, a decrease in pH below 7.35 signals acidosis. (See *Acidosis.*)

Now I get it!

Acidosis

Acidosis, a condition in which pH is below 7.35, occurs when acids (H) accumulate or bases such as bicarbonate are lost.

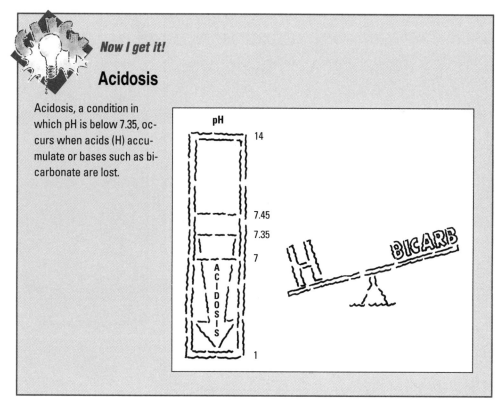

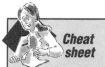

Cheat sheet

Deviation from normal pH

• Compromises well-being, electrolyte balance, activity of critical enzymes, muscle contraction, and basic cellular function
• Usually fatal if below 6.8 or above 7.8
• Indicates alkalosis if above 7.45
• Indicates acidosis if below 7.35

High pH

If the bicarbonate level increases or the hydrogen ion concentration of the blood decreases—the opposite effect of a low pH—pH may increase. In either case, an increase in pH above 7.45 signals alkalosis. (See *Alkalosis*, page 38.)

Regulating acids and bases

A person's well-being depends on his ability to maintain a normal pH. A deviation in the pH can compromise essential body processes, including electrolyte balance, activity of critical enzymes, muscle contraction, and basic cellular function. The body normally maintains pH within a narrow range by carefully balancing acidic and alkaline elements. When one aspect of that balancing act breaks down, the body can't maintain a healthy pH as easily, and problems arise.

Now I get it!

Alkalosis

Alkalosis, a condition in which pH is higher than 7.45, occurs when bases such as bicarbonate accumulate or acids (H) are lost.

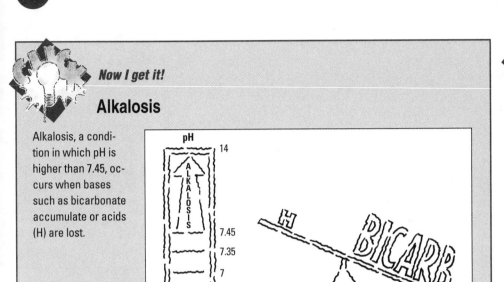

Cheat sheet

Three regulatory systems

- *Chemical buffers*—neutralize the offending acid or base
- *Respiratory system*—regulates retention and excretion of acids
- *Kidneys*—excrete or retain more acids or bases

The big three regulators

The body regulates acids and bases to avoid potentially serious consequences. Therefore, when pH rises or falls, three regulatory systems come into play:

- Chemical buffers act immediately to protect tissues and cells. These buffers instantly combine with the offending acid or base, neutralizing harmful effects until other regulators take over.
- The respiratory system uses hypoventilation or hyperventilation as needed to regulate excretion or retention of acids within minutes of a change in pH.
- The kidneys kick in by excreting or retaining more acids or bases as needed. Renal regulation can restore normal hydrogen ion concentration within hours or days.

Regulation method 1

The body maintains a healthy pH in part through chemical buffers, substances that minimize changes in pH by combining with excess acids or bases. Chemical buffers in the blood, the intracellular fluid, and the interstitial fluid serve as the body's most efficient pH-

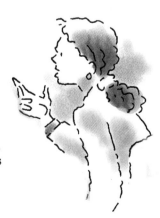

Cheat sheet

Chemical buffer systems

• *Bicarbonate-buffer system*—buffers blood and interstitial fluid; kidneys regulate bicarbonate production, and lungs regulate carbonic acid production

• *Phosphate-buffer system*—reacts with acids and bases to form compounds that alter pH; especially effective in the renal tubules

• *Protein-buffer system*—inside and outside cell; binds with acids and bases to neutralize them

balancing weapon. The main chemical buffers are bicarbonate, phosphate, and protein.

Bicarbonate buffers

The bicarbonate-buffer system is the body's primary buffer system and is mainly responsible for buffering blood and interstitial fluid. This system relies on a series of chemical reactions in which pairs of weak acids and bases (such as carbonic acid and bicarbonate) combine with the stronger acids (such as hydrochloric acid) and bases to weaken them.

Decreasing the strength of potentially damaging acids and bases reduces the danger those chemicals pose to pH balance. The kidneys assist the bicarbonate-buffer system in regulating production of bicarbonate. The lungs assist by regulating the production of carbonic acid, which results from combining carbon dioxide and water.

Phosphate buffers

Like the bicarbonate-buffer system, the phosphate-buffer system also depends on a series of chemical reactions to minimize pH changes. Phosphate buffers react with either acids or bases to form compounds that slightly alter pH, which can provide extremely effective buffering. This system proves especially effective in renal tubules, where phosphates exist in greater concentrations.

Protein buffers

Protein buffers, the most plentiful buffers in the body, work inside and outside cells. They're made up of hemoglobin as well as other proteins. Behaving chemically like bicarbonate buffers, protein

Ages and stages

Acid-base balance in the young and the old

Remember that an infant's kidneys can't acidify urine as well as an adult's can. Also keep in mind that the respiratory system of an older adult may be compromised and less able to regulate acid-base balance. Because ammonia production decreases with age, the kidneys of an older adult can't handle excess acid as well as the kidneys of a younger adult.

buffers bind with acids and bases to neutralize them. In red blood cells, for instance, hemoglobin combines with hydrogen ions to act as a buffer.

Regulation method 2

The respiratory system serves as the second line of defense against acid-base imbalances. The lungs regulate blood levels of carbon dioxide, a gas that combines with water to form carbonic acid. Increased levels of carbonic acid lead to a decrease in pH.

Chemoreceptors in the medulla of the brain sense those pH changes and vary the rate and depth of breathing to compensate. Breathing faster or deeper eliminates more carbon dioxide from the lungs. The more carbon dioxide that's lost, the less carbonic acid that's made and, as a result, pH rises. The body normalizes such a pH change by reducing carbon dioxide excretion, by breathing slower or less deeply. (See *CO_2 and hyperventilation*.)

Check the $Paco_2$

To assess the effectiveness of ventilation, look at the partial pressure of carbon dioxide in arterial blood ($Paco_2$). Normal $Paco_2$ level in the body is 35 to 45 mm Hg. $Paco_2$ values reflect carbon dioxide levels in the blood. As those levels increase, so does $Paco_2$. (See *Acid-base balance in the young and the old*, page 39.)

Twice as good

As a buffer, the respiratory system can maintain acid-base balance twice as effectively as can chemical buffers because it can handle twice the amount of acids and bases. Although the respiratory sys-

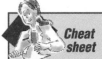

Respiratory system function

- Responds to pH changes in minutes
- Makes temporary adjustments to pH
- Regulates blood carbon dioxide levels by varying the rate and depth of breathing
- Low bicarbonate level—compensates with quicker and deeper breathing so more carbon dioxide is lost
- High bicarbonate level—compensates with slower, shallower breathing so more carbon dioxide is retained

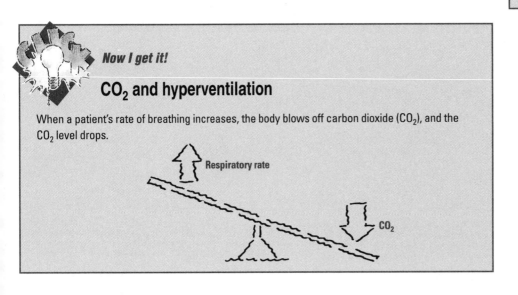

Now I get it!

CO_2 and hyperventilation

When a patient's rate of breathing increases, the body blows off carbon dioxide (CO_2), and the CO_2 level drops.

Respiratory rate

CO_2

tem responds to pH changes within minutes, it can restore normal pH only temporarily. The kidneys are responsible for long-term adjustments to pH.

Regulation method 3

The kidneys serve as yet another mechanism for maintaining acid-base balance in the body. They can reabsorb acids and bases or excrete them into urine. They can also produce bicarbonate to replenish lost supplies. Such adjustments to pH take the kidneys hours to days to complete.

Adjusting the bicarb

The kidneys also regulate the bicarbonate level, which reflects the metabolic component of acid-base balance. Normally, the bicarbonate level is reported with arterial blood gas (ABG) results. The normal bicarbonate level is 22 to 26 mEq/L. Bicarbonate is also reported with serum electrolyte levels as total serum carbon dioxide content.

The kidney keeps working

If the blood contains too much acid or not enough base, the pH drops and the kidneys reabsorb sodium bicarbonate. The kidneys also excrete hydrogen along with phosphate or ammonia. Although urine tends to be acidic because the body usually produces slightly more acids than bases, in such situations urine becomes more acidic than normal.

The reabsorption of bicarbonate and the increased excretion of hydrogen causes more bicarbonate to be formed in the renal tubules and eventually retained in the body. The bicarbonate level in the blood then rises to a more normal level, increasing pH.

In, out, in, out

If the blood contains more base and less acid, pH rises. The kidneys compensate by excreting bicarbonate and retaining more hydrogen ions. As a result, urine becomes more alkaline and the blood bicarbonate level drops. Conversely, if the blood contains less bicarbonate and more acid, pH drops.

The body responds to acid-base imbalances by activating compensatory mechanisms that minimize pH changes. Returning the pH to a normal or near-normal level mainly involves changes in the component—metabolic or respiratory—not primarily affected by the imbalance.

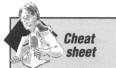
When a lack of bicarbonate causes acidosis, the lungs increase the rate of breathing, which blows off carbon dioxide.

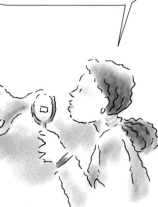

Taking an ABG sample

When a needle puncture is needed to obtain an arterial blood gas (ABG) sample, the radial, brachial, or femoral arteries may be used. However, the angle of penetration varies.

For the radial artery—the artery most commonly used—the needle should enter bevel up at a 45-degree angle, as shown. For the brachial artery, the angle should be 60 degrees; for the femoral artery, 90 degrees.

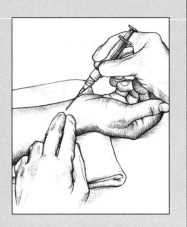

If the body compensates only partially for an imbalance, pH will still be outside the normal range. If the body compensates fully or completely, pH will be back to normal.

Respiratory helps metabolic

If metabolic disturbance is the primary cause of an acid-base imbalance, the lungs can compensate in one of two ways. When a lack of bicarbonate causes acidosis, the lungs increase the rate of breathing, which blows off carbon dioxide and helps to raise the pH to normal. When an excess of bicarbonate causes alkalosis, the lungs decrease the rate of breathing, which retains carbon dioxide and helps lower the pH.

Metabolic helps respiratory

If the respiratory system disturbs the acid-base balance, the kidneys can compensate by altering levels of bicarbonate and hydrogen ions. When the $Paco_2$ is high (a state of acidosis), the kidneys retain bicarbonate and excrete more acid to raise the pH. When the $Paco_2$ level is low (a state of alkalosis), the kidneys excrete bicarbonate and hold on to more acid to lower the pH.

Diagnosing imbalances

A number of tests are used to diagnose acid-base disturbances. Here's a look at the more common ones.

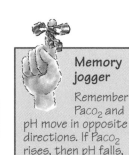

Memory jogger

Remember $Paco_2$ and pH move in opposite directions. If $Paco_2$ rises, then pH falls, and vice versa.

ABG analysis

An ABG analysis is a diagnostic test, which uses a sample of blood obtained from an arterial puncture, that can help you assess the effectiveness of breathing and overall acid-base balance. In addition to helping you identify problems with oxygenation and acid-base imbalances, the test can also help you monitor a patient's response to treatment. (See *Taking an ABG sample.*)

Keep in mind that ABG analysis should be used only in conjunction with a full patient assessment. Only by assessing all information can you gain a clear picture of what's happening.

An ABG analysis involves several separate test results, only three of which relate to acid-base balance: pH, $Paco_2$, and bicarbonate level. The normal ranges for adults are:
- *pH* — 7.35 to 7.45
- *$Paco_2$* — 35 to 45 mm Hg
- *HCO_3^-* — 22 to 26 mEq/L.

The ABC's of ABG

Recall that pH is a measure of the hydrogen ion concentration of the blood; $Paco_2$ is a measure of the partial pressure of carbon dioxide in arterial blood that indicates the effectiveness of breathing. $Paco_2$ levels move in the opposite direction as pH. Bicarbonate, which moves in the same direction as pH, represents the metabolic component of the body's acid-base balance.

Other information routinely reported with ABG results include partial pressure of oxygen dissolved in arterial blood (Pao_2) and arterial oxygen saturation (Sao_2). The normal Pao_2 range is 80 to 100 mm Hg; however, Pao_2 varies with age. After age 60, the Pao_2 may drop below 80 mm Hg without signs of hypoxia. The normal Sao_2 range is 95% to 100%.

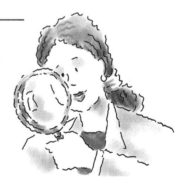

Quick look at ABG results

This is a quick look at how to interpret arterial blood gas (ABG) results:
- Check the pH. Is it normal (7.35 to 7.45), acidotic (below 7.35), or alkalotic (above 7.45)?
- Check $Paco_2$. Is it normal (35 to 45 mm Hg), low, or high?
- Check the bicarbonate level. Is it normal (22 to 26 mEq/L), low, or high?
- Check for signs of compensation. Which value ($Paco_2$ or bicarbonate) more closely corresponds to the change in pH?
- Check Pao_2 and Sao_2. Is the Pao_2 normal (80 to 100 mm Hg), low, or high? Is the Sao_2 normal (95% to 100%), low, or high?

Interpreting ABG results

When interpreting results from an ABG analysis, be consistent in the sequence you use to analyze the information. Here's one step-by-step process you can use. (See *Quick look at ABG results.*)

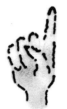

Step 1: Check the pH

First, check the pH. This figure will form the basis for understanding most other figures.

If the pH is abnormal, determine whether it reflects acidosis (below 7.35) or alkalosis (above 7.45). Then figure out whether the cause is respiratory or metabolic.

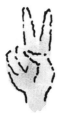

Step 2: Determine the CO$_2$

Remember that the PaCO_2 level provides information about the respiratory component of acid-base balance.

If the PaCO_2 is abnormal, determine whether it's low (less than 35 mm Hg) or high (greater than 45 mm Hg). Then determine whether the abnormal result corresponds with a change in pH. For example, if the pH is high, you would expect the PaCO_2 to be low (hypocapnia), indicating that the problem is primarily respiratory in origin. Conversely, if the pH is low, you would expect the PaCO_2 to be high (hypercapnia), indicating that the problem is respiratory acidosis.

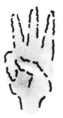

Step 3: Watch the bicarbonate

Next, examine the bicarbonate level, which provides information about the metabolic aspect of acid-base balance.

If the bicarbonate level is abnormal, determine whether it's low (less than 22 mEq/L) or high (greater than 26 mEq/L). Then determine whether the abnormal result corresponds with the change in pH. For example, if the pH is high, you would expect the bicarbonate level to be high, indicating that the problem is primarily metabolic in origin. Conversely, if the pH is low, you would expect the bicarbonate level to be low, indicating that the problem is metabolic acidosis.

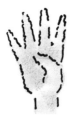

Step 4: Look for compensation

Sometimes you'll see a change in both the PaCO_2 and the bicarbonate level. One value indicates the primary source of the pH change; the other, the body's effort to compensate for the disturbance.

Complete compensation occurs when the body's ability to compensate is so effective that the pH falls within the normal range. Partial compensation, on the other hand, occurs when the pH remains outside the normal range.

Compensation involves opposites. For instance, if results indicate primary metabolic acidosis, compensation will come in the form of respiratory alkalosis. For example, the following ABG results indicate metabolic acidosis with compensatory respiratory alkalosis:
• *pH*—7.27
• *PaCO_2*—7 mm Hg
• *HCO$_3^-$*—10 mEq/L.

The low pH indicates acidosis. However, the PaCO_2 is low, which normally leads to alkalosis, and the bicarbonate level is low, which normally leads to acidosis. The bicarbonate level, then, more closely corresponds with the pH, making the primary cause

Inaccurate ABG results

To avoid altering arterial blood gas (ABG) results, be sure to use proper technique when drawing a sample of arterial blood. Remember:
• A delay in getting the sample to the laboratory or drawing blood for ABG analysis within 15 to 20 minutes of a procedure, such as suctioning or administering a respiratory treatment, could alter results.
• Air bubbles in the syringe could affect the oxygen level.
• Venous blood in the syringe could alter carbon dioxide and oxygen levels and pH.

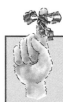

Memory jogger

Remember: Bicarbonate and pH increase or decrease together. When one rises or falls, so does the other.

of the problem metabolic. The resultant decrease in the $Paco_2$ reflects respiratory compensation.

Normal values for pH, $Paco_2$, and HCO_3^- would indicate that the patient's acid-base balance is normal.

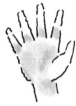

Step 5: Determine Pao_2 and Sao_2

Last, check Pao_2 and Sao_2, which yield information about the patient's oxygenation status.

If the values are abnormal, determine whether they're high (Pao_2 greater than 100 mm Hg) or low (Pao_2 less than 80 mm Hg and Sao_2 less than 95%).

Remember that Pao_2 reflects the body's ability to pick up oxygen from the lungs. A low Pao_2 represents hypoxemia and can cause hyperventilation. The Pao_2 value also indicates when to make adjustments in the concentration of oxygen being administered to a patient. (See *Inaccurate ABG results.*)

Anion gap

You may come across a test result called the anion gap. (See *Crossing the great anion gap.*) Earlier chapters discuss how the strength of cations (positively charged ions) and anions (negatively charged ions) must be equal in the blood to maintain a proper balance of electrical charges. The anion gap result helps you differentiate among various acidotic conditions.

Crossing the great anion gap

This illustration represents the normal anion gap. The gap is calculated by adding the chloride level and the bicarbonate level and then subtracting that total from the sodium level. The value normally ranges from 8 to 14 mEq/L and represents the level of unmeasured anions in extracellular fluid.

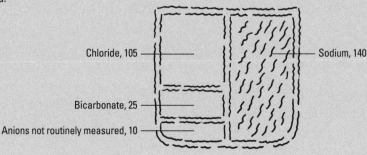

Chloride, 105

Sodium, 140

Bicarbonate, 25

Anions not routinely measured, 10

Look at the main cations and anions and the way they affect acid-base balance.

Identifying the gap

The anion gap refers to the relationship among the body's cations and anions. Sodium accounts for more than 90% of the circulating cations. Chloride and bicarbonate together account for 85% of the counterbalancing anions. (Potassium is generally omitted because it occurs in such low, stable amounts.)

The gap between the two measurements represents the anions not routinely measured, including sulfates, phosphates, proteins, and organic acids, such as lactic acid and ketone acids. Because these anions aren't measured in routine laboratory tests, the anion gap is a way of determining their presence.

Looking into the gap

An increase in the anion gap that's greater than 14 mEq/L indicates an increase in the percentage of one or more unmeasured anions in the bloodstream. Increases can occur with acidotic conditions characterized by higher-than-normal amounts of organic acids. Such conditions include lactic acidosis and ketoacidosis.

The anion gap remains normal for certain other conditions, including hyperchloremic acidosis, renal tubular acidosis, and severe bicarbonate-wasting conditions, such as biliary or pancreatic fistulas and poorly functioning ileal loops.

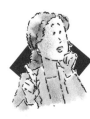

Quick quiz

1. A measurement of $Paco_2$ indicates the effectiveness of:
    A. kidney function.
    B. lung ventilation.
    C. phosphate buffers.

Answer: B. $Paco_2$ reflects how well the respiratory system is helping to maintain acid-base balance.

2. The kidneys respond to acid-base disturbances by:
    A. adjusting $Paco_2$ levels.
    B. producing phosphate buffers.
    C. excreting or reabsorbing hydrogen or bicarbonate.

Answer: C. The kidneys respond to particular acid-base imbalances by excreting or reabsorbing hydrogen or bicarbonate, according to the body's needs.

3. If your patient is breathing rapidly, his body is attempting to:
  A. retain carbon dioxide.
  B. get rid of excess carbon dioxide.
  C. improve the buffering ability of bicarbonate.

Answer: B. High carbon dioxide levels in the blood, measured as $Paco_2$, cause a drop in pH. Chemoreceptors in the brain sense this decrease and stimulate the lungs to hyperventilate, causing the body to eliminate more carbon dioxide.

4. If your patient has a higher-than-normal pH (alkalosis), you would expect to also see:
  A. high $Paco_2$.
  B. low $Paco_2$.
  C. low HCO_3^-.

Answer: B. A low $Paco_2$ means less carbon dioxide (acid) is in the blood, which raises the pH.

5. The laboratory reports the following ABG results for your patient: pH, 7.33; $Paco_2$, 40 mm Hg; and HCO_3^-, 20 mEq/L. You interpret these results as:
  A. respiratory acidosis.
  B. metabolic acidosis.
  C. respiratory alkalosis.

Answer: B. The pH is low, which indicates acidosis. Because the $Paco_2$ is normal and the bicarbonate is low (matching the pH), the primary cause of the problem is metabolic.

6. A Pao_2 level of 49 mm Hg indicates:
  A. acidosis.
  B. hypoxia.
  C. hypercapnia.

Answer: B. A Pao_2 of 49 mm Hg is below the normal range of 80 to 100 mm Hg and therefore indicates hypoxia.

7. A colleague hands you these ABG results: pH, 7.52; $Paco_2$, 47 mm Hg; and HCO_3^-, 36 mEq/L. You interpret these results as:
  A. respiratory acidosis.
  B. respiratory alkalosis with respiratory compensation.
  C. metabolic alkalosis with respiratory compensation.

Answer: C. The pH is alkalotic. Although both $Paco_2$ and HCO_3^- have changed, the HCO_3^- matches the pH. The elevated $Paco_2$ represents the efforts of the respiratory system to compensate for the alkalosis by retaining carbon dioxide.

Scoring

☆☆☆ If you answered all seven questions correctly, congratulations! You did a great job covering all the bases (and acids)!

☆☆ If you answered four to six correctly, great! You certainly didn't hydrogen bomb!

☆ If you answered fewer than four correctly, don't worry! It's never too late to get your PhD in pH!

Part II

Fluid and electrolyte imbalances

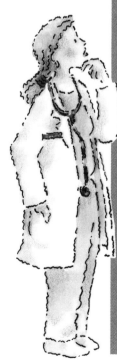

When fluids tip the balance

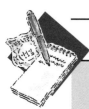

Just the facts

This chapter will help you learn how to assess and care for patients with fluid imbalances. In this chapter, you'll learn:

♦ how to assess a patient's fluid status

♦ which patients are at risk for developing fluid imbalances

♦ what to watch for in a patient with a fluid imbalance

♦ what to teach the patient about his particular fluid imbalance

♦ how to document the care given and teaching done for a patient with a fluid imbalance.

A look at fluid volume

Blood pressure is related to the amount of blood that the heart pumps and the extent of vasoconstriction present. Fluid volume affects these elements and makes blood pressure measurements key in assessing a patient's fluid status. Certain types of pressure, such as pulmonary artery pressure (PAP) and central venous pressure (CVP), are measured through specialized catheters. These measurements also help assess fluid volume status.

To maintain the accuracy of whatever blood pressure measurement system you use, periodically compare the readings of automated and direct measurement systems with manual readings.

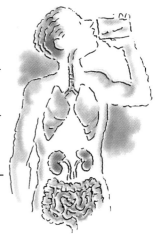

Cuff measurements

A simple blood-pressure measurement, taken with a stethoscope and a sphygmomanometer, is still one of the best tools for assessing fluid volume. It's quick and easy and carries little risk for the patient. Direct and indirect blood pressure measurements are generally related to the amount of blood flowing through the patient's circulatory system.

To measure blood pressure accurately, you must first make sure the cuff is the correct size. The bladder of the cuff should have a width of about 40% of the upper arm circumference.

Position the arm so the brachial artery is at heart level. To properly position a blood pressure cuff, wrap the cuff snugly around the upper arm, above the antecubital space. For adults, place the lower border of the cuff about 1" (2.5 cm) above the antecubital space. For children, place the lower border closer to the antecubital space.

Place the center of the cuff's bladder directly over the medial aspect of the arm, over the brachial artery. Most cuffs have a reference mark to help you position the bladder. After positioning the cuff, palpate the brachial artery and place the bell of the stethoscope directly over the point where you can feel the strongest pulsations. (See *Positioning a blood pressure cuff.*)

Taking BP automatically

You may also have access to an automated blood pressure unit. The unit is designed to take blood pressure measurements repeatedly, which is helpful when you're caring for a patient whose blood pressure is expected to change frequently (for example, a patient with a fluid imbalance). The unit automatically computes and digitally records blood pressure readings.

The cuff automatically inflates to check the blood pressure and deflates immediately afterward. You can program the monitor

Positioning a blood pressure cuff

This illustration shows how to properly position a blood pressure cuff and stethoscope bell.

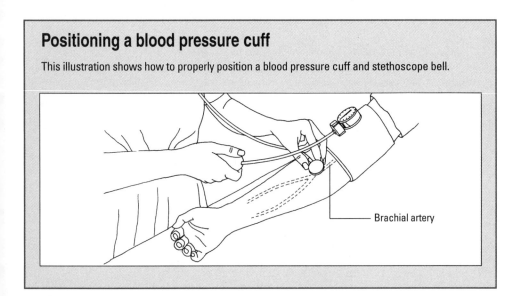

Brachial artery

to inflate the cuff as often as needed and set alarms for high, low, and mean blood pressures. The monitor displays each blood pressure reading until the next reading is taken.

Palpable pressures

If you have trouble hearing the patient's blood pressure, which is common when a patient is hypotensive, palpate the blood pressure to estimate systolic pressure.

To palpate the blood pressure, place a cuff on the upper arm and palpate the brachial pulse or the radial pulse. Inflate the cuff until you no longer feel the pulse. Then slowly deflate the cuff, noting the point at which you feel the pulse again—the systolic pressure. If you palpate a patient's blood pressure at 90 mm Hg, for example, chart it as "90/P" (the P stands for palpable).

The Doppler difference

What should you do if your patient's arm is swollen or his blood pressure is so low you can't feel his pulse? First, palpate his carotid artery to make sure he has a pulse. Then use a Doppler device to obtain a reading of his systolic pressure. (See *How to take a Doppler blood pressure.*)

The Doppler probe uses ultrasound waves directed at the blood vessel to detect blood flow. Through the Doppler unit, you'll be able to hear the patient's blood flow with each pulse.

To obtain a Doppler blood pressure, place a blood pressure cuff on the arm as you normally would. Apply lubricant to the antecubital area where you would expect to find the brachial pulse. Turn the unit on and place the probe lightly on the arm, over the brachial artery. Adjust the volume control and the placement of the probe until you hear the pulse clearly. (See *Correcting problems of blood pressure measurement,* page 54.)

Inflate the blood pressure cuff until the pulse sound disappears. Slowly deflate the cuff and note the point at which the pulse sound returns—the systolic pressure. If you hear the pulse at 80 mm Hg, for instance, record it as "80/D" (the D stands for Doppler).

Direct measurements

Direct measurement is an invasive method of obtaining blood pressure readings. It's indicated when highly accurate or frequent blood pressure measurements are required, as with severe fluid imbalances.

How to take a Doppler blood pressure

When you can't hear or feel a patient's blood pressure, try using a Doppler ultrasound device, as shown below.

Blood pressure cuff

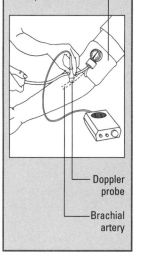

Doppler probe

Brachial artery

It's not working!

Correcting problems of blood pressure measurement

Use this chart to figure out what to do for each possible cause of a falsely high or falsely low blood pressure reading.

Problem and possible cause	What to do
False-high reading	
• Cuff too small	• Make sure the cuff bladder is long enough to completely encircle the extremity.
• Cuff wrapped too loosely, reducing its effective width	• Tighten the cuff.
• Slow cuff deflation causing venous congestion in the arm or leg	• Never deflate the cuff slower than 2 mm Hg/heartbeat.
• Tilted mercury column	• Read pressures with the mercury column vertical.
• Poorly timed measurement—after the patient has eaten, ambulated, appeared anxious, or flexed his arm muscles	• Postpone blood pressure measurement, or help the patient relax before taking pressures.
• Multiple attempts at reading blood pressure in the same arm, causing venous congestion	• Don't attempt to measure blood pressure more than twice in the same arm; wait several minutes between attempts.
False-low reading	
• Incorrect position of the arm or leg	• Make sure the arm or leg is level with the patient's heart.
• Mercury column below eye level	• Read mercury column at eye level.
• Failure to notice auscultatory gap (sound fades out for 10 to 15 mm Hg, then returns)	• Estimate systolic pressure using palpation before actually measuring it. Then check the palpable pressure against the measured pressure.
• Inaudible or low-volume sounds	• Before reinflating the cuff, instruct the patient to raise his arm or leg to decrease venous pressure and amplify low-volume sounds. After inflating the cuff, tell the patient to lower his arm or leg. Then deflate the cuff and listen. If you still fail to detect low-volume sounds, chart the palpable systolic pressure.

Arterial lines

Arterial lines, or A-lines, are inserted into the radial or the brachial artery (or the femoral artery, if needed). A-lines monitor blood pressure continuously and can also be used to sample arterial blood for blood gas analysis or other laboratory tests. Because the lines require a certain level of technology and staff training, patients who have these lines are usually placed in intermediate or critical care units.

Lines under pressure

The catheter is connected to a continuous flush system—a bag of normal saline solution (which may contain heparin) inside a pressurized cuff. This system maintains the patency of the line.

The line is connected to a transducer and then to a bedside monitor. The transducer converts fluid-pressure waves from the catheter into an electronic signal that can be analyzed and displayed on the monitor. Because the patient's blood pressure is displayed continuously, you can instantly note changes in the measurements and respond quickly.

Pulmonary artery catheters

An A-line directly measures blood pressure, whereas a pulmonary artery (PA) catheter directly measures other pressures. PA catheters are usually inserted into the subclavian vein or the internal jugular vein, although the lines are sometimes inserted into a vein in the arm or the leg.

The tip of the catheter is advanced through the vein into the right atrium, then into the right ventricle, and finally into the pulmonary artery. The hubs of the catheter are then connected to a pressurized transducer system that's similar to the system used for an A-line. (See *Pulmonary artery catheter*, page 56.)

Getting a clearer picture

The PA catheter provides a clearer picture of the patient's fluid volume status than other measurement techniques. The catheter allows for measurement of PAP, pulmonary artery wedge pressure (PAWP), cardiac output and CVP—all of which provide information about how the left side of the heart is functioning, including its pumping ability, filling pressures, and vascular volume.

The PAP is the pressure routinely displayed on the monitor. The normal systolic PAP is 15 to 25 mm Hg and reflects pressure from contraction of the right atrium. The normal diastolic PAP is 8 to 15 mm Hg and reflects the lowest pressure in the pulmonary vessels. The mean PAP is 10 to 20 mm Hg.

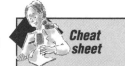

Cheat sheet

Arterial lines

• Typically inserted into the radial or brachial artery
• Used to monitor blood pressure continuously
• Can be used to sample arterial blood for laboratory tests

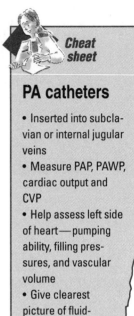

Pulmonary artery catheter

The ports on a pulmonary artery catheter (shown here) can be used for pacing, infusing solutions, or monitoring oxygen saturation, body temperature, cardiac output, or various intraluminal pressures, such as central venous pressure (through the proximal lumen) or pulmonary artery wedge pressure (through the distal lumen).

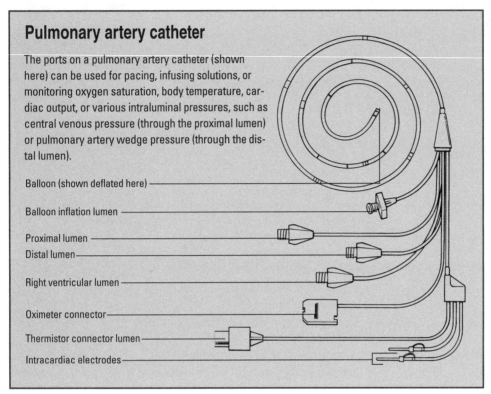

Balloon (shown deflated here)

Balloon inflation lumen

Proximal lumen

Distal lumen

Right ventricular lumen

Oximeter connector

Thermistor connector lumen

Intracardiac electrodes

Cheat sheet

PA catheters

• Inserted into subclavian or internal jugular veins
• Measure PAP, PAWP, cardiac output and CVP
• Help assess left side of heart—pumping ability, filling pressures, and vascular volume
• Give clearest picture of fluid-volume status

Wedging the balloon

When you inflate the small balloon at the catheter tip, blood carries the catheter tip farther into the pulmonary artery. The tip floats inside the artery until it stops—or becomes wedged—in a smaller branch.

When the tip is wedged in a branch of the pulmonary artery, the catheter measures pressures coming from the left side of the heart, a measurement that may prove useful in gauging changes in blood volume. The normal PAWP is 6 to 12 mm Hg.

PAP and PAWP are generally increased in cases of fluid overload and decreased in cases of fluid-volume deficit. That's why a PA catheter is useful when assessing and treating an acutely ill patient with a fluid imbalance.

Cardiac output, too

PA catheters also measure cardiac output, either continuously or after injections of I.V. fluid through the proximal lumen. Cardiac output is the amount of blood that the heart pumps in 1 minute and is calculated by multiplying the heart rate by the stroke volume. (Don't worry, the monitor makes that calculation for you!)

The stroke volume is the amount of blood the ventricle pumps out with each beat, and it's also calculated by the bedside monitor. The normal cardiac output is 4 to 8 L/minute. If a person lacks adequate blood volume, cardiac output is low (assuming the heart can pump normally otherwise). If the person is overloaded with fluid, cardiac output is high.

Estimating CVP

To estimate a patient's central venous pressure (CVP), follow these steps:

1. Place the patient at a 45- to 60-degree angle.
2. Use tangential lighting to observe the internal jugular vein.
3. Note the highest level of visible pulsation.
4. Locate the angle of Louis, or sternal notch, by palpating the point at which the clavicles join the sternum (the suprasternal notch).
5. Place two fingers on the patient's suprasternal notch and slide them down the sternum un-

til they reach a bony protuberance—the angle of Louis. The right atrium lies about 2″ (5 cm) below this point.
6. Measure the distance between the angle of Louis and the highest level of visible pulsation. Normally, this distance is less than 1.2″ (3 cm).
7. Add 2″ to this figure to estimate the distance between the highest level of pulsation and the right atrium. A distance greater than 4″ (10 cm) may indicate elevated CVP.

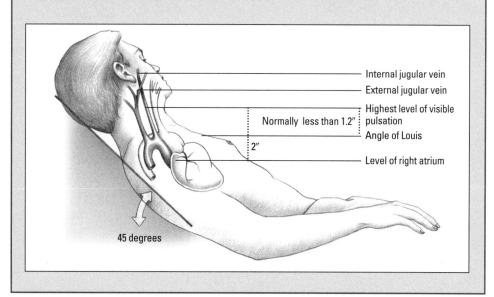

Central venous pressure

A central venous catheter can measure CVP, another useful indication of a patient's fluid status. The term *CVP* refers to the pressure of the blood inside the central venous circulation. The tip of a CVP catheter is usually placed in one of the jugular veins in the neck or in a subclavian vein in the chest.

The normal CVP ranges from 0 to 7 mm Hg (5 to 10 cm H_2O). If CVP is high, it usually means the patient is overloaded with fluid. If it's low, it usually means the patient is low on fluid. (To estimate CVP yourself, see *Estimating CVP*, page 57.)

How the body compensates

Most of the time, the body adequately compensates for minor fluid imbalances and keeps blood pressure readings and other measurements fairly normal. Sometimes, however, the body can't compensate for fluid deficits or excesses. When that happens, any of several problems may result, including dehydration, hypovolemia, hypervolemia, and water intoxication.

Dehydration

The body loses water all the time. A person responds to the thirst reflex by drinking fluids and eating foods that contain water. However, if water isn't adequately replaced, the body's cells can lose water, a condition called dehydration.

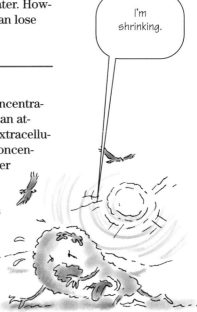

I'm shrinking.

How it happens

Loss of body fluids causes an increase in blood solute concentration (increased osmolality). Serum sodium levels rise. In an attempt to regain fluid balance between intracellular and extracellular spaces, water molecules shift out of cells into more concentrated blood. This process, combined with increased water intake and increased water retention in the kidneys, usually restores the body's fluid volume. (For more information on dehydration, see the *Incredibly Easy* color pages on passive and active transport and hypovolemia.)

Incredibly shrinking cells

Without an adequate supply of water in the extracellular space, fluid continues to shift out of the cells into the extracellular space. The cells begin to shrink as the

(Text continues on page 63.)

Passive transport mechanisms

Substances can move across the cell membrane by passive transport. No energy is required to accomplish this. It occurs through two mechanisms: diffusion and osmosis.

Diffusion
Substances move from an area of higher concentration to an area of lower concentration. Movement continues until distribution is uniform.

Osmosis
Water molecules move from an area of higher concentration to an area of lower concentration.

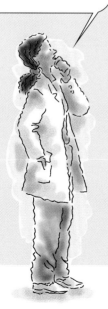

No energy is required for passive transport. And it's a good thing because I have my hands full already!

Diffusion

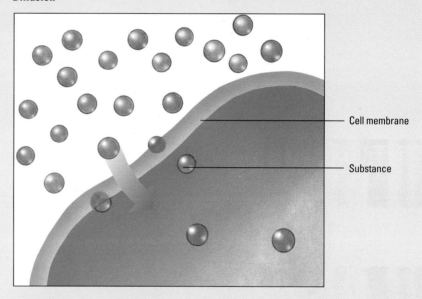

Cell membrane

Substance

Osmosis

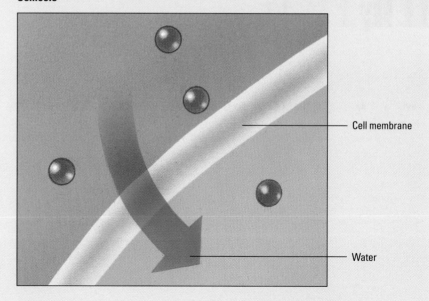

Cell membrane

Water

Hypovolemic shock

In patients with hypovolemic shock, fluid circulating in the blood vessels decreases, lowering cardiac output and leading to hypotension and impaired tissue perfusion. Recognizing hypovolemic shock promptly is crucial. Untreated, this condition can lead to progressive hypoxia, tissue death and, ultimately, cardiac and respiratory arrest.

Jump start for the heart

Sensory nerves in the aortic arch respond to decreased blood pressure by stimulating the sympathetic nervous system, causing tachycardia, increased cardiac contractility, and venous constriction. This temporarily improves cardiac output. Look for a progressive drop in blood pressure accompanied by a rapid, thready pulse.

Meanwhile, in the kidneys

Blood pressure sensors in the kidneys activate the renin-angiotensin-aldosterone system, which causes increased sodium and water retention in the kidneys. This mechanism helps the body preserve fluid.

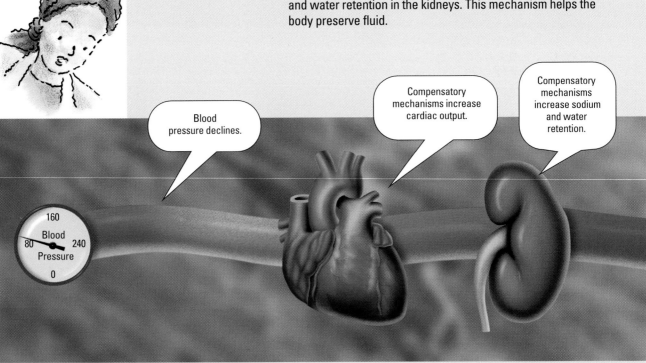

One heck of a hormone

When the brain senses low blood pressure, antidiuretic hormone (ADH) stimulates thirst, a mechanism to increase volume. You may note decreased urine output.

Now, the bad news...

Without prompt treatment, compensatory mechanisms can't maintain circulation for long and blood pressure falls dramatically. When blood pressure falls below 80 mm Hg, tissue perfusion decreases and not enough blood reaches the coronary arteries. Watch for arrhythmias and myocardial ischemia or infarction.

Dangerous complications

Hypoxia from poor tissue perfusion may cause dilation of the arterioles, which causes blood to become trapped in the capillaries. This can lead to disseminated intravascular coagulation. Watch for signs of this life-threatening complication: petechiae, bruising, bleeding, and oozing from the gums.

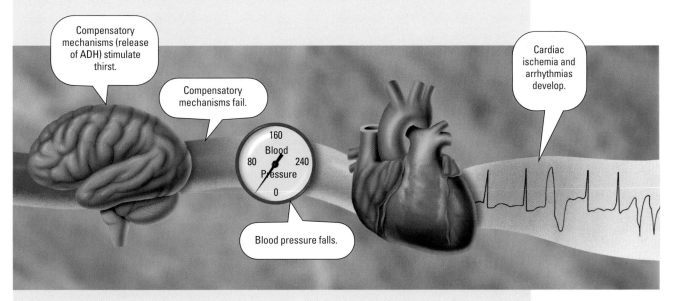

Active transport mechanisms

Active transport usually moves molecules and ions against a concentration gradient, from an area of lower concentration to one of higher concentration. This movement requires energy, usually in the form of adenosine triphosphate (ATP). The sodium-potassium pump and pinocytosis are two examples of active transport.

Sodium-potassium pump

This mechanism moves sodium from inside the cell to outside, where the sodium concentration is greater; potassium moves from outside the cell to inside, where the potassium concentration is greater.

Pinocytosis

In this mechanism, tiny vacuoles take droplets of fluid containing dissolved substances into the cell. The engulfed fluid is used in the cell.

Sodium-potassium pump

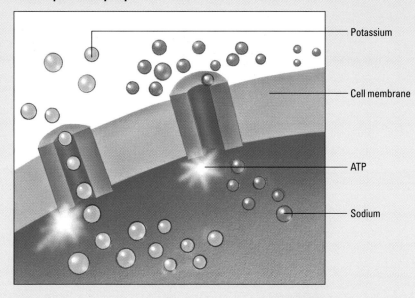

- Potassium
- Cell membrane
- ATP
- Sodium

Pinocytosis

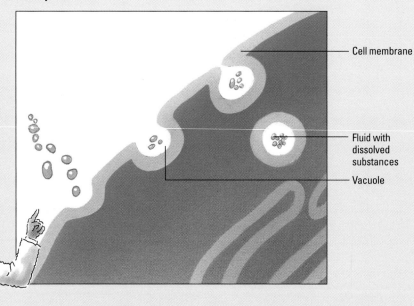

- Cell membrane
- Fluid with dissolved substances
- Vacuole

Energy is needed for active transport.

process continues. Because water is essential for obtaining nutrients, expelling wastes, and maintaining cell shape, cells can't function properly without adequate fluid.

Who is at risk?

Failure to respond adequately to the thirst stimulus increases the risk of dehydration. Confused, comatose, or bedridden patients are particularly vulnerable, as are infants, who can't drink fluid on their own and who have immature kidneys that can't concentrate urine efficiently.

Older patients are also prone to dehydration because they have a lower body-water content, diminished kidney function, and a reduced ability to sense thirst, so they can't correct fluid-volume deficits as easily as younger adults can. A patient may also become dehydrated if he's receiving highly concentrated feedings without enough supplemental water. (See *Different but the same.*)

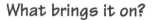

What brings it on?

Any situation that accelerates fluid loss can lead to dehydration. For instance, in diabetes insipidus, the brain fails to secrete antidiuretic hormone (ADH). If the brain doesn't secrete enough ADH, the result is a greater-than-normal diuresis.

A patient with diabetes insipidus produces large amounts of highly dilute urine—as much as 30 L/day. The patient is also thirsty and tends to drink large amounts of fluids, although he generally can't keep up with the diuresis.

Other causes of dehydration include prolonged fever, watery diarrhea, and renal failure and hyperglycemia, which causes the person to produce large amounts of dilute urine.

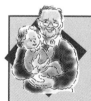

Ages and stages

Different but the same

Elderly patients and very young patients are susceptible to fluid and electrolyte imbalances. Despite the significant age difference, the contributing factors for these imbalances are the same in many cases:

• inability to obtain fluid without help
• inability to express feelings of thirst
• inaccurate assessment of output—for example, if the patient must wear a diaper
• loss of fluid through perspiration because of fever
• loss of fluid through diarrhea and vomiting.

What to look for

As dehydration progresses, watch for changes in mental status. The patient may complain of dizziness, weakness, or extreme thirst. He may have a fever (because less fluid is available for perspiration, which lowers body temperature), dry skin, or dry mucous membranes. Skin turgor may be poor. Because an older patient's skin may lack elasticity, checking skin turgor may be unreliable.

Heart rate may go up, and blood pressure may fall. In severe cases, seizures and coma may result. Also, urine output may fall because less fluid is circulating in the body. The urine is more concentrated unless the person has diabetes insipidus, in which case the urine will probably be pale and produced in large volume. (See *Danger signs of dehydration.*)

What tests show

Diagnostic test results you may see include:
- elevated hematocrit (HCT)
- elevated serum osmolality (above 300 mOsm/kg)
- elevated serum sodium level (above 145 mEq/L)
- urine specific gravity above 1.030.

Because patients with diabetes insipidus have more diluted urine, specific gravity is usually less than 1.005; osmolality, 50 to 200 mOsm/kg.

How dehydration is treated

Treatment for dehydration aims to replace missing fluids. Because a dehydrated patient's blood is concentrated, avoid hypertonic solutions. If the patient can handle oral fluids, encourage them; however, because the serum sodium level is elevated, make sure the fluids given are salt-free.

A severely dehydrated patient will receive I.V. fluids to replace lost fluids. Most patients receive hypotonic, low-sodium fluids, such as dextrose 5% in water (D_5W).

Remember, if you give a hypotonic solution too quickly, the fluid will move from the veins into the cells and cause them to become edematous. Swelling of cells in the brain can create cerebral edema. To avoid such potentially devastating problems, give fluids gradually, over a period of about 48 hours.

Cheat sheet

Signs and symptoms of dehydration

- irritability
- confusion
- dizziness
- weakness
- extreme thirst
- fever
- dry skin and mucous membranes
- sunken eyeballs
- poor skin turgor
- decreased urine output (with diabetes insipidus, urine will be pale and plentiful)
- increased heart rate with falling blood pressure.

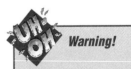

Warning!

Danger signs of dehydration

Begin emergency treatment for dehydration if your patient shows any of these signs:
- impaired mental status
- seizure
- coma.

How you intervene

Monitor at-risk patients closely to detect impending dehydration early. If a patient develops dehydration, here are some things you'll want to do:
• Monitor symptoms and vital signs closely so you can intervene quickly.
• Accurately record the patient's intake and output, including urine and stool.
• Maintain I.V. access as ordered. Monitor I.V. infusions. Watch for signs and symptoms of cerebral edema when your patient is receiving hypotonic fluids. Signs and symptoms include headache, confusion, irritability, lethargy, nausea, vomiting, widening pulse pressure, decreased pulse rate, and seizures. (See *Teaching about dehydration.*)
• Keep in mind that vasopressin may be ordered for patients with diabetes insipidus.
• Monitor serum sodium levels, urine osmolality, and urine specific gravity to assess fluid balance.
• Insert a urinary catheter, as ordered, to monitor output accurately.
• Provide a safe environment for any patient who is confused, dizzy, or at risk for a seizure, and teach his family to do the same.
• Obtain daily weights (same scale, same time of day) to evaluate treatment progress. (See *Documenting dehydration.*)
• Provide skin and mouth care to maintain the integrity of the skin surface and oral mucous membranes.
• Assess the patient for diaphoresis—it can be the source of major water loss.

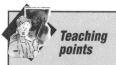

Teaching points

Teaching about dehydration

Be sure to cover these topics and to evaluate your patient's learning:
• explanation of dehydration and its treatment
• warning signs and symptoms
• prescribed medications
• importance of complying with therapy.

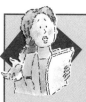

Chart smart

Documenting dehydration

When your patient is dehydrated, you'll want to document the following:
• assessment findings
• intake, output, and daily weight
• I.V. therapy
• patient's response to interventions
• associated diagnostic test results
• patient teaching done and the patient's response.

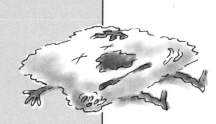

Hypovolemia

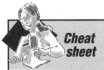

Hypovolemia refers to isotonic fluid loss (which includes loss of fluids and solutes) from the extracellular space. Children and older patients are especially vulnerable to hypovolemia. Some of the initial signs and symptoms of hypovolemia can be subtle as the body tries to compensate for the loss of circulating blood volume. Subtle signs can become more serious and, if not detected early and treated properly, can progress to hypovolemic shock, a common form of shock. (See *Hypovolemic shock*, page 60.)

How hypovolemia happens

Excessive fluid loss (bleeding, for instance) is a risk factor for hypovolemia, especially when combined with reduced fluid intake. Another risk factor is a third-space fluid shift, which occurs when fluid moves out of the intravascular space but not into the intracellular space. For instance, fluid may shift into the abdominal cavity (ascites), the pleural cavity, or the pericardial sac. These third-space fluid shifts may occur as a result of increased permeability of the capillary membrane or a decrease in plasma colloid osmotic pressure.

Extracellular losses

Fluid loss from the extracellular compartment can result from many different things, including:
- abdominal surgery
- diabetes mellitus (with increased urination)
- excessive diuretic therapy
- excessive laxative use
- excessive sweating
- fever
- fistulas
- hemorrhage (bleeding may be frank or occult)
- nasogastric drainage
- renal failure with increased urination
- vomiting and diarrhea.

Third-space shifting

Third-space fluid shifts can result from any number of conditions, including:
- acute intestinal obstruction
- acute peritonitis
- burns (during the initial phase)

Cheat sheet

Understanding hypovolemia

- Hypotonic fluid loss from extracellular space
- May progress to hypovolemic shock if not detected early and treated properly
- Caused by excessive fluid loss or third-space fluid shift
- Treated with fluid replacement (using fluids of same concentration)

- crush injuries
- hip fracture
- hypoalbuminemia
- pleural effusion.

What to look for

If volume loss is minimal (10% to 15% of an average of about 5 L of total circulating blood volume), the body tries to compensate for its lack of circulating volume by increasing the heart rate. You may also note orthostatic hypotension, restlessness, or anxiety. The patient will probably still produce more than 30 ml of urine per hour, but he may have delayed capillary refill and cool, pale skin over the arms and legs. (See *Danger signs of hypovolemia.*)

Weighty evidence

The hypovolemic patient may also lose weight. Acute weight loss can indicate rapid fluid changes. A drop in weight of 5% to 10% can indicate mild to moderate loss; more than 10%, severe loss. As hypovolemia progresses, the patient's symptoms worsen. CVP and PAP may fall as well. Monitor your patient for subtle signs, including orthostatic hypotension

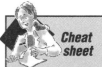

Cheat sheet

Signs and symptoms of hypovolemia

Mild fluid loss
- Orthostatic hypotension
- Restlessness
- Anxiety
- Weight loss

Moderate fluid loss
- Confusion
- Irritability
- Thirst
- Coolness
- Clamminess
- urine output drops to 10 to 30 ml/hour

Warning!

Danger signs of hypovolemia

Avoid surprises. Watch for these signs and symptoms of hypovolemia and impending hypovolemic shock:
- deterioration in mental status (from restlessness and anxiety to unconsciousness)
- thirst
- tachycardia
- delayed capillary refill
- orthostatic hypotension progressing to marked hypotension
- urine output initially more than 30 ml/minute, then urine output drops below 10 ml/hour
- cool, pale skin over arms and legs
- weight loss
- flat jugular veins, decreased central venous pressure
- weak or absent peripheral pulses.

Dazed and confused

With moderate intravascular volume loss (about 25%), the patient may become more confused and irritable and complain of extreme thirst. The pulse usually becomes rapid and thready, and the blood pressure drops. The patient may become cool and clammy, and the urine output may drop to 10 to 30 ml/hour.

Shock!

Severe hypovolemia (40% or more of intravascular volume loss) may lead to hypovolemic shock. In a patient with this condition, cardiac output drops and mental status can deteriorate to unconsciousness. Signs may progress to marked tachycardia and hypotension, with weak or absent peripheral pulses. The skin may become cool and mottled, or even cyanotic. Urine output drops to less than 10 ml/hour.

What tests show

No single diagnostic finding can confirm hypovolemia. Laboratory test values can vary, depending on the underlying cause and other factors. Values usually suggest an increased concentration of blood. Typical laboratory findings include:
• normal or high serum sodium level (> 145 mEq/L), depending on the amount of fluid and sodium lost
• decreased hemoglobin levels and HCT, with hemorrhage
• elevated blood urea nitrogen (BUN) level
• increased urine specific gravity, with the kidneys trying to conserve fluid.

In cases of hypovolemic shock, the patient needs large amounts of I.V. fluids in a short amount of time.

How hypovolemia is treated

Treatment for hypovolemia includes replacing lost fluids with fluids of the same concentration. Such replacement helps normalize blood pressure and restore blood volume. Oral fluids generally aren't enough to adequately treat hypovolemia. Isotonic fluids, such as normal saline solution or lactated Ringer's solution, are given I.V. to expand circulating volume.

Take the fluid challenge

Fluids may initially be administered as a fluid challenge, in which the patient receives large amounts of I.V. fluids in a short amount of time. For hypovolemic shock, an emergency condition, multiple fluid challenges are essential. Numerous I.V. infusions

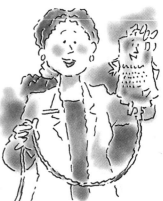

should be started with the shortest, largest-bore catheters possible, because they offer less resistance to fluid flow than long, skinny catheters.

Infusions of normal saline solution or lactated Ringer's solution are given rapidly, commonly followed by an infusion of plasma proteins such as albumin. If a patient is hemorrhaging, he'll need a blood transfusion. He may also need a drug such as dopamine, a vasopressor, to support his blood pressure.

Oxygen therapy should be initiated to ensure sufficient tissue perfusion. Surgery may be required to control bleeding.

How you intervene

Nursing responsibilities for a hypovolemic patient include the following.

Intervene stat!

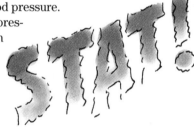

- Make sure the patient has a patent airway.
- Apply and adjust oxygen therapy as ordered.
- Lower the head of the bed to slow a declining blood pressure.
- If the patient is bleeding, apply direct continuous pressure to the area and elevate it, if possible. Assist with other interventions to stop bleeding.
- If the blood pressure doesn't respond to interventions as expected, look again for a site of bleeding that might have been missed. Remember, a patient can lose a large amount of blood internally from a

Teaching points

Teaching about hypovolemia

If your patient has hypovolemia, teach him about the following points and then evaluate his learning:
- nature of the condition and its causes
- warning signs and symptoms and when he should report them
- treatment and the importance of compliance
- importance of changing positions slowly, especially when going from a supine position to a standing position, to avoid orthostatic hypotension
- measuring blood pressure and pulse rate
- prescribed medications.

fractured hip or pelvis. Furthermore, fluids alone may not be enough to correct hypotension associated with a hypovolemic condition. A vasopressor such as dopamine may be needed to raise blood pressure.

• Maintain patent I.V. access. Use short, large-bore catheters to allow for faster infusion rates.

• Administer I.V. fluid, a vasopressor, and blood as prescribed. An autotransfuser, which allows for reinfusion of the patient's own blood, may be required.

• Draw blood for typing and crossmatching, as ordered, to prepare for transfusion.

• Closely monitor the patient's mental status and vital signs, including orthostatic blood pressure measurements, when appropriate. Watch for arrhythmias.

• If available, monitor hemodynamics (cardiac output, CVP, PAP, and PAWP), to judge how well the patient is responding to treatment. (See *Hemodynamic values in hypovolemic shock.*)

• Monitor the quality of peripheral pulses and skin temperature and appearance to assess for continued peripheral vascular constriction.

• Obtain and record results from diagnostic tests, such as a complete blood count, electrolyte levels, arterial blood gas (ABG) analyses, a 12-lead electrocardiogram, and chest X-rays.

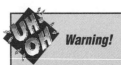

Warning!

Hemodynamic values in hypovolemic shock

Hemodynamic monitoring helps you evaluate the patient's cardiovascular status in hypovolemic shock. Look for these values:

• central venous pressure below the normal range of 5 to 10 cm H_2O

• pulmonary artery pressure below the normal mean of 10 to 20 mm Hg

• pulmonary artery wedge pressure below the normal mean of 6 to 12 mm Hg

• cardiac output below the normal range of 4 to 8 L/minute.

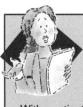

Chart smart

Documenting hypovolemia

With a patient who is hypovolemic, you'll document:
• mental status
• vital signs
• strength of peripheral pulses
• appearance and temperature of skin
• I.V. therapy
• blood products infused
• doses of vasopressors used
• breath sounds and oxygen therapy used
• hourly urine output
• laboratory results
• daily weight
• interventions and the patient's response
• patient teaching.

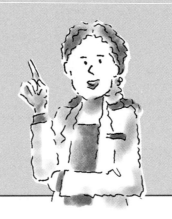

• Offer emotional support to the patient and his family. (See *Teaching about hypovolemia,* page 69.)
• Encourage the patient to drink fluids as appropriate.
• Insert a urinary catheter, as ordered, to measure urine output. Measure output hourly if indicated. (See *Documenting hypovolemia.*)
• Auscultate the patient for breath sounds periodically to monitor for signs of fluid overload, a potential complication of I.V. therapy. Excess fluid in the lungs may cause a crackling sound on auscultation.
• Observe the patient for development of such complications as disseminated intravascular coagulation, myocardial infarction, or adult respiratory distress syndrome.
• Weigh patient daily to monitor progress of treatment.
• Provide effective skin care to prevent skin breakdown.

Hypervolemia

Hypervolemia is an excess of isotonic fluid (water and sodium) in the extracellular compartment. Osmolality is usually unaffected because fluid and solutes are gained in equal proportion. The body has compensatory mechanisms to deal with hypervolemia but when they fail, the signs and symptoms of hypervolemia develop.

How it happens

Extracellular fluid volume may increase in either the interstitial or intravascular compartments. Usually, the body can compensate and restore fluid balance by fine-tuning circulating levels of aldosterone, ADH, and atrial natriuretic peptide (hormone produced by the atrial muscle of the heart) to cause the kidneys to release additional water and sodium.

However, if hypervolemia is prolonged or severe or the patient has poor heart function, the body can't compensate for the extra volume. Heart failure and pulmonary edema may result. Fluid will be forced out of the blood vessels and will move into the interstitial space, causing edema of the tissues.

Elderly patients and patients with impaired renal or cardiovascular function are especially prone to developing hypervolemia.

The rising tide

Hypervolemia results from excessive sodium or fluid intake, fluid or sodium retention, or a shift in fluid from the interstitial space into the intravascular space. It may also result from acute or chronic renal failure with low urine output.

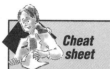

Cheat sheet

Understanding hypervolemia

• Excess isotonic fluid gain in the extracellular space (in either interstitial or intravascular compartments)
• *Mild to moderate fluid gain:* 5% to 10% weight increase
• *Severe fluid gain:* more than 10% weight increase
• *Prolonged or severe or in patients with poor heart function:* can lead to heart failure and pulmonary edema
• *Elderly patients and patients with impaired renal or cardiovascular function:* increased susceptibility

Factors that cause excessive sodium or fluid intake include:
• I.V. replacement therapy using normal saline solution or lactated Ringer's solution
• blood or plasma replacement
• high intake of dietary sodium.

Factors that cause fluid and sodium retention include:
• heart failure
• cirrhosis of the liver
• nephrotic syndrome
• corticosteroid therapy
• hyperaldosteronism
• low intake of dietary protein.

Factors that cause fluids to shift into the intravascular space include:
• remobilization of fluids after burn treatment
• administration of hypertonic fluids, such as mannitol or hypertonic saline solution
• use of plasma proteins such as albumin.

Cheat sheet

Signs and symptoms of hypervolemia

• tachypnea
• dyspnea
• crackles
• rapid, bounding pulse
• hypertension (unless the heart is failing)
• increased CVP, PAP, and PAWP
• distended neck and hand veins
• acute weight gain
• edema
• S_3 gallop.

What to look for

Because no single diagnostic test confirms hypervolemia, signs and symptoms are key to diagnosis. Cardiac output increases as the body tries to compensate for the excess volume. The pulse becomes rapid and bounding. Blood pressure, CVP, PAP, and PAWP rise. As the heart fails, blood pressure and cardiac output drop. An S_3 gallop develops with heart failure. You'll see distended veins, especially in the hands and neck. If you have the patient raise his hand above the level of his heart, his hand veins will remain distended for more than 5 seconds.

Edema's many faces

Edema results as hydrostatic (fluid-pushing) pressure builds in the vessels. Fluid is forced into the tissues. Edema may first be visible only in dependent areas, such as the sacrum and buttocks, when the patient is lying down and in the legs and feet when the patient is standing, but then the edema becomes generalized. *Anasarca* is the term used to describe severe, generalized edema. Edematous skin looks puffy, even around the eyes, and feels cool and pits when touched. The patient gains weight as a result of fluid retention (each 17 oz of fluid gained translates to a 1-lb weight gain).

An increase in weight of 5% to 10% indicates mild to moderate fluid gain; an increase of more than 10%, a more severe fluid gain.

Overload!

Edema may also occur in the lungs. As the left side of the heart becomes overloaded and pump efficiency declines, fluid backs up into the lungs.

Hydrostatic pressure forces the fluid out of the pulmonary blood vessels (just as in other blood vessels) and into the interstitial and alveolar areas. Pulmonary edema results. In a patient with this condition, you'll hear crackles on auscultation. The patient will become short of breath and tachypneic with a frequent, sometimes frothy, cough. ABG results will reflect pulmonary edema. (See *How pulmonary edema develops*, page 74.)

What tests show

In a patient with hypervolemia, you may see the following diagnostic test results:
- low HCT because of hemodilution
- normal serum sodium level
- lower serum potassium and BUN levels because of hemodilution (higher levels may indicate renal failure or impaired renal perfusion)
- low oxygen level (with early tachypnea, partial pressure of arterial carbon dioxide may be low, causing a drop in pH and respiratory alkalosis)
- pulmonary congestion on chest X-rays.

How hypervolemia is treated

Treatment for hypervolemia includes restriction of sodium and fluid intake and administration of medications to prevent complications, such as heart failure and pulmonary edema. The cause of the hypervolemia should also be treated. Diuretics are given to promote excess fluid loss from the body. (See *Evaluating pitting edema*.)

If the patient has pulmonary edema, additional drugs, such as morphine and nitroglycerin, may be given to dilate blood vessels, which in turn reduces pulmonary congestion and the amount of blood returning to the heart. Heart failure is treated with digoxin, which strengthens cardiac contractions and slows the heart rate. Oxygen and bedrest are also used to support the patient.

When the kidneys aren't working properly, diuretics may be inadequate to rid the body of extra fluid. The patient may require hemodialysis or continuous arteriovenous hemofiltration. (See *Understanding CAVH*, page 75.)

Evaluating pitting edema

Edema can be evaluated using a scale of +1 to +4. Press your fingertip firmly into the skin over a bony surface for a few seconds. Then note the depth of the imprint your finger leaves on the skin.

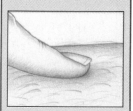

A slight imprint indicates +1 pitting edema.

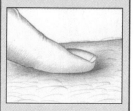

A deep imprint, with the skin slow to return to its original contour, indicates +4 pitting edema.

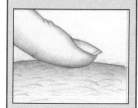

When the skin resists pressure but appears distended, the condition is called brawny edema. In brawny edema, the skin swells so much that fluid can't be displaced.

Now I get it!

How pulmonary edema develops

Excess fluid volume that lasts a long time can cause pulmonary edema. The illustrations here show how that process occurs.

Normal

Normal pulmonary fluid movement depends on the equal force of two opposing pressures—hydrostatic pressure and plasma oncotic pressure from protein molecules in the blood.

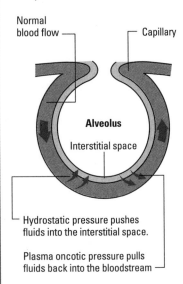

Normal blood flow

Capillary

Alveolus

Interstitial space

Hydrostatic pressure pushes fluids into the interstitial space.

Plasma oncotic pressure pulls fluids back into the bloodstream

Congestion

Abnormally high pulmonary hydrostatic pressure (indicated by increased pulmonary artery wedge pressure) forces fluid out of the capillaries and into the interstitial space, causing pulmonary congestion.

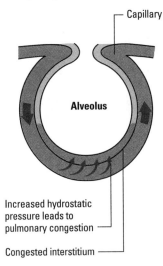

Capillary

Alveolus

Increased hydrostatic pressure leads to pulmonary congestion

Congested interstitium

Edema

When the amount of interstitial fluid becomes excessive, fluid is forced into the alveoli. Pulmonary edema results. Fluid fills the alveoli and prevents the exchange of gases.

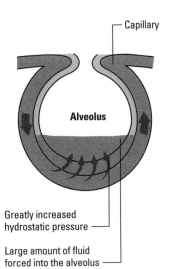

Capillary

Alveolus

Greatly increased hydrostatic pressure

Large amount of fluid forced into the alveolus

How you intervene

Caring for a patient with hypervolemia requires a number of nursing actions, many of which are listed below.

Assess

• Assess the patient's vital signs and hemodynamic status, noting his response to therapy. Watch for signs of hypovolemia due to overcorrection. Remember that elderly, pediatric, and otherwise

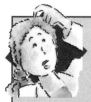

It's not working!

Understanding CAVH

If your hypervolemic patient isn't responding to diuretics, his kidney function may be poor. Dialysis is typically the next step, but if your patient can't tolerate this procedure, continuous arterio-venous hemofiltration (CAVH) may be used.

What it does

By circulating blood through a special filter, CAVH removes plasma water and dissolved solutes while conserving cellular and protein components. In addition to being efficient, CAVH offers these advantages:
• allows arterial blood sampling and arterial blood pressure control
• maintains serum osmolality by avoiding rapid fluid removal
• circulates less blood out of the body than hemodialysis
• allows measurement of serum electrolyte, lactate, glucose, urea, and creatinine levels.

How it works

In CAVH, the patient's arterial blood pressure serves as a natural pump, driving blood through the arterial line. The illustration below shows the standard setup for CAVH. The patient's blood enters the hemofilter from an arterial line, flows through the hemofilter, and returns to the patient through a venous line. The filtered fluid, called ultrafiltrate, drains by gravity into a collection bag.

Filtration replacement fluid (less fluid than the amount removed) may be infused at the venous access port and returned to the patient along with the purified blood. This procedure allows the patient to gradually lose up to 15 L of fluid per day.

> In CAVH, the patient's arterial blood pressure is a natural pump.

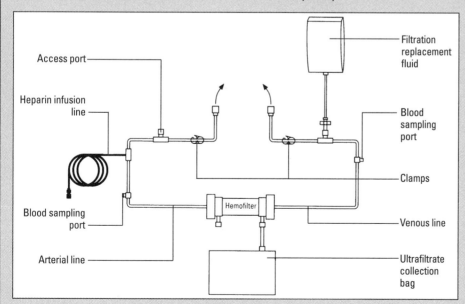

compromised patients are at higher risk for complications with therapy.

• Monitor respiratory patterns for worsening distress, such as increased tachypnea or dyspnea.

• Watch for distended veins in the hands or neck.

• Record intake and output hourly.

• Listen to breath sounds regularly to assess for pulmonary edema. Note crackles or rhonchi.

• Follow ABG results and watch for a drop in the oxygen level or changes in acid-base balance.

• Monitor other laboratory test results for changes, including potassium levels (decreased with use of most diuretics) and HCT.

• Raise the head of the bed (if blood pressure allows) to facilitate breathing, and administer oxygen as ordered.

• Make sure the patient restricts fluids if necessary. Alert the family and staff to ensure compliance. (See *Teaching about hypervolemia.*)

• Insert a urinary catheter, as ordered, to more accurately monitor output before starting diuretic therapy.

• Maintain I.V. access, as ordered, for the administration of medications such as diuretics. If the patient is prone to hypervolemia, use an infusion pump with any infusions to prevent administration of too much fluid.

• Give prescribed diuretics and other medications and monitor for effectiveness and adverse reactions.

• Watch for edema, especially in dependent areas.

• Check for an S_3 heart sound that can be heard when the ventricles are volume overloaded.

Chart smart

Documenting hypervolemia

When your patient has hypervolemia, you'll want to document:

• your assessment, including vital signs, hemodynamic status, pulmonary status, and edema
• oxygen therapy in use
• intake and output
• interventions, such as administration of a diuretic, and patient's response
• daily weight and the type of scale used
• pertinent laboratory results
• dietary or fluid restrictions
• safety measures implemented
• patient teaching.

Teaching points

Teaching about hypervolemia

If your patient has hypervolemia, teach him about the following points and evaluate his learning:

• nature of the condition and its causes
• warning signs and symptoms and when he should report them
• treatment and the importance of compliance
• measuring blood pressure and pulse rate
• restricting intake of sodium and fluids
• importance of being weighed regularly
• prescribed medications
• referral to dietitian, if appropriate.

Maintain

- Provide frequent mouth care.
- Obtain daily weight and evaluate trends.
- Provide skin care because edematous skin is prone to breakdown.
- Offer emotional support to the patient and his family.
- Document your assessment and interventions. (See *Documenting hypervolemia.*)

Water intoxication

Water intoxication occurs when excess fluid moves from the extracellular space to the intracellular space. Here's the lowdown on this condition.

How it happens

Excessive low-sodium fluid in the extracellular space is hypotonic to the cells; the cells are hypertonic to the fluid. In that instance, fluid shifts — by osmosis — into the cells, which have comparatively less fluid and more solutes. That fluid shift, which causes the cells to swell, occurs as a means of balancing the concentration of fluid between the two spaces, a condition called water intoxication.

Holding on to water

By causing the body to hold on to electrolyte-free water (despite low plasma osmolality [dilute plasma] and high fluid volume) syndrome of inappropriate antidiuretic hormone (SIADH) secretion can cause water intoxication. SIADH can result from central nervous system or pulmonary disorders, head trauma, certain medications, tumors, and some surgeries. (We'll talk more about SIADH when we discuss sodium imbalances in Chapter 5.)

Water intoxication can also occur with rapid infusions of hypotonic solutions such as D_5W. Excessive use of tap water as a nasogastric tube irrigant or enema also increases water intake.

Psychogenic polydipsia, a psychological disturbance, is another cause. It occurs when a person continues to drink water or other fluids in large amounts, even when they aren't needed. The condition is especially dangerous if the person's kidneys don't function well.

What to look for

Signs and symptoms of water intoxication reflect low sodium levels and increased intracranial pressure (ICP) as brain cells swell. Although headache and personality changes are the first indications, be suspicious of any change in behavior or level of consciousness, such as confusion, irritability, or lethargy. The patient may also experience nausea, vomiting, cramping, muscle weakness, twitching, thirst, dyspnea on exertion, and dulled sensorium.

Late signs of increased ICP include pupillary and vital sign changes, such as bradycardia and widened pulse pressure. A patient with water intoxication may develop seizures and coma. Any weight gain reflects additional cellular fluid.

What tests show

In a patient with water intoxication, you may see the following diagnostic test results:
• serum sodium level < 125 mEq/L
• serum osmolality < 280 mOsm/kg.

How water intoxication is treated

Treatment for water intoxication includes correcting the underlying cause, restricting both oral and parenteral fluid intake, and avoiding the use of hypotonic I.V. solutions, such as D_5W, until serum sodium levels rise. Hypertonic solutions are used only in severe situations to draw fluid out of the cells and must be accompanied by close patient monitoring. The original cause of the intoxication should also be addressed.

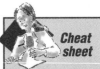

Cheat sheet

Understanding water intoxication

Excess fluid movement from the extracellular space to the intracellular space causes increased ICP and may lead to seizures and coma.

Causes
• SIADH
• Rapid infusion of a hypotonic solution
• Excessive use of tap water as an NG tube irrigant or enema
• Psychogenic polydipsia

Test results
• Low serum sodium levels
• Low serum osmolality

▶ *Teaching points*

Teaching about water intoxication

Make sure you teach your patient the following points about water intoxication and evaluate his learning:

• nature of the condition and its causes
• need for fluid restriction
• warning signs and symptoms and when he should report them
• prescribed medications
• need for being weighed regularly.

How you intervene

The best treatment for water intoxication is prevention. However, if your patient develops water intoxication, you'll want to take the following nursing actions.
• Closely assess his neurologic status; watch for deterioration, especially changes in personality or level of consciousness.
• Monitor vital signs and intake and output to evaluate the patient's progress.
• Maintain oral and I.V. fluid restrictions, as prescribed.
• Alert the dietitian and the patient's family to the restrictions.
• Post a sign in the patient's room to alert staff to fluid restrictions. (See *Teaching about water intoxication.*)
• Insert an I.V. catheter and maintain it, as ordered; infuse hypertonic solutions with care, using an infusion pump.
• Closely observe the patient's response to therapy.
• Weigh patient daily to detect retention of excess water.
• Monitor laboratory test results such as serum sodium levels.
• Provide a safe environment for the patient with an alteration in neurologic status and teach his family to do the same.
• Institute seizure precautions in severe cases.
• Document your assessment and interventions. (See *Documenting water intoxication.*)

Chart smart

Documenting water intoxication

When your patient has water intoxication, you'll want to document:
• all assessment findings
• intake and output, noting fluid restrictions
• safety measures
• types of seizure activity and treatment
• laboratory results
• daily weight
• nursing interventions and patient's response
• patient teaching.

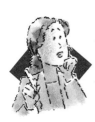

Quick quiz

1. Populations at risk for dehydration include:
    A. infants.
    B. adolescents.
    C. patients with SIADH.

Answer: A. Patients at risk for dehydration are those who either have an impaired thirst mechanism or can't respond to the thirst reflex. Infants fall into this category.

2. Checking for orthostatic hypotension allows the nurse to detect early signs of:
    A. hypovolemia.
    B. low serum osmolality.
    C. high serum osmolality.

Answer: A. Changes in blood pressure and pulse are two initial changes seen with hypovolemia.

3. Of the following, the first step you should take for a patient with hypovolemic shock is to:
   A. assess for dehydration.
   B. administer I.V. fluids.
   C. insert a urinary catheter.

Answer: B. Hypovolemic shock is an emergency that requires rapid infusions of I.V. fluids.

4. A sign of hypervolemia is:
   A. a rapid, bounding pulse.
   B. clear, watery sputum.
   C. severe hypertension.

Answer: A. Excess fluid in the intravascular space causes a rapid, bounding pulse. When hypervolemia progresses, it can fill the lungs with fluid and cause pulmonary edema, as indicated by the presence of pink, frothy sputum.

5. Water intoxication can be caused by:
   A. administering too much hypertonic fluid.
   B. administering too much hypotonic fluid.
   C. encouraging fluid intake.

Answer: B. Administering too much hypotonic fluid can cause water to shift from the blood vessels into the cells, leading to water intoxication and cellular edema.

6. If your critically ill patient's fluid volume decreases, you would expect to see:
   A. high blood pressure and low oxygen saturation.
   B. increased cardiac output and distended neck veins.
   C. decreased CVP and PAWP.

Answer: C. With a decrease in circulating volume, the CVP and PAWP will generally drop, as will blood pressure, cardiac output, and PAP.

Scoring

☆☆☆ If you answered all six questions correctly, way to go! Your fluidity leaves us breathless!

☆☆ If you answered four or five correctly, great going! Your A-lines are A+!

☆ If you answered fewer than four correctly, that's OK. We think your third-space fluid shifts are swell!

5

When sodium tips the balance

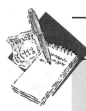

Just the facts

This chapter discusses the important role sodium plays in keeping the body functioning normally. In this chapter, you'll learn:

♦ how sodium contributes to fluid and electrolyte balance

♦ how the body regulates sodium balance

♦ what causes, signs, symptoms, and treatments are associated with sodium imbalances

♦ how to care for the patient with a sodium imbalance.

A look at sodium

Sodium is one of the most important elements in the body. It accounts for 90% of extracellular fluid cations (positively charged ions) and is the most abundant solute in extracellular fluid. Almost all sodium in the body is found in this fluid.

The body needs sodium to maintain proper extracellular fluid osmolality (concentration). Sodium attracts fluid and helps preserve the extracellular fluid volume and fluid distribution in the body. It also helps transmit impulses in nerve and muscle fibers and combines with chloride and bicarbonate to regulate acid-base balance. Because the electrolyte compositions of serum and interstitial fluid are essentially equal, sodium concentration in extracellular fluid is measured in serum levels. The normal range for the serum sodium level is 135 to 145 mEq/L. As a comparison, the amount of sodium inside a cell is 10 mEq/L.

Sodium is vital to life!

Balancing act

What a person eats and how the intestines absorb it determine a body's sodium level. Sodium requirements vary according to the individual's size and age. The minimum daily requirement is 0.5 to 2.7 g; however, the salty American diet provides at least 6 g/day. Even so, sodium levels stay fairly constant because the more sodium a person takes in, the more sodium the kidneys excrete. (See *Dietary sources of sodium.*)

Sodium is also excreted through the GI tract and in sweat. When you think *sodium*, think *water*—the two are that closely related in the body. The normal range of serum sodium levels reflects the relationship between sodium and water. If sodium intake suddenly increases, extracellular fluid concentration also rises, and vice versa.

Not too much!

The body makes adjustments when the sodium level rises. Increased serum sodium levels cause the individual to feel thirsty and the posterior pituitary gland to release antidiuretic hormone (ADH). (For more information about ADH, see chapter 1, Balancing Fluids.) ADH causes the kidneys to retain water, which dilutes the blood and normalizes serum osmolality.

When serum osmolality decreases and thirst and ADH secretion are suppressed, the kidneys excrete more water to restore normal osmolality. (See *Regulating sodium and water.*)

Aldosterone also regulates extracellular sodium balance via a feedback loop. The adrenal cortex secretes aldosterone, which stimulates the renal tubules to conserve water and sodium when the body's sodium level is low, thus helping to normalize extracellular fluid sodium levels.

The pump explained

Normally, extracellular sodium levels are very high compared to intracellular sodium levels. The body contains an active transport mechanism, called the sodium-potassium pump, which helps maintain normal sodium levels. This is how the pump works.

In diffusion, a substance moves from an area of higher concentration to one of lower concentration. Sodium ions, normally most abundant outside the cells, tend to diffuse inward, and potassium ions, normally most abundant inside the cells, tend to diffuse outward. To combat this ionic diffusion and maintain normal sodium and potassium levels, the sodium-potassium pump is constantly at work in every body cell.

However, moving sodium out of the cell and potassium back in can't happen without some help. Each ion links with a carrier be-

Dietary sources of sodium

Major dietary sources of sodium include:
- canned soups and vegetables
- cheese
- ketchup
- processed meats
- salt
- salty snack foods
- seafood.

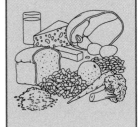

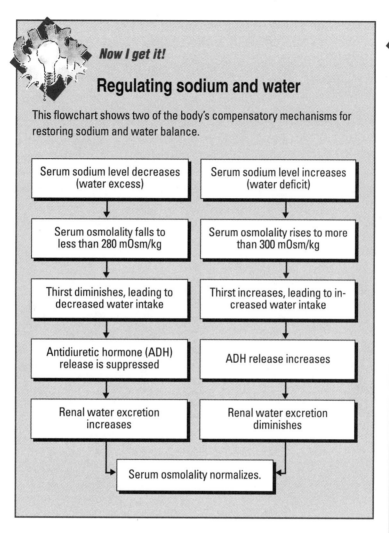

Now I get it!

Regulating sodium and water

This flowchart shows two of the body's compensatory mechanisms for restoring sodium and water balance.

Serum sodium level decreases (water excess)	Serum sodium level increases (water deficit)
↓	↓
Serum osmolality falls to less than 280 mOsm/kg	Serum osmolality rises to more than 300 mOsm/kg
↓	↓
Thirst diminishes, leading to decreased water intake	Thirst increases, leading to increased water intake
↓	↓
Antidiuretic hormone (ADH) release is suppressed	ADH release increases
↓	↓
Renal water excretion increases	Renal water excretion diminishes

Serum osmolality normalizes.

Sodium balance

- Maintained by ADH secreted from the posterior pituitary gland
- Depends on what's eaten and how it's absorbed by the intestines
- *Increased sodium intake:* increased extracellular fluid volume
- *Decreased sodium intake:* decreased extracellular fluid volume.
- *Increased sodium levels:* increased thirst, release of ADH, retention of water by the kidneys, dilution of blood.
- *Decreased sodium levels:* suppression of thirst, suppression of ADH secretion, excretion of water by the kidneys

cause it can't get through the cell wall alone. This movement requires energy, which comes from adenosine triphosphate (made up of phosphorus, another electrolyte), magnesium, and an enzyme. These substances help release sodium from the cell and draw potassium into the cell.

The sodium-potassium pump allows the body to carry out its essential functions and helps prevent cellular swelling from too many ions inside the cell attracting excessive amounts of water. The pump also creates an electrical charge in the cell from the movement of ions, permitting transmission of neuromuscular impulses. (See *Sodium-potassium pump*, page 84.)

Now I get it!

Sodium-potassium pump

This illustration shows how the sodium-potassium pump carries ions when their concentrations change.

Normal placement
More sodium (Na) ions normally exist outside cells than inside. More potassium (K) ions exist inside cells than outside.

Increased permeability
Certain stimuli increase the membrane's permeability. Sodium ions diffuse inward; potassium ions diffuse outward.

Energy source
The cell links each ion with a carrier molecule that helps the ion return through the cell wall. Energy for the ion's return trip comes from adenosine triphosphate (ATP), magnesium (Mg), and an enzyme commonly found in cells.

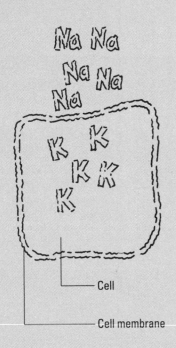

Cell

Cell membrane

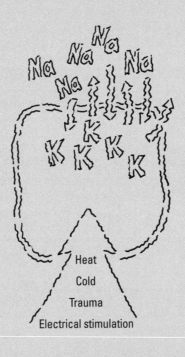

Heat
Cold
Trauma
Electrical stimulation

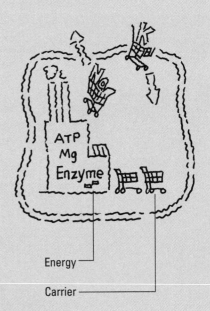

Energy

Carrier

Hyponatremia

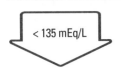

< 135 mEq/L

Hyponatremia, a common electrolyte imbalance, refers to a sodium deficiency in relation to body water. In other words, body fluids are diluted and cells swell from decreased extracellular fluid osmolality. Severe hyponatremia can lead to seizures, coma, and permanent neurologic damage.

How it happens

Normally, the body gets rid of excess water by secreting less ADH; less ADH causes diuresis. For that to happen, the nephrons must be functioning normally, receiving and excreting excess water and reabsorbing sodium.

Hyponatremia develops when this regulatory function goes haywire. Serum sodium levels decrease, and fluid shifts occur. When the blood vessels contain more water and less sodium, fluid moves by osmosis from the extracellular area into the more concentrated intracellular area. With more fluid in the cells and less in the blood vessels, cerebral edema and hypovolemia (fluid volume deficit) can occur. (See *Fluid movement in hyponatremia*.)

Now I get it!

Fluid movement in hyponatremia

This illustration shows fluid movement in hyponatremia. When serum osmolality decreases because of decreased sodium concentration, fluid moves by osmosis from the extracellular area to the intracellular area.

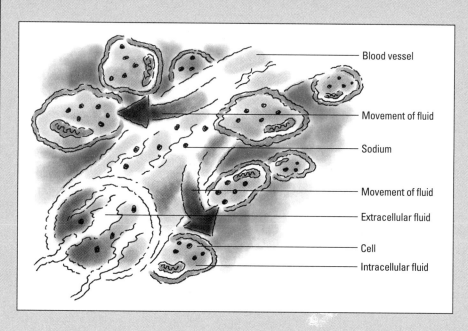

- Blood vessel
- Movement of fluid
- Sodium
- Movement of fluid
- Extracellular fluid
- Cell
- Intracellular fluid

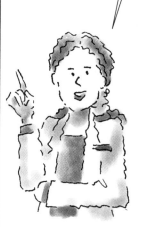

In hyponatremia, fluid moves by osmosis.

Deplete and dilute

Hyponatremia occurs from sodium loss, water gain (dilutional hyponatremia), or inadequate sodium intake (depletional hyponatremia). It may be classified according to whether extracellular fluid volume is abnormally decreased (hypovolemic hyponatremia), abnormally increased (hypervolemic hyponatremia), or equal to intracellular fluid volume (isovolumic hyponatremia).

Both sides lose

In hypovolemic hyponatremia, sodium loss is greater than water loss. Causes may be nonrenal or renal. Nonrenal causes include vomiting, diarrhea, fistulas, gastric suctioning, excessive sweating, cystic fibrosis, burns, and wound drainage. Renal causes include osmotic diuresis, salt-losing nephritis, adrenal insufficiency, and diuretic use.

Diuretics cause sodium loss and volume depletion from the blood vessels, causing the individual to feel thirsty and his kidneys to retain water. Drinking large quantities of water can worsen hyponatremia. Sodium deficits can also become more pronounced if the patient is on a sodium-restricted diet. Diuretics can cause potassium loss, which is also linked to hyponatremia. (See *Drug culprits.*)

Both sides gain

In hypervolemic hyponatremia, both water and sodium levels increase in the extracellular area, but the water gain is more impressive. Serum sodium levels are diluted and edema also occurs. Causes include heart failure, liver failure, nephrotic syndrome, excessive administration of hypotonic I.V. fluids, and hyperaldosteronism.

Only water gains

In isovolumic hyponatremia, sodium levels may appear low because too much fluid is in the body. However, these patients have no physical signs of fluid volume excess, and total body sodium remains stable. Causes include glucocorticoid deficiency (causing inadequate fluid filtration by the kidneys), hypothyroidism (causing limited water excretion), and renal failure.

Disturbing the balance

Another cause of isovolumic hyponatremia is syndrome of inappropriate antidiuretic hormone (SIADH) secretion, which causes excessive release of ADH and disturbs fluid and electrolyte balance. This syndrome is a major cause of low sodium levels. ADH is released when the body doesn't need it, which results in water retention and sodium excretion. (See *What happens in SIADH*, page 88.)

Drug culprits

Drugs can cause hyponatremia by potentiating the action of antidiuretic hormone or by causing syndrome of inappropriate antidiuretic hormone secretion. Diuretics may also cause hyponatremia by inhibiting sodium reabsorption in the kidney.

Anticonvulsants
- Carbamazepine

Antidiabetics
- Chlorpropamide
- Tolbutamide (rarely)

Antineoplastics
- Cyclophosphamide
- Vincristine

Antipsychotics
- Fluphenazine
- Thioridazine
- Thiothixene

Diuretics
- Bumetanide
- Ethacrynic acid
- Furosemide
- Thiazides

Sedatives
- Barbiturates
- Morphine

SIADH occurs with:
- cancers, especially of the duodenum and pancreas and oat cell carcinoma of the lung
- central nervous system (CNS) disorders, such as trauma, tumors, and stroke
- pulmonary disorders, such as tumors, asthma, and chronic obstructive pulmonary disease
- medications, such as certain oral antidiabetics, chemotherapeutic drugs, psychoactive drugs, diuretics, synthetic hormones, and barbiturates.

The patient is treated for the underlying cause of SIADH and for hyponatremia. For instance, if a tumor caused the syndrome, the patient would receive cancer treatment; if a medication caused it, the drug would be stopped. The low sodium levels are treated with fluid restrictions (about 1 qt [1 L]/day) and diuretics such as furosemide.

The patient may receive oral urea or follow a high-sodium diet to increase the kidneys' excretion of solutes (water will follow). Medications, such as demeclocycline or lithium, may be used to block ADH in the renal tubule. If fluid restriction doesn't raise sodium levels, a hypertonic saline solution may be given.

It's important to treat the underlying cause of SIADH.

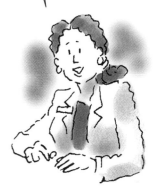

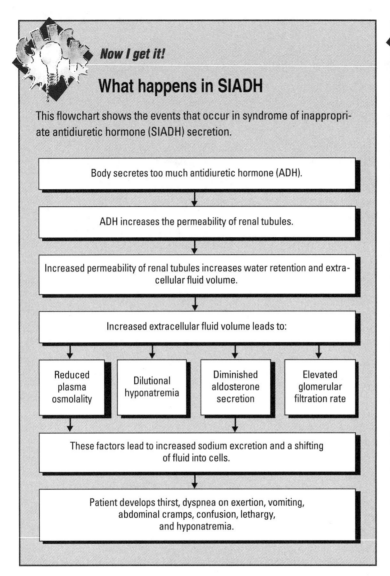

Now I get it!

What happens in SIADH

This flowchart shows the events that occur in syndrome of inappropriate antidiuretic hormone (SIADH) secretion.

Body secretes too much antidiuretic hormone (ADH).

↓

ADH increases the permeability of renal tubules.

↓

Increased permeability of renal tubules increases water retention and extra-cellular fluid volume.

↓

Increased extracellular fluid volume leads to:

↓

| Reduced plasma osmolality | Dilutional hyponatremia | Diminished aldosterone secretion | Elevated glomerular filtration rate |

↓

These factors lead to increased sodium excretion and a shifting of fluid into cells.

↓

Patient develops thirst, dyspnea on exertion, vomiting, abdominal cramps, confusion, lethargy, and hyponatremia.

Cheat sheet

Key facts about hyponatremia

• Caused by inadequate sodium intake, excessive sodium loss, or water gain
• Serum sodium level less than 135 mEq/L
• Signs and symptoms vary greatly among patients
• Results in decreased serum osmolality
• *Fluid shifts into intracellular areas:* neurologic symptoms related to cerebral edema
• Stupor and coma may occur if serum sodium level drops to 110 mEq/L.

What to look for

As you look for signs of hyponatremia, remember that they vary from patient to patient. They also vary depending on how quickly the sodium level drops. If the level drops quickly, the patient will be more symptomatic than if the level drops slowly. Patients with sodium levels above 125 mEq/L may not show signs of hyponatremia—but, again, this depends on how quickly sodium levels drop.

When signs occur, they're primarily neurologic. The patient may complain of a headache, nausea, or abdominal cramps. He may experience muscle twitching, tremors, or weakness. Changes in level of consciousness (LOC) may start as a shortened attention span and progress to lethargy or confusion. If sodium levels drop to 110 mEq/L, the patient's neurologic status will deteriorate further, leading to stupor and even coma. He may also develop seizures.

Patients with hypovolemia may have poor skin turgor and dry, cracked mucous membranes. Assessment of vital signs shows a weak, rapid pulse and low blood pressure or orthostatic hypotension. Central venous pressure (CVP), pulmonary artery pressure (PAP), and pulmonary artery wedge pressure may be decreased.

Patients with hypervolemia (fluid volume excess) may have edema, hypertension, weight gain, and rapid, bounding pulse. The CVP and PAP in these patients may be elevated.

What tests show

You'll probably note these diagnostic test results in your patient with hyponatremia:
- serum osmolality less than 280 mOsm/kg (dilute blood)
- serum sodium level less than 135 mEq/L (low sodium level in blood)
- urine specific gravity less than 1.010
- increased urine specific gravity and elevated urine sodium levels (above 20 mEq/L) in patients with SIADH
- elevated hematocrit and plasma protein levels.

How hyponatremia is treated

Generally, treatment varies with the cause and severity of hyponatremia. For example, hormone therapy may be needed to treat underlying endocrine disorders.

For mild cases...

Therapy for mild hyponatremia associated with hypervolemia or isovolemia usually consists of restricted fluid intake and, possibly, oral sodium supplements. If hypovolemia is related to hyponatremia, isotonic I.V. fluids such as normal saline solution may be given to restore volume. High-sodium foods may also be offered to the patient.

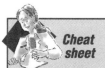
Cheat sheet

Signs and symptoms of hyponatremia

Signs and symptoms of hyponatremia include:
- abdominal cramps
- altered LOC, such as lethargy and confusion
- headache
- muscle twitching, tremors, weakness
- nausea.

Signs and symptoms of hypovolemia with depletional hyponatremia include:
- dry mucous membranes
- orthostatic hypotension
- poor skin turgor
- tachycardia.

Signs and symptoms of hypervolemia with dilutional hyponatremia include:
- hypertension
- rapid, bounding pulse
- weight gain.

For more severe cases...

When serum sodium levels fall below 110 mEq/L, treatment in the intensive care unit may include infusion of a hypertonic saline solution (such as 3% or 5% saline). Monitor the patient carefully during the infusion for signs of circulatory overload or worsening neurologic status. A hypertonic saline solution causes water to shift out of cells, which may lead to intravascular volume overload and serious brain damage (osmotic demyelination), especially in the pons.

Fluid overload can be fatal if it isn't treated. To prevent overload, the hypertonic sodium chloride solution is infused slowly and in small volumes. Furosemide is usually administered at the same time.

Hypervolemic patients shouldn't receive hypertonic sodium chloride solutions, except in rare instances of severe symptomatic hyponatremia. During treatment, monitor serum sodium levels and related diagnostic tests to follow the patient's progress.

How you intervene

Watch patients at risk for hyponatremia. They include those with heart failure, cancer, or GI disorders with fluid losses. Review your patient's medications, noting those that are associated with hyponatremia. For patients who develop hyponatremia, you'll want to take the following actions.

Monitor

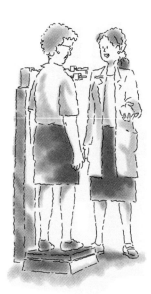

• Monitor and record vital signs, especially blood pressure and pulse, and watch for orthostatic hypertension and tachycardia.
• Monitor neurologic status frequently. Report any deterioration in LOC. Assess patient for lethargy, muscle twitching, seizures, and coma.
• Accurately measure and record intake and output.
• Weigh the patient daily to monitor the success of fluid restriction.
• Assess skin turgor at least every 8 hours for signs of dehydration.
• Watch for and report extreme changes in serum sodium levels and accompanying serum chloride levels. Also monitor other test results, such as urine specific gravity and serum osmolality.

Administer and maintain

• Restrict fluid intake as ordered. (Fluid restriction is the primary treatment for dilutional hyponatremia.) Post a sign about fluid restriction in the patient's room and make sure the staff, the patient,

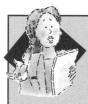

Chart smart

Documenting hyponatremia

If your patient has hyponatremia, make sure you chart the following:

- assessment findings (including neurologic status)
- vital signs
- daily weight
- types of seizures, if any
- intake and output
- serum sodium level and any other pertinent laboratory results
- medications given and I.V. therapy implemented

- nursing interventions and patient response
- patient compliance with fluid restrictions and dietary changes
- patient teaching provided and patient response to the teaching
- safety measures taken to protect the patient

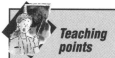

Teaching points

Teaching about hyponatremia

Make sure you cover these topics with your patient and then evaluate his learning:
- explanation of hyponatremia, including causes and treatment
- drug therapy and possible adverse effects
- dietary changes and fluid restrictions (if any)
- signs and symptoms and when to report them
- need to monitor weight daily.

and his family are aware of the restrictions. (See *Teaching about hyponatremia.*)

• Administer oral sodium supplements, if prescribed, to treat mild hyponatremia. If the doctor has instructed the patient to increase his intake of dietary sodium, teach him about foods high in sodium.

• For severe hyponatremia, make sure a patent I.V. line is in place. Then administer prescribed I.V. isotonic or hypertonic saline solutions cautiously to avoid inducing hypernatremia, brain injury, or volume overload from an excessive or too rapid infusion. Watch closely for signs of hypervolemia (dyspnea, crackles, engorged neck or hand veins), and report them immediately. Use an infusion pump to ensure that the patient receives only the prescribed volume of fluid.

• Keep the patient safe while he undergoes treatment. Provide a safe environment for a patient who has altered thought processes and reorient him as needed. If seizures are likely, pad the bed's side rails and keep suction equipment and an airway handy. (See *Documenting hyponatremia.*)

Hypernatremia

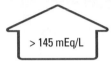

> 145 mEq/L

Hypernatremia, which is less common than hyponatremia, refers to an excess of sodium relative to body water. Severe hypernatremia can lead to seizures, coma, and permanent neurologic damage.

How it happens

Thirst is the body's main defense against hypernatremia. The hypothalamus (with its osmoreceptors) is the brain's thirst center. High serum osmolality (increased solute concentrations in the blood) stimulates the hypothalamus and initiates the sensation of thirst.

The drive to respond to thirst is so strong that severe, persistent hypernatremia occurs only in people who can't drink voluntarily, such as infants, confused elderly patients, or immobile or unconscious patients. Hypothalamic disorders, such as a lesion on the hypothalamus, may cause a disturbance of the thirst mechanism but this condition is rare.

Striving for balance

The body strives to maintain a normal sodium level by secreting ADH from the posterior pituitary gland. This hormone causes water to be retained, which helps to lower serum sodium levels.

The cells also play a role in maintaining sodium balance. When serum osmolality increases because of hypernatremia, fluid moves by osmosis from inside the cell to outside the cell, to balance the concentrations in the two compartments. (For more information, see chapter 1, Balancing Fluids.)

As fluid leaves them, the cells become dehydrated—especially those of the CNS. When this occurs, patients may show signs of neurologic impairment. They may also show signs of hypervolemia (fluid overload) from increased extracellular fluid volume in the blood vessels. (See *Fluid movement in hypernatremia.*)

Increased concentration

A water deficit can cause hypernatremia—that is, more sodium relative to water in the body. Excessive intake of sodium can also cause it. Regardless of the cause, body fluids become hypertonic (more concentrated).

Too little water can cause hypernatremia

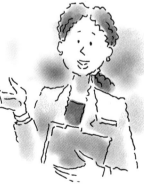

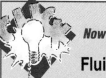

Now I get it!

Fluid movement in hypernatremia

With hypernatremia, the body tries to maintain balance by shifting fluid from the inside of cells to the outside of them. This illustration shows fluid movement in hypernatremia.

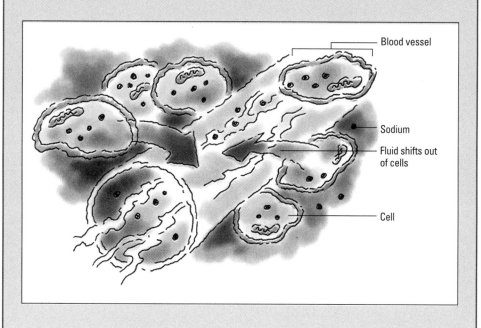

Blood vessel

Sodium

Fluid shifts out of cells

Cell

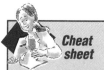

Cheat sheet

Key facts about hypernatremia

- Caused by water loss, inadequate water intake, or sodium gain (rarely from failure of the thirst mechanism)
- Increased risk for infants, immobile and comatose patients
- Always results in increased osmolality
- Fluid shifts out of the cells
- Must be corrected slowly to prevent a rapid shift of water back into the cells, which could cause cerebral edema

Water deficit

A water deficit may occur alone or with a sodium loss (but more water will be lost than sodium). In either case, serum sodium levels are elevated. This elevation is more dangerous in debilitated patients and others with a deficient water intake.

Insensible water losses of several liters per day can result from fever and heat stroke, with older adults and athletes being equally susceptible. Significant water losses also occur in patients with pulmonary infections, who lose water vapor from the lungs with hyperventilation, and in patients with extensive burns. Severe watery diarrhea is another cause of water loss and subsequent hypernatremia; it can be especially dangerous in children. Patients with hyperosmolar hyperglycemic nonketotic syndrome can also develop hypernatremia due to severe water losses from osmotic diuresis. Urea diuresis occurs with administration of high-protein feedings or high-protein diets without adequate water supplementation, and can lead to hypernatremia. (See *Infants and children at risk.*)

Thirst to an extreme

Patients with diabetes insipidus have extreme thirst and enormous urinary losses, in many cases more than 4 gal (15 L)/day. Usually, they can drink enough fluids to match the urinary losses; otherwise, severe dehydration and hypernatremia occur. Diabetes insipidus may result from a lack of ADH from the brain (central diabetes insipidus) or a lack of response from the kidneys to ADH (nephrogenic diabetes insipidus).

Central diabetes insipidus may result from a tumor or head trauma (injury or surgery) or be idiopathic (no known cause). It responds well to vasopressin (another name for ADH). Nephrogenic diabetes insipidus doesn't respond well to vasopressin and is more likely to occur with electrolyte imbalance, such as hypokalemia, or with certain medications such as lithium.

Excessive sodium intake

In addition to water losses from the body, sodium gains can also cause hypernatremia. Several factors can contribute to a high sodium intake, including salt tablets, food, and medications such as sodium polystyrene sulfonate (Kayexalate).

Excessive parenteral administration of sodium solutions, such as hypertonic saline solutions or sodium bicarbonate preparations, can also cause hypernatremia. Other causes of increased sodium levels include inadvertent introduction of hypertonic saline solution into maternal circulation during therapeutic abortion, near drowning in salt water, and excessive amounts of adrenocortical hormones, as in Cushing's syndrome and hyperaldosteronism, which affects water and sodium balance. (See *Drugs associated with hypernatremia.*)

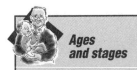

Ages and stages

Infants and children at risk

Hypernatremia is more common in infants and children for two key reasons:

1   Patients in this age group tend to lose more water as a result of diarrhea, vomiting, inadequate fluid intake, and fever.

2   Their intake of water is generally inadequate because they have difficulty swallowing and lack access.

What to look for

The most important signs of hypernatremia are neurologic because fluid shifts have a significant effect on brain cells. Remember that the body can tolerate a high sodium level that develops over time better than one that occurs rapidly. You may see restlessness or agitation, weakness, lethargy, confusion, stupor, seizures, and coma.

You may also observe signs of neuromuscular irritability such as twitching, and the patient may have a low-grade fever and flushed skin. He may complain of intense thirst from stimulation of the hypothalamus from increased osmolality.

Other signs vary depending on the cause of the high sodium levels. If a sodium gain has occurred, fluid may be drawn into the blood vessels and the patient will appear hypervolemic, with an elevated blood pressure, bounding pulse, and dyspnea.

If water loss occurs, fluid will leave the blood vessels and you'll notice signs of hypovolemia, such as dry mucous membranes, oliguria, and orthostatic hypotension (blood pressure drop and heart rate increase with position changes).

What tests show

Now that you know how hypernatremia progresses, you'll better understand its effect on the results of these common diagnostic findings:
• serum sodium level greater than 145 mEq/L
• urine specific gravity greater than 1.030 (except in diabetes insipidus, where urine specific gravity is decreased)
• serum osmolality greater than 300 mOsm/kg.

How hypernatremia is treated

Treatment for hypernatremia varies with the cause. The underlying disorder must be corrected, and serum sodium levels and related diagnostic tests must be monitored. If too little water in the body is causing the hypernatremia, treatment may include oral fluid replacement. Note that the fluids should be given gradually over 48 hours to avoid shifting water into brain cells.

Remember, as sodium levels rise in the blood vessels, fluid shifts out of the cells—including the brain cells—to dilute the blood and equalize concentrations. If too much water is introduced into the body too quickly, water moves into brain cells and they get bigger, causing cerebral edema.

Drugs associated with hypernatremia

The drugs listed below can cause high sodium levels. Ask your patient if any of these are part of his drug therapy:
• antacids with sodium bicarbonate
• antibiotics such as ticarcillin disodium-clavulanate potassium (Timentin)
• salt tablets
• sodium bicarbonate injections (such as those given during cardiac arrest)
• I.V. sodium chloride preparations
• sodium polystyrene sulfonate (Kayexalate).

Memory jogger

To help you remember some common signs and symptoms of hypernatremia, think of the word SALT.

Skin flushed

Agitation

Low-grade fever

Thirst

Cheat sheet

Signs and symptoms of hypernatremia

Signs and symptoms of hypernatremia include:
- agitation
- confusion
- flushed skin
- lethargy
- low-grade fever
- restlessness
- signs and symptoms of hypervolemia including bounding pulse, dyspnea, and hypertension (with sodium gain)
- signs and symptoms of hypovolemia, including dry mucous membranes, oliguria, and orthostatic hypotension (with water loss)
- twitching
- weakness.

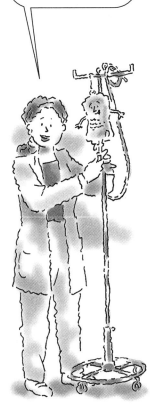

I.V. fluids may be needed for patients who can't drink enough.

If the patient can't drink enough fluids, he'll need I.V. fluid replacement. He may receive salt-free solutions (such as dextrose 5% in water) to return serum sodium levels to normal, followed by infusion of half-normal saline solution to prevent hyponatremia and cerebral edema. Other treatments include restricting sodium intake and administering diuretics along with oral or I.V. fluid replacement to increase sodium loss.

Treatment for diabetes insipidus may include vasopressin, hypotonic I.V. fluids, and thiazide diuretics to decrease free water loss from the kidneys. The underlying cause should also be treated.

How you intervene

Try to prevent hypernatremia in high-risk patients (such as those recovering from surgery near the pituitary gland) by observing them closely. Also find out if they're taking medications that may cause hypernatremia. If your patient does develop hypernatremia, take the following measures.

Assess, replenish, and restore

- Monitor and record vital signs, especially blood pressure and pulse.
- If the patient needs I.V. fluid replacement, monitor fluid delivery and his response to the therapy. Watch for signs of cerebral edema

and check his neurologic status frequently. Report any deterioration in LOC.

• Carefully measure and record intake and output. Weigh the patient daily to check for body fluid loss.

• Assess skin and mucous membranes for signs of breakdown and infection as well as water loss from perspiration.

• Monitor the patient's serum sodium level and report any increase. Monitor urine specific gravity and other laboratory test results.

• If the patient can't take oral fluids, recommend the I.V. route to the doctor. If the patient can drink and is alert and responsible, involve him in his treatment. Give him a target amount of fluid to drink each shift, mark cups with the volume they hold, leave fluids within easy reach, and provide paper and pen to record amounts. If family members will be helping the patient drink, give them specific instructions as well. (See *Teaching about hypernatremia*.)

• Insert and maintain a patent I.V. as ordered. Use an infusion pump to control delivery of I.V. fluids to prevent cerebral edema.

• Assist with oral hygiene. Lubricate the patient's lips frequently with a water-based lubricant and provide mouthwash or gargle if he's alert. Good mouth care helps keep mucous membranes moist and decreases mouth odor.

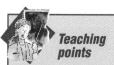

Teaching points

Teaching about hypernatremia

Make sure you cover these topics with your patient and then evaluate his learning:

• explanation of hypernatremia, including causes and treatment

• importance of restricting sodium intake, including both dietary sources and over-the-counter medications that contain sodium

• drug therapy and possible adverse effects

• signs and symptoms and when to report them.

Chart smart

Documenting hypernatremia

When documenting information about your patient with hypernatremia, you'll want to include:

• assessment findings (including neurologic status)

• vital signs

• types of seizures, if any

• daily weight

• serum sodium level and other pertinent laboratory test results

• intake and output

• medications given and I.V. therapy implemented

• notification of the doctor when the patient's condition changes

• nursing interventions and patient response

• patient compliance with fluid restrictions and dietary changes

• patient teaching provided and patient response to the teaching

• safety measures taken to protect the patient (seizure precautions).

• Provide a safe environment for confused or agitated patients. If seizures are likely, pad the bed's side rails and keep an artificial airway and suction equipment handy. Reorient the patient as needed, and reduce environmental stimuli. (See *Documenting hyper-natremia*, page 97.)

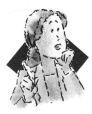

Quick quiz

1. In addition to its responsibility for fluid balance, sodium is also responsible for:

  A. good eyesight and vitamin balance.
  B. bone structure.
  C. impulse transmission.

Answer: C. Sodium is the main extracellular cation responsible for regulating fluid balance in the body. It's also involved in impulse transmission in nerve and muscle fibers.

2. Signs and symptoms of hyponatremia include:

  A. change in LOC, abdominal cramps, and muscle twitching.
  B. headache, rapid breathing, and high energy level.
  C. chest pain, fever, and pericardial rub.

Answer: A. The signs and symptoms include change in LOC, abdominal cramps, and muscle twitching. A patient with hypo-natremia may also exhibit headache, nausea, coma, blood pressure changes, and tachycardia.

3. The minimum daily requirement of sodium for an average adult is:

  A. 2 g.
  B. 5 g.
  C. 8 g.

Answer: A. Although the minimum daily requirement is 2 g, most people in the United States consume more than 6 g/day.

4. Increased serum sodium levels cause thirst and the release of:
    A.   potassium into the cells.
    B.   fluid into the interstitium.
    C.   ADH into the bloodstream.

Answer: C. Higher blood sodium levels prompt the release of ADH from the posterior pituitary.

5. The sodium-potassium pump transports sodium ions:
    A.   into cells.
    B.   out of cells.
    C.   into and out of cells in equal amounts.

Answer: B. Normally most abundant outside of cells, sodium tends to diffuse inward. The sodium-potassium pump returns sodium to the extracellular area. Potassium ions tend to diffuse out of the cells and require transport back into the cell.

6. You're teaching a patient with hypernatremia that he needs to restrict his intake of sodium. Which foods high in sodium should you tell him to avoid?
    A.   Bananas, peaches, and broccoli
    B.   Canned soups, ketchup, and cheese
    C.   Milk, nuts, and liver

Answer: B. Major dietary sources of sodium include: canned soups and vegetables, cheese, ketchup, processed meats, salt, salty snack foods, and seafood.

7. Which of the following causes isovolumic hyponatremia?
    A.   hyperthyroidism.
    B.   syndrome of inappropriate antidiuretic hormone secretion.
    C.   heart failure.

Answer: B. Causes of isovolumic hyponatremia include glucocorticoid deficiency, hypothyroidism, renal failure, and syndrome of inappropriate antidiuretic hormone secretion.

8. Drugs that may cause high sodium levels include:
    A.   antacids.
    B.   diuretics.
    C.   antipsychotics.

Answer: A. If taken on a regular basis, antacids with sodium bicarbonate may cause high sodium levels.

Scoring

☆☆☆   If you answered all eight questions correctly, congratulations! You're a Sodium Somebody!

☆☆   If you answered six or seven correctly, good job. You're a pillar of strength and intelligence (and not salt)!

☆   If you answered fewer than six correctly, don't fret. You'll strike the proper balance in the following chapters!

When potassium tips the balance

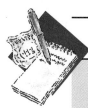

Just the facts

This chapter discusses the important role potassium plays in keeping the cells, nerves, and muscles functioning properly. In this chapter, you'll learn:

♦ how potassium contributes to fluid and electrolyte balance

♦ how the body regulates serum potassium levels

♦ how potassium imbalances are treated

♦ how to care for patients with potassium imbalances

♦ how to document care given to patients with potassium imbalances.

A look at potassium

The major cation (ion with a positive charge) in the intracellular fluid, potassium plays a critical role in many metabolic cell functions. Only 2% of the body's potassium is found in extracellular fluid; 98% is in intracellular fluid. That significant difference affects nerve impulse transmission.

Diseases, injuries, medications, and therapies can all disturb potassium levels. Small, untreated alterations in serum potassium levels can seriously affect neuromuscular and cardiac functioning.

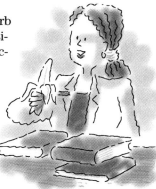

Bananas are loaded with potassium!

How it happens

Potassium directly affects how well the body's cells, nerves, and muscles function by:
• maintaining cells' electrical neutrality and osmolality
• aiding neuromuscular transmission of nerve impulses

• assisting skeletal and cardiac muscle contraction and electrical conductivity
• affecting acid-base balance in relationship to the hydrogen ion (another cation). (See *Potassium's role in acid-base balance.*)

Normal serum potassium levels range from 3.5 to 5 mEq/L. In the cell, the potassium level (usually not measured) is much higher, at 140 mEq/L. Potassium must be ingested daily because the body can't conserve it. The recommended daily requirement for adults is about 40 mEq; the average daily intake is 60 to 100 mEq. (See *Dietary sources of potassium.*)

Extracellular fluid also gains potassium when cells are destroyed, releasing intracellular potassium, and when potassium shifts out of the intracellular fluid into the extracellular fluid.

Losing potassium

About 80% of the potassium taken in is excreted in urine, with each liter of urine containing 20 to 40 mEq of the electrolyte. Any remaining potassium is excreted in feces and sweat.

Extracellular potassium loss also occurs when potassium moves from the extracellular fluid to the intracellular fluid and when cells undergo anabolism. Three additional factors that affect potassium levels include the sodium-potassium pump, renal regulation, and pH level.

Pumpin' sodium and potassium

The sodium-potassium pump is an active transport mechanism that moves ions across the cell membrane against a concentration gradient. Specifically, the pump moves sodium from the cell into the extracellular fluid and maintains high intracellular potassium levels by pumping potassium into the cell.

Regulatin' those renals

The body also rids itself of excess potassium by way of the kidneys. As serum potassium levels rise, the renal tubules excrete more potassium, leading to increased potassium loss in the urine.

Sodium and potassium have a reciprocal relationship. The kidneys reabsorb sodium and excrete potassium when the hormone aldosterone is secreted. The kidneys have no effective mechanism to combat loss of potassium and may excrete it even when the serum potassium level is low.

Free trade

A change in pH may affect serum potassium levels because hydrogen ions and potassium ions freely exchange across plasma cell membranes. For example, in acidosis, excess hydrogen ions move into cells and push potassium into the extracellular fluid. Thus,

Dietary sources of potassium

Here are some major sources of potassium:
• chocolate
• dried fruit, nuts, and seeds
• fruits, such as oranges, bananas, apricots, and cantaloupe
• meats
• vegetables, especially potatoes, mushrooms, tomatoes, and carrots.

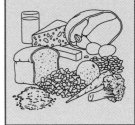

Now I get it!

Potassium's role in acid-base balance

The illustrations below show the movement of potassium ions in response to changes in extracellular hydrogen ion concentration. Hydrogen ion concentration changes with acidosis and alkalosis.

Normal balance

Under normal conditions, the potassium ion (K) content in intracellular fluid is much greater than in extracellular fluid. Hydrogen ion (H) concentration is low in both compartments.

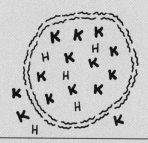

Acidosis

In acidosis, hydrogen ion content in extracellular fluid increases and the ions move into the intracellular fluid. To keep the intracellular fluid electrically neutral, an equal number of potassium ions leave the cell, which causes hyperkalemia.

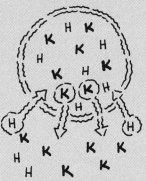

Alkalosis

In alkalosis, more hydrogen ions are present in intracellular fluid than in the extracellular fluid. Therefore, hydrogen ions move from the intracellular fluid into the extracellular fluid. To keep the intracellular fluid electrically neutral, potassium ions move from the extracellular fluid into the intracellular fluid, which causes hypokalemia.

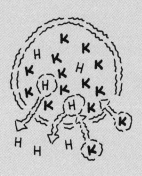

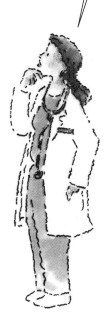

Potassium ions really get around!

acidosis can cause hyperkalemia as potassium moves out of the cell to maintain balance. Likewise, alkalosis can cause hypokalemia, as potassium moves into the cell to maintain balance.

Hypokalemia

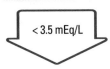

< 3.5 mEq/L

In hypokalemia, the serum potassium level drops below 3.5 mEq/L. Because the normal range for a serum potassium level is narrow (3.5 to 5 mEq/L), a slight decrease has profound consequences.

How it happens

Remember that the body can't conserve potassium. Inadequate intake and excessive output of potassium can cause a moderate drop in its level, upsetting the balance and causing a potassium deficiency in the body.

Conditions, such as prolonged intestinal suction, recent ileostomy, and villous adenoma can cause a decrease in the body's overall potassium level. In certain situations, potassium shifts from the extracellular space to the intracellular space and hides in the cells. Because the cells contain more potassium than usual, less can be measured in the blood.

Not enough intake

Inadequate potassium intake causes a drop in the body's overall potassium level. That could mean a person isn't eating enough potassium-rich foods or is receiving potassium-deficient I.V. fluids.

Too much output

Intestinal fluids contain large amounts of potassium. Severe GI fluid losses from suction, lavage, or prolonged vomiting can deplete the body's potassium supply. As a result, potassium levels drop. Diarrhea, fistulas, laxative abuse, and severe diaphoresis also contribute to potassium loss.

Potassium can also be depleted through the kidneys. Diuresis that occurs with a newly functioning transplanted kidney can lead to hypokalemia. High urine glucose levels cause osmotic diuresis, and potassium is lost through the urine. Other potassium losses are seen in renal tubular acidosis, magnesium depletion, Cushing's syndrome, and periods of high stress.

Drugs can upset the balance

Drugs, such as diuretics (especially thiazide and furosemide), corticosteroids, insulin, cisplatin, and certain antibiotics (gentamicin,

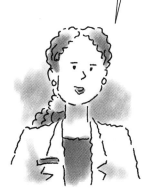

Remember that the body can't conserve potassium.

carbenicillin, and amphotericin B, for instance), also cause potassium loss. (See *Drugs associated with hypokalemia.*)

Excessive secretion of insulin, whether endogenous or exogenous, may shift potassium into the cells. Insulin can be released from the body and cause hypokalemia in patients receiving large amounts of dextrose solutions. Potassium levels also drop when adrenergics, such as epinephrine or albuterol, are used to treat asthma.

Diseases can wreak havoc, too

Conditions (such as vomiting) that lead to the loss of gastric acids can cause alkalosis and hypokalemia. Alkalosis moves potassium ions into the cell as hydrogen ions move out.

Other disorders associated with hypokalemia are hepatic disease, hyperaldosteronism, acute alcoholism, heart failure, malabsorption syndrome, nephritis, and Bartter's syndrome.

What to look for

The signs and symptoms of a low potassium level reflect how important the electrolyte is to normal body functions.

Neuromuscular alerts

Skeletal muscle weakness, especially in the legs, is a sign of a moderate loss of potassium. Weakness progresses, and paresthesia develops. Leg cramps occur. Deep tendon reflexes may be decreased or absent. Paralysis could involve the respiratory muscles.

> **Memory jogger**
>
> To help you remember some of the signs and symptoms of hypokalemia, think of the word SUCTION. (Keep in mind that hypokalemia can be caused by a loss of stomach contents from nasogastric suctioning.)
>
> Skeletal muscle weakness
>
> U wave (electrocardiogram changes)
>
> Constipation, ileus
>
> Toxic effects of digoxin (from hypokalemia)
>
> Irregular, weak pulse
>
> Orthostatic hypotension
>
> Numbness (paresthesia)

Drugs associated with hypokalemia

These drugs can deplete potassium and cause hypokalemia:
• adrenergics, such as albuterol and epinephrine
• antibiotics, such as amphotericin B, carbenicillin, and gentamicin
• cisplatin
• corticosteroids
• diuretics, such as furosemide and thiazide
• insulin
• laxatives (when used excessively).

Because potassium affects cell function, hypokalemia can lead to rhabdomyolysis, a breakdown of muscle fibers leading to myoglobin in the urine. As hypokalemia affects smooth muscle, the patient may develop anorexia, nausea, and vomiting.

Read this intestinal tract

The patient may experience intestinal problems, such as decreased bowel sounds, constipation, and paralytic ileus. He may also have difficulty concentrating urine (when hypokalemia is prolonged) and pass large volumes of urine.

ECG alerts

Cardiac problems can result from a low potassium level. The pulse may be weak and irregular. The patient may have orthostatic hypotension. The electrocardiogram (ECG) may show a flattened T wave, a depressed ST segment, and a characteristic U wave.

Cardiac arrest can result from hypokalemia. A patient taking digoxin, especially if he's also taking a diuretic, should be watched closely for hypokalemia, which can potentiate the action of the digoxin and cause a toxic reaction. (See *Danger signs of hypokalemia.*)

What tests show

The following test results may help confirm the diagnosis of hypokalemia:
- serum potassium level less than 3.5 mEq/L
- elevated pH and bicarbonate levels
- slightly elevated serum glucose level
- characteristic ECG changes.

How hypokalemia is treated

Treatment for hypokalemia focuses on restoring a normal potassium balance, preventing serious complications, and removing or treating the underlying causes. Treatment varies depending on the severity of the imbalance.
- The patient should be placed on a high-potassium diet.
- However, increasing the intake of dietary potassium may be insufficient to treat less acute hypokalemia. The patient may need oral potassium supplements using potassium salts, in which case potassium chloride is preferred.
- Patients who have severe hypokalemia or who can't take oral supplements may need I.V. potassium replacement therapy.

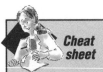

Cheat sheet

Signs and symptoms of hypokalemia

Common signs and symptoms of hypokalemia include:
- anorexia
- constipation
- cramps
- decreased bowel sounds
- ECG changes
- hyporeflexia
- muscle weakness
- nausea
- orthostatic hypotension
- paresthesia
- polyuria
- vomiting
- weak, irregular pulse.

Whether through a peripheral or a central catheter, I.V. potassium must be administered with care to prevent serious complications.

Bouncing back to balanced

After the serum potassium level is back to normal, the patient may receive a sustained-release oral potassium supplement and may need to increase his dietary intake of potassium. A patient taking a diuretic may be switched to a potassium-sparing diuretic to prevent excessive loss of potassium in the urine.

How you intervene

Careful monitoring and skilled interventions can help prevent hypokalemia and spare your patient from its associated complications. For patients who are at risk for developing hypokalemia or who have hypokalemia already, you'll want to perform these actions.

Assess and monitor

• Monitor vital signs, especially pulse and blood pressure, because hypokalemia is commonly associated with hypovolemia, which can cause orthostatic hypotension.
• Check heart rate and rhythm and ECG tracings in patients with a serum potassium level less than 3 mEq/L (severe hypokalemia) because hypokalemia is commonly associated with hypovolemia, and hypovolemia will create tachyarrhythmias.
• Assess the patient's respiratory rate, depth, and pattern. Hypokalemia may weaken or paralyze respiratory muscles. Notify the doctor immediately if respirations become shallow and rapid. Keep a manual resuscitation bag at the bedside of a patient with severe hypokalemia. (See *When treatment doesn't work*, page 108.)
• Monitor serum potassium levels. Changes in serum potassium levels can lead to serious cardiac complications.
• Assess patient for clinical evidence of hypokalemia, especially if he's receiving a diuretic or digoxin. A patient who has hypokalemia and takes digoxin is at increased risk for digoxin toxicity because the body has less potassium with which to work (potassium is needed to balance the level of the digoxin in the blood).
• Monitor and document fluid intake and output. About 40 mEq of potassium is lost in each liter of urine. Diuresis can put the patient at risk for potassium loss.
• Check for signs of hypokalemia-related metabolic alkalosis, including irritability and paresthesia.

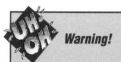

Warning!

Danger signs of hypokalemia

• Arrhythmias
• Cardiac arrest
• Digoxin toxicity
• Muscle paralysis
• Paralytic ileus
• Respiratory arrest

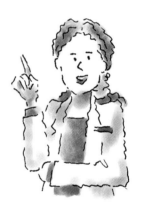

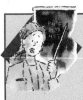

> **Teaching points**
>
> # Teaching about hypokalemia
>
> Make sure you cover these topics with your patient and then evaluate his learning:
> • explanation of hypokalemia, including its signs, symptoms, and complications
> • causes and risk factors
> • prevention of future episodes
> • medication, including dosages and possible adverse effects
> • need for a potassium-rich diet
> • warning signs and symptoms to report to the doctor.

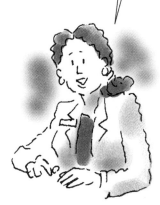

These guidelines will lead you to I.V. success.

I.V. guidelines

• Insert and maintain patent I.V. access as ordered. When choosing a vein, remember that I.V. potassium preparations can irritate peripheral veins and cause discomfort.
• Administer I.V. potassium replacement solutions as prescribed. (See *Guidelines for I.V. potassium administration.*)
• Monitor heart rate and rhythm and ECG tracings of patients receiving potassium infusions of more than 5 mEq/hour or a concentration of more than 40 mEq/L of fluid.
• Administer I.V. potassium infusions cautiously. Make sure that infusions are diluted and mixed thoroughly in adequate amounts of fluid. Use premixed potassium solutions when possible.
• Watch the I.V. infusion site for infiltration.

> **It's not working!**
>
> # When treatment doesn't work
>
> If you're having trouble raising a patient's potassium level, step back and take a look at the entire fluid and electrolyte picture.
> • Is the patient still experiencing diuresis or suffering losses from the GI tract or the skin? If so, he's losing fluid and potassium.
> • Is the patient's magnesium level normal, or does he need supplementation? Keep in mind that low magnesium levels make it hard for the kidneys to conserve potassium.

Guidelines for I.V. potassium administration

Following are some guidelines for administering I.V. potassium and for monitoring patients receiving it. Remember that potassium only needs to be replaced I.V. if hypokalemia is severe or if the patient can't take oral potassium supplements.

Administration

• When adding the potassium preparation to an I.V. solution, mix well. Don't add it to a hanging container; the potassium will pool, and the patient will receive a highly concentrated bolus. Use premixed potassium when possible.

• To prevent or reduce toxic effects, I.V. infusion concentrations shouldn't exceed 40 to 60 mEq/L. Rates are usually 10 mEq/hour. More rapid infusions may be used in severe cases; however, rapid infusion requires closer monitoring of cardiac status. The maximum adult dose generally shouldn't exceed 200 mEq/24 hours unless prescribed.

• Use infusion devices when administering potassium solutions in order to control flow rate.

• NEVER administer potassium by I.V. push or bolus; doing so can cause cardiac arrhythmias and cardiac arrest.

Patient monitoring

• Monitor the patient's cardiac rhythm during rapid I.V. potassium administration to prevent toxic effects from hyperkalemia. Report any irregularities immediately.

• Evaluate the results of treatment by checking serum potassium levels and assessing the patient for signs and symptoms of toxic reaction, such as muscle weakness and paralysis.

• Watch the I.V. site for signs and symptoms of infiltration, phlebitis, or tissue necrosis.

• Monitor the patient's urine output and notify the doctor if volume is inadequate. Urine output should exceed 30 ml/hour to avoid hyperkalemia.

• Never give potassium by I.V. push or as a bolus. It could be fatal.

• To prevent gastric irritation from oral potassium supplements, administer the supplements in at least 4 oz (118 ml) of fluid or with food.

• To prevent a quick load of potassium from entering the body, don't crush slow-release tablets.

• Use the same care when giving an oral supplement as you would when administering an I.V. supplement.

• Provide a safe environment for the patient who is weak from hypokalemia. Explain any imposed activity restrictions. (See *Teaching about hypokalemia.*)

• Check for signs of constipation, such as abdominal distention and decreased bowel sounds. Although medication may be prescribed to combat constipation, don't use laxatives that promote potassium loss. (See *Documenting hypokalemia,* page 110.)

• Emphasize the importance of taking potassium supplements as prescribed, especially when the patient is also taking digoxin or a diuretic. If appropriate, teach the patient to recognize and report

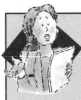

Chart smart

Documenting hypokalemia

Include these topics when documenting the condition of your patient with hypokalemia:
- assessment findings
- vital signs (including arrhythmias)
- serum potassium level and other pertinent laboratory data
- intake and output
- doctor notification
- potassium supplements given and method of administration
- nursing interventions and patient's response
- safety measures implemented
- patient teaching provided and patient's response to the teaching.

signs and symptoms of digoxin toxicity, such as pulse irregularities, anorexia, nausea, and vomiting.
- Make sure the patient can identify the signs and symptoms of hypokalemia.

Hyperkalemia

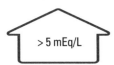

> 5 mEq/L

Hyperkalemia occurs when the serum potassium level rises above 5 mEq/L. Because the normal serum potassium range is so narrow (3.5 to 5 mEq/L), a slight increase can have profound consequences. Although less common than hypokalemia, hyperkalemia is more serious. Other treatments are commonly the cause of hyperkalemia.

How it happens

Remember, potassium is gained through intake and lost by excretion. If either is altered, hyperkalemia can result.

The kidneys, which excrete potassium, are vital in preventing a toxic buildup of this electrolyte. Acid-base imbalances can alter potassium balance as well. Acidosis moves potassium outside the cell as hydrogen ions shift into the cell. Cell injury results in release, or spilling, of potassium into the serum, which is reflected in the patient's laboratory test results.

Too much intake

Increased dietary intake of potassium (especially with decreased urine output) can cause the potassium level to rise. Excessive use of salt substitutes (most of which use potassium as a substitute for sodium) further compounds the situation. Potassium supplements, whether oral or I.V., raise the potassium level. Excessive doses can lead to hyperkalemia.

Watch transfusions and drugs

The serum potassium level of donated blood increases the longer the blood is stored. Therefore, a patient's potassium level may rise if he's given a large volume of donated blood that's nearing its expiration date.

Certain medications are associated with high potassium levels, such as beta-adrenergic blockers (which inhibit potassium shifts into cells), potassium-sparing diuretics such as spironolactone, and some antibiotics such as penicillin G potassium. Chemotherapy, which causes cell death (and sometimes renal injury), can lead to hyperkalemia.

Angiotensin-converting enzyme inhibitors and nonsteroidal anti-inflammatory drugs are thought to cause hyperkalemia by influencing aldosterone secretion, which promotes potassium excretion in the kidneys. When administering any medication that can cause renal injury (such as an aminoglycoside), monitor the patient for hyperkalemia. (See *Drugs associated with hyperkalemia.*)

Too little output

Potassium excretion is diminished with acute or chronic renal failure. Any disease that can cause kidney damage (diabetes, sickle cell disease, or systemic lupus erythematosus, for instance) can lead to hyperkalemia. Addison's disease and hypoaldosteronism can also decrease potassium excretion from the body.

Injury moves it out

When a burn, severe infection, trauma, crush injury, or intravascular hemolysis has injured a cell, potassium may leave the cell.

Chemotherapy causes cell lysis and the release of potassium. Metabolic acidosis and insulin deficiency decrease the movement of potassium into cells. (See *Make sure the results are real,* page 113.)

What to look for

Signs and symptoms of hyperkalemia reflect its effects on neuromuscular and cardiac functioning in the body. Paresthesia, an early symptom, and irritability signal hyperkalemia.

Drugs associated with hyperkalemia

The following drugs are associated with increased potassium levels:

• angiotensin-converting enzyme inhibitors
• antibiotics
• beta-adrenergic blockers
• chemotherapeutic drugs
• nonsteroidal anti-inflammatory drugs
• potassium (in excessive amounts)
• spironolactone.

Cheat sheet

Signs and symptoms of hyperkalemia

Common signs and symptoms of hyperkalemia include:
- abdominal cramping
- diarrhea
- electrocardiogram changes (first noted as a tall, tented T wave)
- hypotension
- irregular pulse rate
- irritability
- muscle weakness, especially of the lower extremities
- nausea
- paresthesia.

Cheat sheet

Key facts about hyperkalemia

- Most dangerous of the electrolyte disorders
- Commonly accompanies metabolic acidosis
- *Underlying mechanisms:* increased intake of potassium, decreased urine excretion of potassium, shift of potassium out of the cells to extracellular fluid.
- *Best clinical indicators:* serum potassium levels and electrocardiogram tracings
- *Serum potassium levels exceeding 7 mEq/L:* possible serious cardiac arrhythmias leading to cardiac arrest

Neuromuscular alerts

Hyperkalemia may cause skeletal muscle weakness that, in turn, may lead to flaccid paralysis. Muscle weakness tends to spread from the legs to the trunk and involves respiratory muscles. Hyperkalemia also causes smooth-muscle hyperactivity, particularly in the GI tract, which can result in nausea, abdominal cramping, and diarrhea, an early sign.

Cardiac alerts

Other possible complications include a decreased heart rate, irregular pulse, decreased cardiac output, hypotension and, possibly, cardiac arrest.

The tall, tented T wave is a prominent ECG characteristic of the patient with hyperkalemia. Other ECG changes include a flattened P wave, prolonged PR interval, widened QRS complex, and depressed ST segment. The condition can also lead to heart block, ventricular arrhythmias, and asystole. The more serious arrhythmias become especially dangerous when serum potassium levels reach 7 mEq/L or more.

What tests show

The following test results help confirm the diagnosis and determine the severity of hyperkalemia:
- serum potassium level greater than 5 mEq/L
- decreased arterial pH, indicating acidosis
- ECG abnormalities.

Make sure the results are real

When a laboratory test result indicates that your patient has a high serum potassium level, and the result just doesn't seem to make sense, make sure it's a true result. If the sample was drawn using poor technique, the results may be falsely high. Some of the causes of high potassium levels that don't truly reflect the patient's serum potassium level include:
• drawing the sample above an I.V. infusion containing potassium
• using a recently exercised extremity for the venipuncture site
• causing hemolysis (cell damage) as the specimen is obtained.

How hyperkalemia is treated

Treatment for hyperkalemia is aimed at lowering the potassium level and treating its cause. The severity of hyperkalemia dictates how it will be treated.

For mild cases...

Mild hyperkalemia may be treated with a loop diuretic to increase potassium loss from the body or to resolve any acidosis present. Dietary potassium is restricted. Medications associated with high potassium level should be readjusted or stopped. Underlying disorders leading to the high potassium level are treated.

For moderate to severe cases...

With moderate to severe hyperkalemia, other measures may be undertaken. If the patient has renal failure, a diuretic may not be effective. For acute symptomatic hyperkalemia, hemodialysis may be required.

Sodium polystyrene sulfonate (Kayexalate), a cation-exchange resin, is a common treatment for hyperkalemia. Sorbitol, or another osmotic substance, should be given with this medication to promote its excretion. Kayexalate can be given orally, through a nasogastric tube, or as a retention enema (may require repeated treatments). The onset of action may take several hours; the duration of action is 4 to 6 hours. As the medication sits in the intestines, sodium moves across the bowel wall into the blood, and potassium moves out of the blood into the intestines. Loose stools remove potassium from the body.

Emergency measures

More severe hyperkalemia is treated as an emergency. Closely monitor the patient's cardiac status. ECGs are obtained to follow progress.

Closely watch the cardiac status of a patient with severe hypokalemia.

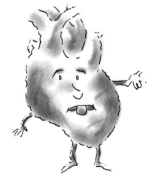

To counteract the myocardial effects of hyperkalemia, administer 10% calcium gluconate (usually 10 ml) I.V. over 3 minutes. The patient must be connected to a cardiac monitor. However, calcium gluconate isn't a treatment for hyperkalemia itself, and the hyperkalemia must still be treated because the effects of calcium last only a short time.

A patient with acidosis may receive sodium bicarbonate (usually 50 mEq) I.V., which helps decrease serum potassium level by temporarily shifting potassium into the cells. The drug becomes effective within 15 to 30 minutes and lasts 1 to 3 hours.

Another way to move potassium into the cells and lower the serum level is to administer 10 units of regular insulin I.V. The drug becomes active within 15 to 60 minutes and lasts 4 to 6 hours. It's given with I.V. hypertonic dextrose (10% to 50%).

How you intervene

Patients at risk for hyperkalemia require frequent monitoring of serum potassium and other electrolyte levels. Those at risk include patients with acidosis or renal failure and those receiving a potassium-sparing diuretic, an oral potassium supplement, or an I.V. potassium preparation. If a patient develops hyperkalemia, take these nursing actions.

Assess and monitor

• Assess vital signs. Anticipate cardiac monitoring if the patient's serum potassium level exceeds 6 mEq/L. A patient with ECG changes may need aggressive treatment to prevent cardiac arrest.
• Monitor the patient's intake and output. Report an output of less than 30 ml/hour. An inability to excrete potassium adequately may lead to dangerously high potassium levels. (See *The next step.*)

▶ *Teaching points*

Teaching about hyperkalemia

Make sure you cover these topics with your patient and then evaluate his learning:
• explanation of hyperkalemia, including its signs, symptoms, and complications
• medication, including dosage and potential for hypokalemia
• need for a potassium-restricted diet and importance of avoiding salt substitutes
• prevention of future episodes of hyperkalemia
• warning signs and symptoms to report to the doctor.

• Prepare to administer a slow calcium gluconate I.V. infusion in acute cases to counteract the myocardial depressant effects of hyperkalemia.
• For a patient receiving repeated insulin and glucose treatment, check for clinical signs and symptoms of hypoglycemia, including muscle weakness, syncope, hunger, and diaphoresis.
• Keep in mind when giving Kayexalate that serum sodium levels may rise. Watch for signs of heart failure.
• Monitor bowel sounds and the number and character of bowel movements. Hyperactive bowel sounds result from the body's attempt to maintain homeostasis by causing significant potassium excretion through the bowels.
• Monitor serum potassium level and related laboratory test results. Keep in mind that patients with serum potassium levels exceeding 6 mEq/L require cardiac monitoring because asystole may occur as hyperkalemia makes depolarization of cardiac muscle easier and shortens repolarization times.

Administer and follow up

• Administer prescribed medications and monitor the patient for their effectiveness and for adverse effects.
• Encourage the patient to retain Kayexalate enemas for 30 to 60 minutes. Monitor the patient for hypokalemia when administering this drug on 2 or more consecutive days.
• If the patient has diarrhea and can't retain the enema liquid, try an indwelling rectal catheter, inflating the balloon after insertion into the patient's rectum.
• If the patient has acute hyperkalemia that doesn't respond to other treatments, prepare him for dialysis.
• If the patient has muscle weakness, implement safety measures. Advise him to ask for help before attempting to get out of bed and walk. Continue to evaluate muscle strength.
• Administer prescribed antidiarrheals and monitor the patient's response.
• Help the patient select foods that don't stimulate peristalsis. (See *Teaching about hyperkalemia*.)
• If the patient has hyperkalemia and needs a transfusion, obtain fresh blood.
• Watch for signs of hypokalemia after treatment.
• Document all care given and the patient's response. (See *Documenting hyperkalemia*, page 116.)
• Explain the signs and symptoms of hyperkalemia, including muscle weakness, diarrhea, and pulse irregularities. Urge the patient to report such signs and symptoms to the doctor.
• Describe the signs of hypokalemia to patients taking medications to lower serum potassium levels.

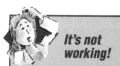

It's not working!

The next step

If you can't bring down your patient's potassium level as expected, consider the following questions:
• Is the patient taking an antacid? Antacids containing magnesium or calcium can interfere with ion exchange resins.
• Is the patient's renal status worsening?
• Is the patient taking a medication that could raise the potassium level?
• Is the patient receiving old donated blood during transfusions?

Chart smart

Documenting hyperkalemia

When your patient has hyperkalemia, you'll want to document the following information:
• assessment findings
• vital signs (including arrhythmias)
• serum potassium level and other pertinent laboratory test results
• intake and output
• doctor notification
• medications administered
• nursing interventions and patient's response
• safety measures implemented
• patient teaching provided and patient's response to the teaching.

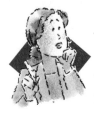

Quick quiz

1. Potassium is responsible for:
    A.   building muscle mass.
    B.   building bone structure and strength.
    C.   maintaining the heartbeat.

Answer: C. Potassium is vital for proper cardiac function because it facilitates cardiac muscle contraction and electrical conductivity. Alterations in the serum potassium level should be recognized and treated as early as possible.

2. When the hormone aldosterone is secreted, the kidneys reabsorb:
    A.   sodium.
    B.   potassium.
    C.   magnesium.

Answer: A. The kidneys reabsorb sodium and excrete potassium when aldosterone is secreted.

3. Neuromuscular signs and symptoms of hypokalemia include:
   A. confusion and irritability.
   B. diminished deep tendon reflexes.
   C. Parkinsonian-type tremors.

Answer: B. Deep tendon reflexes may be decreased or absent in hypokalemia. Also, leg cramps may occur, and respiratory muscles may be paralyzed.

4. Medications to be given when treating severe hyperkalemia include:
   A. methylprednisolone and mannitol.
   B. mannitol and regular insulin.
   C. 10% calcium gluconate and regular insulin.

Answer: C. Calcium gluconate helps to stabilize cardiac cell membranes, though it doesn't lower a high potassium level itself. Regular insulin, in conjunction with hypertonic dextrose, causes potassium to move into the cells, thus lowering the serum potassium level.

5. A hallmark ECG characteristic of the patient with hyperkalemia is the presence of:
   A. irregular PR intervals.
   B. narrowed QRS complexes.
   C. tall, tented T waves.

Answer: C. Tall, tented T waves are a hallmark of hyperkalemia, a condition that can also lead to heart block, ventricular arrhythmias, and asystole.

6. An 83-year-old patient with heart failure develops hypokalemia as a result of her diuretic therapy. You suggest that she increase her dietary intake of potassium. Which foods should she consume?
   A. Chocolate, mushrooms, and bananas
   B. Canned soups, peas, and milk
   C. Apples, whole wheat bread, and oatmeal

Answer: A. Major dietary sources of potassium include: chocolate, dried fruit, nuts and seeds, oranges, bananas, apricots, cantaloupes, potatoes, mushrooms, tomatoes, and carrots.

7. When administering I.V. potassium for severe hypokalemia, you should:
   A.   administer potassium by I.V. push or bolus.
   B.   add the potassium to the hanging container.
   C.   prepare a solution for infusion with a concentration that doesn't exceed 40 to 60 mEq/L.

Answer: C. To prevent or reduce toxic effects, the I.V. infusion concentration shouldn't exceed 40 to 60 mEq/L.

Scoring

☆☆☆   If you answered all seven questions correctly, wow! You're Top Banana!

☆☆   If you answered five or six correctly, super! You've great potassium power!

☆   If you answered fewer than five correctly, hang in there. You'll raise your fluid level yet!

When magnesium tips the balance

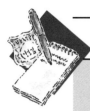

Just the facts

This chapter describes how to care for patients who have a deficiency or an excess of magnesium. In this chapter, you'll learn:

♦ why magnesium is so important

♦ why your patient's serum magnesium level might be a challenge to interpret

♦ what causes the serum magnesium level to be above normal or below normal and what to do if either imbalance occurs.

A look at magnesium

After potassium, magnesium is the most abundant cation (positively charged ion) in the intracellular fluid. The bones contain about 60% of the body's magnesium; extracellular fluid contains less than 1%. Intracellular fluid holds the rest.

What it does

Magnesium performs many important functions in the body. For example, it:
• promotes enzyme reactions within the cell during carbohydrate metabolism
• helps the body produce and use adenosine triphosphate for energy
• takes part in protein synthesis
• influences vasodilation, helping the cardiovascular system function normally

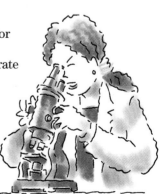

• helps sodium and potassium ions cross the cell membrane (this explains why magnesium affects sodium and potassium ion levels both inside and outside the cell).

Regulating muscle movements

Magnesium also regulates muscle contractions, making it especially vital to the neuromuscular system. By acting on the myoneural junctions—the sites where nerve and muscle fibers meet—magnesium affects the irritability and contractility of cardiac and skeletal muscle.

What does calcium have to do with it?

Magnesium has another function that's worth remembering: It influences the body's calcium level through its effect on parathyroid hormone (PTH). PTH, you might recall, maintains a constant calcium level in extracellular fluid.

Interpreting magnesium levels

You'll need to keep the magnesium-calcium connection in mind when assessing a patient's laboratory values. However, that isn't the only thing you'll need to consider.

Your patient's serum magnesium level *itself* may be misleading. Normally, the body's total serum magnesium level is 1.6 to 2.6 mEq/L. (See *At different levels.*)

But the level may not accurately reflect your patient's *actual* magnesium stores. That's because most magnesium is found within cells, where it measures about 40 mEq/L. In serum, magnesium levels are relatively low.

Ties that bind

Here's another reason why interpreting a patient's serum magnesium level can pose a challenge. More than half of circulating magnesium moves in a free, ionized form. Another 30% binds with a protein—mostly albumin—and the remainder binds with other substances.

Ionized magnesium is physiologically active and must be regulated to maintain homeostasis. However, this form alone can't be measured, so a patient's measured levels reflect the total amount of circulating magnesium.

To complicate matters, magnesium levels are linked to albumin levels. A patient with a low serum albumin level will have a low total serum magnesium level—even if the level of ionized magnesium remains unchanged. That's why serum albumin levels need to be measured with serum magnesium levels.

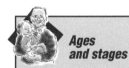

Ages and stages

At different levels

Don't forget that magnesium levels in newborns and children are different from those of adults. In newborns, magnesium levels range from 1.4 to 2.9 mEq/L; in children, 1.6 to 2.6 mEq/L.

Serum calcium and certain other laboratory values also come into play when assessing and treating magnesium imbalances. Because magnesium is mainly an intracellular electrolyte, changes in the levels of other intracellular electrolytes, such as potassium and phosphorus, can affect serum magnesium levels, too.

How the body regulates magnesium

The GI and urinary systems regulate magnesium through absorption, excretion, and retention—that is, through dietary intake and output in urine and feces. A well-balanced diet should provide roughly 25 mEq (or 300 to 350 mg) of magnesium daily. (See *Dietary sources of magnesium.*) Of this amount, about 40% is absorbed in the small intestine.

The body's balancing act

The body tries to adjust to any changes in the magnesium level. For instance, if the serum magnesium level drops, the GI tract may absorb more magnesium and, if the magnesium level rises, the GI tract excretes more in the feces.

The kidneys, for their part, balance magnesium by altering its reabsorption at the proximal tubule and loop of Henle. So, if serum magnesium levels climb, the kidneys excrete the excess in the urine. Diuretics heighten this effect. The reverse occurs, too: If serum magnesium levels fall, the kidneys conserve magnesium. That conservation is so efficient that the daily loss of circulating ionized magnesium can be restricted to just 1 mEq.

Dietary sources of magnesium

Most healthy people can get all the magnesium they need by eating a well-balanced diet that includes foods rich in magnesium. Here are the "lucky 7" foods high in magnesium:

- chocolate
- dry beans and peas
- green, leafy vegetables
- meats
- nuts
- seafood
- whole grains.

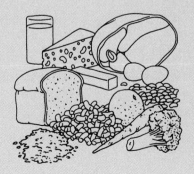

Hypomagnesemia

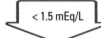

< 1.5 mEq/L

Hypomagnesemia occurs when the body's serum magnesium level falls below 1.5 mEq/L. Although sometimes overlooked, this imbalance is relatively common, affecting about 10% of all hospitalized patients. As you might expect, the condition is most common among critically ill patients. (See *Danger signs of low magnesium levels.*)

Most symptoms of hypomagnesemia occur when the magnesium level drops below 1 mEq/L. At its worst, hypomagnesemia can lead to:
• respiratory muscle paralysis
• complete heart block
• coma.

How it happens

Any condition that impairs either of the body's magnesium regulators—the GI system or the urinary system—can lead to a magnesium shortage. These conditions fall into four main categories:
• poor dietary intake of magnesium
• poor magnesium absorption by the GI tract
• excessive magnesium loss from the GI tract
• excessive magnesium loss from the urinary tract.

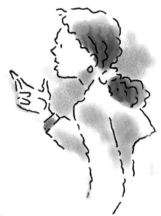

Warning!

Danger signs of low magnesium levels

Suspect that your patient with hypomagnesemia is *really* in trouble if he has any of these late-developing danger signs or symptoms:
• cardiac arrhythmias
• digoxin toxicity
• laryngeal stridor
• respiratory muscle weakness
• seizures.

The price of alcohol

Chronic alcoholics are at risk for hypomagnesemia because they tend to eat a poor diet. What's worse, alcohol overuse causes the urinary system to excrete more magnesium than normal. Alcoholics can also lose magnesium through poor intestinal absorption or from frequent or prolonged vomiting.

At risk!

Patients who can't take magnesium orally are at high risk for developing a magnesium deficiency unless they get adequate supplementation. These include patients receiving prolonged I.V. fluid therapy, total parenteral nutrition (TPN), or enteral feeding formulas that contain insufficient magnesium.

Patients who have diabetes mellitus are also at risk for magnesium loss due to osmotic diuresis.

Absorption problems

If a patient's dietary intake seems adequate but his serum magnesium level remains low, poor GI absorption may be the culprit. For instance, malabsorption syndromes, steatorrhea, ulcerative colitis, and Crohn's disease can diminish magnesium absorption. Surgery to treat these disorders can also reduce absorption. Bowel resection, for example, reduces potential absorption sites by decreasing the surface area within the GI tract.

Other conditions that can cause hypomagnesemia from poor GI absorption include cancer, pancreatic insufficiency, and excessive calcium or phosphorus in the GI tract.

GI problems

Fluids in the GI tract (especially the lower part) contain magnesium. That's why a person who loses a great deal of these fluids — from prolonged diarrhea or fistula drainage, for example — can have a magnesium deficiency. A patient who abuses laxatives or who has a nasogastric tube connected to suction is also at risk. In the latter case, the magnesium is lost from the upper, not the lower, GI tract.

In acute pancreatitis, magnesium forms soaps with fatty acids. This process takes some of the magnesium out of circulation, causing serum levels to drop.

Urinary problems

Greater excretion of magnesium in urine can also lead to a low serum magnesium level. Conditions that boost such excretion include:

• primary aldosteronism (overproduction of aldosterone, an adrenal hormone)
• hyperparathyroidism (hyperfunction of the parathyroid glands) or hypoparathyroidism (hypofunction of the parathyroid glands)
• diabetic ketoacidosis (DKA)
• use of amphotericin B, cisplatin, cyclosporine, pentamidine isethionate, or aminoglycoside antibiotics, such as tobramycin or gentamicin
• prolonged administration of loop or thiazide diuretics (see *Drugs associated with hypomagnesemia*)
• impaired renal absorption of magnesium resulting from diseases such as glomerulonephritis, pyelonephritis, and renal tubular acidosis.

Other causes

Magnesium levels may also drop dramatically in patients who are pregnant (second and third trimester); patients who are receiving magnesium-free, sodium-rich I.V. fluids to induce extracellular fluid expansion; and patients who have:
• excessive loss of body fluids (for example, from sweating, breast-feeding, diuretic abuse, or chronic diarrhea)
• hemodialysis
• hypercalcemia
• hypothermia
• inappropriate secretion of antidiuretic hormone
• sepsis
• serious burns
• wounds requiring debridement
• any condition that predisposes them to excessive calcium or sodium in the urine.

What to look for

Signs and symptoms of hypomagnesemia can range from mild to life-threatening and can involve the:
• central nervous system (CNS)
• neuromuscular system
• cardiovascular system
• GI system.
    Generally speaking, your patient's signs and symptoms may resemble those you'd see with a potassium or calcium imbalance. However, you can't always count on detecting hypomagnesemia from clinical findings alone. Occasionally, a patient remains symptom-free even though his serum magnesium level measures less than 1.5 mEq/L. (See *Identifying hypomagnesemia*.)

Drugs associated with hypomagnesemia

Because certain drugs can cause or contribute to hypomagnesemia, you should monitor your patient's serum magnesium levels if he's receiving:
• an aminoglycoside antibiotic, such as amikacin, gentamicin, streptomycin, or tobramycin
• amphotericin B
• cisplatin
• cyclosporine
• insulin
• a laxative
• a loop or thiazide diuretic, such as bumetanide, furosemide, or torsemide
• pentamidine isethionate.

Irritating the CNS

A low serum magnesium level irritates the CNS. Such irritation can lead to:
- altered level of consciousness (LOC)
- ataxia
- confusion
- delusions
- depression
- emotional lability
- hallucinations
- insomnia
- psychosis
- seizures
- vertigo.

When magnesium moves out

The body compensates for a low serum magnesium level by moving magnesium out of the cells. Such movement can take an especially high toll on the neuromuscular system. As cells become magnesium starved, skeletal muscles grow weak and nerves and muscles become hyperirritable.

The three Ts and hyperactive DTRs

Watch your patient for neuromuscular signs of hypomagnesemia, such as:
- tremors
- twitching
- tetany
- hyperactive deep tendon reflexes (DTRs). (See *Grading DTRs*, page 126.)

Respiratory muscles may be affected, too, resulting in breathing difficulties. Some patients also experience laryngeal stridor, foot or leg cramps, and paresthesia.

Check these signs

If you suspect hypomagnesemia, you'll also want to test your patient for hypocalcemia by checking for these signs:
- Chvostek's sign — facial twitching when the facial nerve is tapped
- Trousseau's sign — carpal spasm when the upper arm is compressed. (For more information about these signs, see chapter 8, When calcium tips the balance.)

Hard on the heart

You'll recall that magnesium promotes cardiovascular function. So if you're thinking that hypomagnesemia must affect the heart and

---

Identifying hypomagnesemia

Consult the list of signs and symptoms below whenever you need to assess your patient for hypomagnesemia.
- *Central nervous system:* altered level of consciousness, confusion, hallucinations
- *Neuromuscular:* muscle weakness, leg and foot cramps, hyperactive deep tendon reflexes, tetany, Chvostek's and Trousseau's signs
- *Cardiovascular:* tachycardia, hypertension, characteristic electrocardiogram changes
- *GI:* dysphagia, anorexia, nausea, vomiting

Grading DTRs

If you suspect your patient has hypomagnesemia, you'll want to test his deep tendon reflexes (DTRs) to determine whether his neuromuscular system is irritable—a clue that his magnesium level is too low. When grading your patient's DTRs, use the following scale:

0	Absent
+	Present but diminished
++	Normal
+++	Increased but not necessarily abnormal
++++	Hyperactive, clonic

To record the patient's reflex activity, draw a stick figure and mark the strength of the response at the proper locations. This figure indicates normal DTR activity.

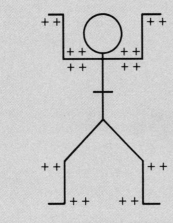

blood vessels, you're right. A drop in the magnesium level can irritate the myocardium—with potentially disastrous consequences.

Wrongful rhythms

Myocardial irritability can lead to cardiac arrhythmias, which can cause a drop in cardiac output. Arrhythmias are especially likely to develop in patients with coexisting potassium and calcium imbalances. Arrhythmias triggered by a low serum magnesium level include:

• atrial fibrillation
• heart block
• paroxysmal atrial tachycardia
• premature ventricular contractions

(Text continues on page 131.)

How electrolyte imbalances affect ECGs

Electrical impulses move through the heart's conduction system to create rhythmic contractions. Normal electrical activity in the heart depends on normal serum electrolyte concentrations.

The electrolytes sodium, potassium, and calcium, with the help of magnesium, shift back and forth across myocardial cell membranes. This shifting of electrolytes causes alternating periods of activity (depolarization) and rest (repolarization), which allow for normal myocardial function. Electrolyte imbalances cause trademark changes in electrocardiogram (ECG) readings and in altered myocardial function. This special section details changes in two critical electrolytes: magnesium and potassium.

Hypermagnesemia

Magnesium

Hypermagnesemia (serum magnesium > 2.5 mEq/L) can be caused by excessive magnesium administration or renal failure. The condition can cause a prolonged PR interval and the ECG changes shown below. If left untreated, hypermagnesemia can lead to sinoatrial or atrioventricular (AV) heart block and, finally, cardiac arrest.

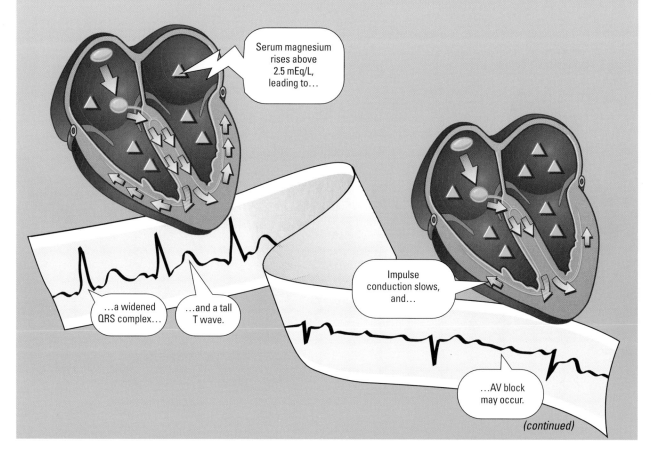

Serum magnesium rises above 2.5 mEq/L, leading to…

…a widened QRS complex…

…and a tall T wave.

Impulse conduction slows, and…

…AV block may occur.

(continued)

Hyperkalemia

Potassium

Hyperkalemia (serum potassium > 5.5 mEq/L) may be caused by renal failure or excessive potassium administration. Excess potassium alters the heart's electrical activity and leads to depressed conduction. Among the earliest signs of hyperkalemia is a tall, tented T wave, as shown below. AV or ventricular block may develop. Other possible ECG abnormalities include a flattened P wave, a prolonged PR interval, a widened QRS complex as ventricular conduction slows, and a depressed ST segment.

If left untreated, severe hyperkalemia (serum potassium > 9 mEq/L) occurs, causing the the P wave to disappear, the QRS complex to widen, and sine waves to form. Hyperkalemia may end in lethal arrhythmias.

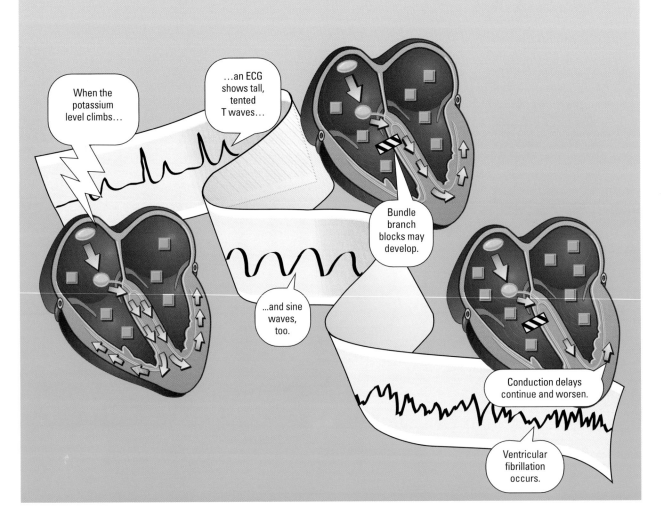

Hypokalemia

Potassium

Hypokalemia (serum potassium < 3.5 mEq/L) can be caused by diuresis or loss of other body fluids. An abnormally low potassium level affects the heart's electrical activity. Ventricular repolarization is prolonged. ECG changes include a prominent U wave — a hallmark of hypokalemia.

As the potassium level decreases, ectopic impulses form and conduction disturbances increase. Atrial and ventricular arrhythmias may develop. As ectopy becomes more frequent, the patient is at risk for potentially fatal arrhythmias. Examples of hypokalemic ECG changes are shown here.

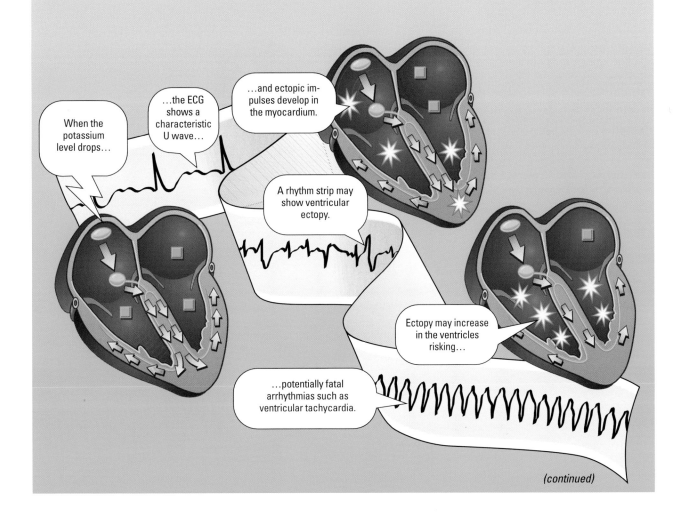

When the potassium level drops…

…the ECG shows a characteristic U wave…

…and ectopic impulses develop in the myocardium.

A rhythm strip may show ventricular ectopy.

Ectopy may increase in the ventricles risking…

…potentially fatal arrhythmias such as ventricular tachycardia.

(continued)

Hypomagnesemia

Magnesium

Hypomagnesemia (serum magnesium < 1.5 mEq/L) may be caused by malnutrition or excessive loss of body fluids. Its effects on the electrical activity of the heart include ECG changes (shown below), such as a slightly widened QRS complex, a prolonged QT interval (which increases myocardial vulnerability to a stimulus), and a depressed ST segment.

Dangerously low magnesium levels make myocardial cells more excitable, which may trigger such life-threatening arrhythmias as ventricular tachycardia, torsades de pointes, and ventricular fibrillation.

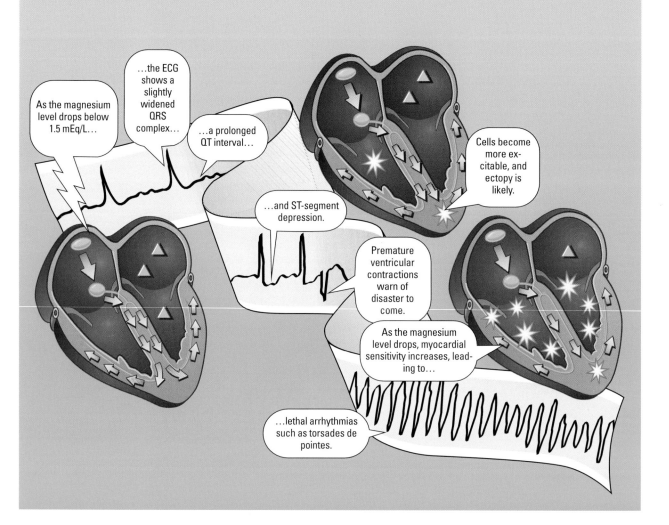

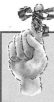

- supraventricular tachycardia
- torsades de pointes
- ventricular fibrillation
- ventricular tachycardia.

Because of the risk of arrhythmia, patients with severe hypomagnesemia (serum levels below 1 mEq/L) should undergo continuous cardiac monitoring.

General electrocardiogram (ECG) changes that can occur with a low serum magnesium level include:
- prolonged PR interval
- widened QRS complex
- prolonged QT interval
- depressed ST segment
- broad, flattened T wave
- prominent U wave.

The plot may turn toxic

If your patient with hypomagnesemia is receiving digoxin, watch him closely for signs and symptoms of digoxin toxicity — another condition that can trigger arrhythmias. A low magnesium level may increase the body's retention of digoxin. Suspect digoxin toxicity if your patient has:
- anorexia
- arrhythmias
- nausea
- vomiting
- yellow-tinged vision.

Tough times for the GI tract

A patient who doesn't have a sufficient amount of magnesium in the bloodstream may suffer such GI problems as:
- anorexia
- dysphagia
- nausea and vomiting.

These conditions can lead to poor dietary magnesium intake or loss of magnesium through the GI tract, which in turn worsen the patient's condition.

What tests show

Diagnostic test results that point to hypomagnesemia include:
- a serum magnesium level below 1.5 mEq/L (possibly with a below-normal serum albumin level)
- other electrolyte abnormalities, such as a below-normal serum potassium or calcium level
- characteristic ECG changes
- elevated serum levels of digoxin in a patient receiving the drug.

How hypomagnesemia is treated

Treatment for hypomagnesemia depends on the underlying cause of the condition and the patient's clinical findings. For patients with mild magnesium shortages, dietary replacement and teaching alone may correct the imbalance. Some doctors also prescribe an oral supplement, such as magnesium chloride, which is preferable to magnesium oxide because the latter is poorly absorbed and can cause alkalosis. Because it may take a few days to replenish magnesium stores inside the cell, magnesium replacement may be necessary for several days after the serum magnesium level returns to normal.

Patients with more severe hypomagnesemia may need I.V. or deep I.M. injections of magnesium sulfate. Before magnesium administration, renal function should be assessed. If renal function is impaired, magnesium levels should be monitored closely. (See *Check the label.*)

How you intervene

The best treatment for hypomagnesemia is prevention, so keep a watchful eye on patients at risk for this imbalance such as those who can't tolerate oral intake. For patients who have already been diagnosed with hypomagnesemia, take the following actions.

Check the label

When you prepare a magnesium sulfate injection, keep in mind that the drug comes in various concentrations, such as 10%, 12.5%, and 50%. Check the label (such as the one shown here) to make sure you're using the correct concentration. The label shows other dosage information as well.

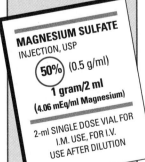

MAGNESIUM SULFATE
INJECTION, USP
50% (0.5 g/ml)
1 gram/2 ml
(4.06 mEq/ml Magnesium)
2-ml SINGLE DOSE VIAL FOR
I.M. USE, FOR I.V.
USE AFTER DILUTION

Assess

- Assess the patient's mental status and report changes.
- Evaluate the patient's neuromuscular status regularly by checking for hyperactive DTRs, tremors, and tetany. Check for Chvostek's and Trousseau's signs if hypocalcemia is also suspected.
- Check the patient for dysphagia before he's given food, oral fluids, or oral medications. Hypomagnesemia may impair his ability to swallow.

Monitor

- Monitor and record your patient's vital signs. Report findings that indicate hemodynamic instability.
- Monitor the patient's respiratory status. A magnesium deficiency can cause laryngeal stridor and compromise the airway.
- Connect your patient to a cardiac monitor if his magnesium level is below 1 mEq/L. Watch the rhythm strip closely for arrhythmias.
- Monitor patients who have lost an excessive amount of fluid (for example, due to prolonged diarrhea or fistula drainage). Patients who have experienced excessive fluid loss are at risk for magnesium deficiency.
- Urine output should be monitored at least every 4 hours. Magnesium generally isn't administered if urine output is less than 10 ml in 4 hours.
- Assess vital signs every 15 minutes. If patient is experiencing respiratory distress, assess him for a sharp decrease in blood pressure.
- If the patient is receiving digoxin, monitor him closely for signs and symptoms of digoxin toxicity (such as nausea, vomiting, and bradycardia). Magnesium deficiency enhances the pharmacologic action of digoxin
- If the patient is receiving a medication, such as an aminoglycoside, amphotericin B, cisplatin, cyclosporine, gentamicin, insulin, a laxative, a loop or thiazide diuretic, pentamidine isethionate, or torsemide, monitor his serum magnesium levels closely. Certain medications can contribute to low serum magnesium levels.
- Monitor the patient's serum electrolyte levels, and notify the doctor if the serum potassium level or calcium level is low. Both hypocalcemia and hypokalemia can cause hypomagnesemia.
- Monitor patients who are receiving nothing by mouth and receiving I.V. fluids without magnesium salts for weeks. Prolonged administration of magnesium-free fluids can result in low serum magnesium levels.

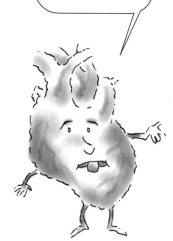

Hypocalcemia and hypokalemia can cause hypomagnesemia.

Prepare

- Institute seizure precautions.
- If a seizure occurs, report the type of seizure, its length, and the patient's behavior during the seizure. Reorient him as needed.
- Keep emergency equipment nearby for airway protection.

Maintain and administer

- Ensure your patient's safety at all times.
- Reorient the patient as needed.
- To ease your patient's anxiety, tell him what to expect before each procedure. (See *Teaching about low magnesium levels.*)
- Establish I.V. access and maintain a patent I.V. line in case your patient needs I.V. magnesium replacement or I.V. fluids.
- When preparing an infusion of magnesium sulfate, keep in mind that I.V. magnesium sulfate comes in various concentrations (such as 10%, 12.5%, and 50%). Clarify a doctor's order that specifies only the number of ampules or vials to give. A proper order states how many grams or milliliters of a particular concentration to administer, the volume of desired solution for dilution, and the length of time for infusion. (See *Infusing magnesium sulfate.*)
- Administer magnesium supplements as needed and ordered.

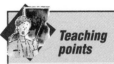

Teaching about low magnesium levels

When teaching a patient about his hypomagnesemia, include the following points and evaluate his learning:
- explanations about hypomagnesemia, its risk factors, and its treatment
- prescribed medications
- avoidance of drugs that deplete magnesium in the body, such as diuretics and laxatives
- consumption of high-magnesium diet
- danger signs and when to report them
- referral to appropriate support groups such as Alcoholics Anonymous.

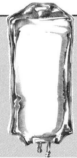

Infusing magnesium sulfate

If the doctor prescribes magnesium sulfate to boost your patient's serum magnesium level, you'll need to take some special precautions. Read on for details.
- Using an infusion pump, administer magnesium sulfate *slowly*—no faster than 150 mg/minute. Injecting a bolus dose too rapidly can trigger cardiac arrest.
- Monitor your patient's vital signs and deep tendon reflexes during magnesium sulfate therapy. Every 15 minutes, check for signs and symptoms of magnesium excess, such as hypotension and respiratory distress.
- Check the patient's serum magnesium level after each bolus dose or at least every 6 hours if he has a continuous I.V. drip.
- Stay especially alert for an above-normal serum magnesium level if your patient's renal function is impaired.
- Place the patient on continuous cardiac monitoring. Observe him closely, especially if he's also receiving digoxin.
- Monitor urine output before, during, and after magnesium sulfate infusion. Notify the doctor if output measures less than 100 ml over 4 hours.
- Keep calcium gluconate on hand to counteract adverse reactions. Have resuscitation equipment nearby and be prepared to use it if the patient goes into cardiac or respiratory arrest.

Chart smart

Documenting hypomagnesemia

Here's a list of key points to document when caring for a patient with hypomagnesemia:
- vital signs
- heart rhythm
- neurologic, neuromuscular, and cardiac assessment findings
- magnesium sulfate or other drugs administered
- fluid intake and output
- seizures and safety measures used
- your interventions and patient's response
- pertinent laboratory values, including serum electrolyte, albumin and, if appropriate, digoxin levels
- doctor notification
- patient teaching.

• During magnesium replacement, check the cardiac monitor frequently and assess the patient closely for signs of magnesium excess, such as hypotension and respiratory distress. Keep calcium gluconate at the bedside in case such signs occur.

• Maintain an accurate record of your patient's fluid intake and output. Report any decrease in urine output. (See *Documenting hypomagnesemia.*)

Hypermagnesemia

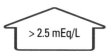

> 2.5 mEq/L

Having too much magnesium in the serum can be just as bad as having too little. Hypermagnesemia occurs when the body's serum magnesium level rises above 2.5 mEq/L.

How it happens

Hypermagnesemia results from the conditions opposite those that bring on a magnesium shortage. Its main causes are impaired magnesium excretion (for example, from renal dysfunction) and excessive magnesium intake.

Retaining too much

Renal dysfunction is the most common cause of hypermagnesemia. Just as some renal conditions boost magnesium excretion to cause *hypo*magnesemia, others can make the body retain too much magnesium, causing *hyper*magnesemia. Causes of poor renal excretion of magnesium include:
• advancing age, which tends to reduce renal function
• renal failure
• Addison's disease
• adrenocortical insufficiency
• untreated DKA.

Too much intake

Magnesium buildup is common in patients with renal failure who use magnesium-containing antacids or laxatives. (See *Drugs and supplements associated with hypermagnesemia.*)

Other causes of excessive magnesium intake include:
• hemodialysis with a magnesium-rich dialysate
• TPN solutions that contain too much magnesium
• continuous infusion of magnesium sulfate to treat conditions, such as seizures, pregnancy-induced hypertension, or preterm labor. (The fetus of a woman receiving magnesium sulfate may develop a higher serum magnesium level, too.)

What to look for

Just as an abnormally low serum magnesium level overstimulates the neuromuscular system, an abnormally high one depresses it. So expect neuromuscular signs and symptoms opposite those of hypomagnesemia, such as:
• decreased muscle and nerve activity
• hypoactive DTRs
• generalized weakness (for instance, a patient who has a weak hand grasp or difficulty repositioning himself in bed); in severe cases, weakness progresses to flaccid paralysis
• occasional nausea and vomiting. (See *Signs and symptoms of hypermagnesemia.*)

Drowsy patient? Suspect high magnesium levels

Because excess magnesium depresses the CNS, the patient may appear drowsy and lethargic. His LOC may even diminish to the point of coma.

Hypermagnesemia can pose a danger to the respiratory system — and to life itself — if it weakens the respiratory muscles. Typically, slow, shallow, depressed respirations are indicators of

---

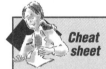
Cheat sheet

Warning!

Signs and symptoms of hypermagnesemia

Use this chart to compare total serum magnesium levels with the typical signs and symptoms that may appear.

Total serum magnesium level	Signs and symptoms
3 mEq/L	• Feelings of warmth • Flushed appearance • Mild hypotension • Nausea and vomiting
4 mEq/L	• Diminished deep tendon reflexes • Muscle weakness
5 mEq/L	• Somnolence • Electrocardiogram changes • Bradycardia • Worsening hypotension
7 mEq/L	• Loss of deep tendon reflexes
8 mEq/L	• Respiratory compromise
12 mEq/L	• Heart block • Coma
15 mEq/L	• Respiratory arrest
20 mEq/L	• Cardiac arrest

such muscle weakness. Eventually, the patient may suffer respiratory arrest and require mechanical ventilation.

A high serum magnesium level may also trigger serious heart problems — among them a weak pulse, bradycardia, heart block, and cardiac arrest. Arrhythmias may lead to diminished cardiac output.

A high serum magnesium level also causes vasodilation, which lowers the blood pressure and may make your patient feel flushed and warm all over.

What tests show

To help confirm the diagnosis of hypermagnesemia, look for a serum magnesium level above 2.5 mEq/L and these telltale ECG changes: prolonged PR interval, widened QRS complex, and tall T wave. (See *How electrolyte imbalances affect ECGs*, pages 127 to 130.)

How hypermagnesemia is treated

After hypermagnesemia is confirmed, the doctor works to correct both the magnesium imbalance and its underlying cause.

Fluid up, magnesium level down

If the patient has normal renal function, expect the doctor to order oral or I.V. fluids. Increased fluid intake raises the patient's urine output, ridding his body of excess magnesium. If the patient doesn't respond to increased fluid intake, the doctor may order a loop diuretic to promote magnesium excretion.

What if it gets worse?

In an emergency, expect to give calcium gluconate, a magnesium antagonist. (You'll probably give 10 to 20 ml of a 10% solution.) Some patients with toxic levels of magnesium in the blood also need mechanical ventilation to relieve respiratory depression.

Patients who have severe renal dysfunction may need hemodialysis with magnesium-free dialysate to lower the serum magnesium level. (See *If treatment doesn't work.*)

Memory jogger

To remember the signs and symptoms of hypermagnesemia, think *RENAL*, because poor renal excretion is a major cause of this electrolyte imbalance. Here's a letter-by-letter rundown.

Reflexes decreased (plus weakness and paralysis)

Electrocardiogram changes (bradycardia) and hypotension

Nausea and vomiting

Appearance flushed

Lethargy (plus drowsiness and coma)

It's not working!

If treatment doesn't work

What should you do if your patient's laboratory test results continue to show that his serum magnesium level is above normal, despite treatment?

Your first step is to notify the doctor. Expect to prepare the patient for peritoneal dialysis or hemodialysis using magnesium-free dialysate. The patient needs to get rid of the excess magnesium fast—especially if his renal function is failing.

How you intervene

Whenever possible, take steps to prevent hypermagnesemia by identifying high-risk patients. Those at risk include:
- elderly people
- those with renal insufficiency or failure
- pregnant women in preterm labor or with pregnancy-induced hypertension
- neonates whose mothers received magnesium sulfate during labor
- those receiving magnesium sulfate to control seizures
- those with a high intake of magnesium or magnesium-containing products, such as antacids or laxatives
- those with adrenal insufficiency
- those with severe DKA
- those who are dehydrated
- those with hypothyroidism.

If your patient already has hypermagnesemia, you may need to take the following actions.
- Monitor your patient's vital signs frequently. Stay especially alert for hypotension and respiratory depression, which are indicators of hypermagnesemia. Notify the doctor immediately if the patient's respiratory status deteriorates. (See *Teaching about hypermagnesemia.*)
- Check for flushed skin and diaphoresis.
- Assess the patient's neuromuscular system, including DTRs and muscle strength. (See *Testing the patellar reflex*, page 140.)
- Monitor laboratory tests and report abnormal results. Monitor serum electrolyte levels and other laboratory test results that reflect renal function, such as blood urea nitrogen and creatinine levels. Monitor the patient for hypocalcemia, which may accompany hypermagnesemia, because a low serum calcium level suppresses PTH secretion.
- Monitor urine output. The kidneys excrete most of the body's magnesium.
- Evaluate the patient for changes in mental status. If the patient's LOC decreases, institute safety measures. Reorient the patient if he's confused.

Prepare

- Prepare the patient for continuous cardiac monitoring. Assess ECG tracings for pertinent changes.
- Be prepared to administer resuscitation drugs, maintain a patent airway, and provide calcium gluconate, as ordered, in case of a hypermagnesemia emergency.

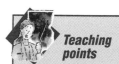

Teaching points

Teaching about hypermagnesemia

Make sure you cover these topics with your patient, and then evaluate his learning:
- explanation of hypermagnesemia
- risk factors
- hydration requirements
- dietary modification, if needed
- prescribed medications
- warning signs and symptoms
- need to avoid medications that contain magnesium
- dialysis, if needed.

Testing the patellar reflex

One way to gauge your patient's magnesium status is to test her patellar reflex, one of the deep tendon reflexes that the serum magnesium level affects. To test the reflex, strike the patellar tendon just below the patella with the patient sitting or lying in a supine position, as shown. Look for leg extension or contraction of the quadriceps muscle in the front of the thigh.

If the patellar reflex is absent, notify the doctor immediately. This finding may mean your patient's serum magnesium level is 7 mEq/L or higher.

Sitting
Have the patient sit on the side of the bed with her legs dangling freely, as shown here. Then test the reflex.

Supine position
Flex the patient's knee at a 45-degree angle, and place your nondominant hand behind it for support. Then test the reflex.

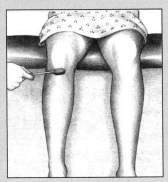

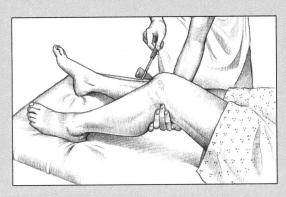

Documenting hypermagnesemia

Here's a list of key points to document when caring for a patient with hypermagnesemia:

- vital signs
- electrocardiogram changes
- signs and symptoms of hemodynamic instability
- deep tendon reflex assessment
- I.V. fluid therapy
- drugs administered
- safety measures
- your interventions and the patient's responses
- pertinent laboratory values, including serum electrolyte and albumin levels
- intake and output
- doctor notification
- patient teaching.

- If the patient's magnesium level becomes dangerously high, prepare him for dialysis as ordered.
- Be prepared to provide mechanical ventilation, which may be needed for patients with compromised respiratory function.
- Be prepared to provide a temporary pacemaker, which may be inserted for patients with bradyarrhythmias.

Maintain

- Establish I.V. access and maintain a patent I.V. line.
- Provide adequate fluids, both I.V. and oral, if prescribed, to help your patient's kidneys excrete excess magnesium. When giving large volumes of fluids, remember to keep accurate intake and output records and to watch closely for signs of fluid overload and kidney failure. Both conditions can arise quickly. (See *Documenting hypermagnesemia*.)
- Avoid giving your patient medications that contain magnesium. To make sure no other staff members give them, flag the patient's

chart and medication administration record with a note that says, "No magnesium products."
• Restrict the patient's dietary magnesium intake as needed.

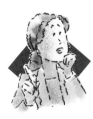

Quick quiz

1. Magnesium is an important electrolyte because it:
   A.   helps control urine volume.
   B.   promotes the production of growth hormone.
   C.   facilitates neuromuscular transmission.

Answer: C. Magnesium acts at the myoneural junction and is vital to nerve and muscle activity.

2. Your patient with Crohn's disease develops tremors while receiving TPN. Suspecting she might have hypomagnesemia, you assess her neuromuscular system. You should expect to see:
   A.   Homans' sign.
   B.   elevated serum potassium.
   C.   hyperactive DTRs.

Answer: C. In a patient with hypomagnesemia, expect to see hyperactive DTRs—because hypomagnesemia increases neuromuscular excitability.

3. When teaching your patient with hypomagnesemia about a proper diet, you should recommend that he consume plenty of:
   A.   seafood.
   B.   fruits.
   C.   corn products.

Answer: A. Magnesium is found in seafood as well as in chocolate, dry beans and peas, green leafy vegetables, meats, nuts, and whole grains.

4. The doctor prescribes I.V. magnesium sulfate for your patient with hypomagnesemia. Before giving the magnesium preparation, you review the doctor's order to make sure it specifies the:
   A.   number of grams or milliliters to give.
   B.   number of ampules to give.
   C.   number of vials to give.

Answer: A. Magnesium sulfate comes in several different concentrations. The doctor's order should specify the number of grams or milliliters of a particular concentration, plus either the amount of solution to use for dilution or the duration of the infusion.

5. Your patient is diagnosed with hypermagnesemia. To treat this imbalance, the doctor is likely to order:

    A.   magnesium citrate.

    B.   magnesium sulfate diluted in fluids.

    C.   oral and I.V. fluids.

Answer: C. Both oral and I.V. fluids may be used to treat hypermagnesemia. By causing diuresis, the fluids promote excretion of excess magnesium by the kidneys.

6. Your hemodialysis patient needs a laxative. When you see that the doctor has ordered magnesium citrate, you decide to question the order because:

    A.   this magnesium salt would be too strong for the patient.

    B.   magnesium administration could worsen the patient's condition.

    C.   magnesium citrate must be given orally.

Answer: B. Magnesium citrate is a poor laxative choice for a patient with a renal impairment whose kidneys can't excrete magnesium properly. The patient could develop hypermagnesemia.

Scoring

☆☆☆ If you answered all six questions correctly, you should be twitching with pride. You're a magnesium magician!

☆☆ If you answered four or five correctly, excellent! You're ready to become a magnesium magician's assistant!

☆ If you answered fewer than four correctly, try not to worry. You're now enrolled as a first-year learner in Magical Magnesium College of Fine Electrolytes.

When calcium tips the balance

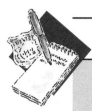

Just the facts

This chapter describes how to care for patients who have a deficiency or an excess of calcium. In this chapter, you'll learn:

♦ how calcium works in the body

♦ what the relationship is between calcium and albumin

♦ how parathyroid hormone helps to regulate calcium levels

♦ how to assess a patient for signs of calcium imbalance

♦ how to care for a patient with hypocalcemia or hypercalcemia.

A look at calcium

Calcium is a positively charged ion, or cation, found in both the extracellular fluid and the intracellular fluid. About 99% of the body's calcium is found in the bones and the teeth. Only 1% is found in serum and in soft tissue. That 1% is what matters when measuring calcium levels in the blood.

What it does

Calcium is involved in numerous body functions. Together with phosphorus, calcium is responsible for the formation and structure of bones and teeth. It helps to maintain cell structure and function and plays a role in cell membrane permeability and impulse transmission.

This cation affects the contraction of cardiac muscle, smooth muscle, and skeletal muscle. Calcium also participates in the blood-clotting process.

Measuring calcium

Calcium can be measured in two ways. The most commonly ordered test is a total serum calcium level, which measures the total amount of calcium in the blood. The normal range for the total serum calcium level is 8.9 to 10.1 mg/dl.

The second test measures the various forms of calcium in extracellular fluid. About 41% of all extracellular calcium is bound to protein; 9% is bound to citrate or other organic ions. About half is ionized (or free) calcium, the only active form of calcium. Ionized calcium carries out most of the ion's physiologic functions. The normal range for the ionized calcium level is 4.5 to 5.1 mg/dl. (See *Calcium levels.*)

Because nearly half of all calcium is bound to the protein albumin, serum protein abnormalities can influence total serum calcium levels. For example, in hypoalbuminemia, the total serum calcium level decreases. However, ionized calcium levels—the more important of the two levels—remain unchanged. So when considering total serum calcium levels, you should also consider serum albumin levels. (See *Calculating calcium and albumin levels.*)

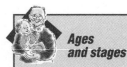

Ages and stages

Calcium levels

Children have higher serum calcium levels than adults. In fact, serum levels can rise as high as 7 mg/dl during periods of increased bone growth.

Also, the normal range for calcium levels is narrower for the elderly. For elderly males, the range is 2.3 to 3.7 mg/dl; for elderly females, the range is 2.8 to 4.1 mg/dl.

How the body regulates calcium

Both intake of dietary calcium and existing stores of calcium affect calcium levels in the body. For adults, the range for the recommended daily requirement of calcium is 800 to 1,200 mg/day. Requirements vary for children, pregnant patients, and patients being treated for osteoporosis.

Calcium is found in large quantities in dairy products but can also be found in green, leafy vegetables. (See *Dietary sources of calcium.*) Calcium is absorbed in the small intestine and is excreted in the urine and feces.

Bones help out

Several factors influence calcium levels in the body. The first is parathyroid hormone (PTH). When serum calcium levels are low, the parathyroid glands release PTH, which draws calcium from the bones and promotes the transfer of calcium (along with phosphorus) into the plasma. That transfer increases serum calcium levels.

PTH also promotes kidney reabsorption of calcium and stimulates the intestines to absorb the mineral. Phosphorus is excreted at the same time. In hypercalcemia, where too much calcium exists in the blood, the body suppresses the release of PTH.

Calcium is found in large quantities in dairy products.

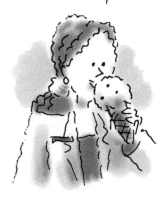

Calculating calcium and albumin levels

For every 1 g/dl that a noncritically ill patient's serum albumin level drops, his total calcium level decreases by 0.8 mg/dl. To see what your patient's calcium level would be if his serum albumin level were normal—and to help determine if treatment is justified—just do a little math.

Correcting a level

The normal albumin level is 4 g/dl. The formula for correcting a patient's calcium level is:

$$\text{Total serum calcium level} + 0.8 (4 - \text{albumin level})$$
$$=$$
$$\text{corrected calcium level}$$

Sample problem

For example, if a patient's serum calcium level is 8.2 mg/dl and his albumin level is 3 g/dl, what would his corrected calcium be?

$$8.2 + 0.8 (4 - 3) = 9 \text{ mg/dl}$$

The corrected calcium level is in normal range and probably wouldn't be treated.

Dietary sources of calcium

Here's a list of the most common dietary sources of calcium:

- bonemeal
- dairy products, such as milk, cheese, and yogurt
- green leafy vegetables
- legumes
- molasses
- nuts
- whole grains.

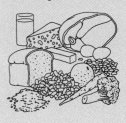

Enter calcitonin

Calcitonin also helps to regulate calcium levels. Calcitonin, a hormone, is produced in the thyroid gland and acts as an antagonist to PTH.

When calcium levels are too high, the thyroid releases calcitonin. High levels of the hormone inhibit bone resorption, which causes a decrease in the amount of calcium available from bone. This causes a decrease in the serum calcium level.

Calcitonin also decreases absorption of calcium and enhances its excretion by the kidneys.

And now, vitamin D

Another factor that influences calcium levels is vitamin D. Vitamin D is ingested with foods, particularly dairy products. Also, when the skin is exposed to ultraviolet light, it synthesizes the vitamin.

Vitamin D (the active form, not the inactive one) promotes calcium absorption through the intestines, calcium resorption from bone, and kidney reabsorption of calcium, all of which raise the serum calcium level. (See *Calcium in balance*, page 146.)

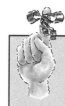

Memory jogger

To help you remember the roles of calcitonin and parathyroid hormone (PTH), think of this memory jogger: *Parathyroid pulls, calcitonin keeps.*
PTH pulls calcium out of the bone.
Calcitonin keeps it there.

Phosphorus follows

Phosphorus also affects serum calcium levels. Phosphorus inhibits calcium absorption in the intestines, the opposite effect of vitamin D. When calcium levels are low and the kidneys retain calcium, phosphorus is excreted.

An inverse relationship between calcium and phosphorus exists in the body. When calcium levels rise, phosphorus levels drop. The opposite is also true: When calcium levels drop, phosphorus levels rise.

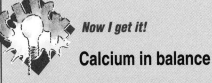

Now I get it!

Calcium in balance

Extracellular calcium levels are normally kept constant by several interrelated processes that move calcium ions into and out of extracellular fluid. Calcium enters the extracellular space through resorption of calcium ions from bone, through the absorption of dietary calcium in the GI tract, and through reabsorption of calcium from the kidneys. Calcium leaves extracellular fluid as it's excreted in feces and urine and deposited in bone tissues. This illustration shows how calcium moves throughout the body.

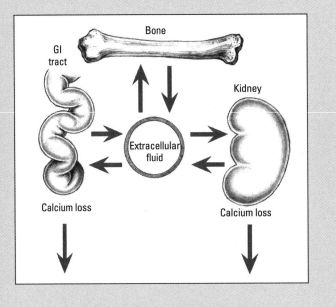

Serum pH helps...inversely

The serum pH also has an inverse relationship with the ionized calcium level. If the serum pH level rises (the blood becomes alkaline), more calcium binds with protein and the ionized calcium level drops. Thus, a patient with alkalosis will typically have hypocalcemia.

The opposite is true for acidosis. When the pH level drops, less calcium binds to protein and the ionized calcium level rises. When all those regulatory efforts fail to control the level of calcium in the body, one of two conditions may result: hypocalcemia or hypercalcemia.

Hypocalcemia

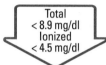

Total
< 8.9 mg/dl
Ionized
< 4.5 mg/dl

Hypocalcemia occurs when calcium levels fall below the normal range—that is, when serum calcium levels fall below 8.9 mg/dl or ionized calcium levels fall below 4.5 mg/dl.

How it happens

Hypocalcemia can occur when a person doesn't take in enough calcium, when the body doesn't absorb the mineral properly, or when excessive amounts of calcium are lost from the body. A decreased level of ionized calcium can also cause hypocalcemia.

When you need calcium

Inadequate intake of calcium can put a patient at risk for hypocalcemia. Alcoholics—with their typically poor nutritional intake, poor calcium absorption, and low magnesium level (magnesium affects PTH secretion)—are especially prone.

A breast-fed infant can have low calcium and vitamin D levels if his mother's intake of those nutrients is inadequate. Also, anyone who doesn't receive sufficient exposure to sunlight may suffer from vitamin D deficiency and subsequently lower calcium levels.

When malabsorption hits

Hypocalcemia can result when calcium isn't absorbed properly from the GI tract, a condition commonly caused by malabsorption. Malabsorption can result from increased intestinal motility from severe diarrhea, laxative abuse, or chronic malabsorption syndrome.

Absorption is also affected by a lack of vitamin D in the diet. Renal failure may harm the kidneys' ability to activate vitamin D.

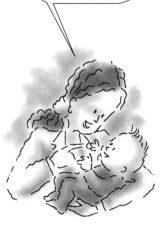

A breast-fed infant can have low calcium and vitamin D levels if his mother's intake is inadequate.

Anticonvulsants, such as phenobarbital and phenytoin (Dilantin), can interfere with vitamin D metabolism and calcium absorption.

A high phosphorus level in the intestines can interfere with absorption, as can a reduction in gastric acidity, which decreases the solubility of calcium salts.

Excess calcium loss

Pancreatic insufficiency can cause malabsorption of calcium and a subsequent loss of calcium in the feces. Acute pancreatitis can cause hypocalcemia as well, although the mechanism isn't well understood. PTH or possibly the combining of free fatty acids and calcium in pancreatic tissue may be involved.

Hypocalcemia can also occur when PTH secretion is reduced or eliminated. Thyroid surgery, surgical removal of the parathyroid gland, removal of a parathyroid tumor, or injury or disease of the parathyroid gland (such as hypoparathyroidism) can all reduce or prevent PTH secretion.

Hypocalcemia can also result from medications, such as calcitonin and mithramycin, because these drugs decrease calcium resorption from bone.

Kidneys take out calcium

The kidneys may excrete excess calcium and cause hypocalcemia. Diuretics, especially loop diuretics such as furosemide (Lasix) and ethacrynic acid (Edecrin), increase renal excretion of calcium as well as water and other electrolytes.

Edetate disodium (disodium EDTA), which is used to treat lead poisoning, can combine with calcium and carry it out of the body when excreted. Other causes of hypocalcemia include severe burns and infections. Burned or diseased tissues trap calcium ions from extracellular fluid, thereby reducing serum calcium levels.

Still more causes

A low magnesium level (hypomagnesemia) can affect the function of the parathyroid gland and cause a decrease in calcium reabsorption in the GI tract and the kidneys. Drugs that lower serum magnesium levels, such as cisplatin and gentamicin, may decrease calcium absorption from bone. (See *Drugs associated with hypocalcemia.*)

Remember also that a low serum albumin level (hypoalbuminemia) can cause low calcium levels. Hyperphosphatemia (a high level of phosphorus in the blood) can cause calcium levels to fall as phosphorus levels rise. Excess phosphorus combines with calcium to form salts, which are then deposited in tissues.

Drugs associated with hypocalcemia

Drugs that can cause hypocalcemia include:
• anticonvulsants, especially phenytoin and phenobarbital
• calcitonin
• drugs that lower serum magnesium levels (such as cisplatin and gentamicin)
• edetate disodium (disodium EDTA)
• loop diuretics
• mithramycin
• phosphates (oral, I.V., rectal).

Ages and stages

Hypocalcemia in elderly patients

Several factors contribute to hypocalcemia in elderly patients. Such factors include:
- inadequate dietary intake of calcium
- poor calcium absorption (especially in postmenopausal women lacking estrogen)
- reduced activity or inactivity. Inactivity causes a loss of calcium from the bone and osteoporosis, in which serum levels may be normal but bone stores of the mineral are depleted.

When phosphates are administered orally, I.V., or rectally, the phosphorus binds with calcium and serum calcium levels drop. Infants receiving cow's milk are predisposed to hypocalcemic tetany because of the high levels of phosphorus in the milk.

Alkalosis can cause calcium to bind to albumin, thereby decreasing ionized calcium levels. Citrate, added to stored blood to prevent clotting, binds with calcium and renders it unavailable for use. Therefore, patients receiving massive blood transfusions are at risk for hypocalcemia. That risk holds true for pediatric patients as well. (See *Hypocalcemia in elderly patients.*)

What to look for

Signs and symptoms of hypocalcemia reflect calcium's effects on nerve transmission and muscle and heart function. The neurologic effects of a low calcium level include anxiety, confusion, and irritability. These symptoms can progress to seizures.

Neuromuscular symptoms may develop. The patient may experience paresthesia of the toes, fingers, or face, especially around the mouth. He may also experience twitching, muscle cramps, or tremors. Laryngeal and abdominal muscles are particularly prone to spasm. An increase in nerve excitability can lead to tetany. At such times, you may be able to elicit positive Trousseau's or Chvostek's signs. (See *Checking for Trousseau's and Chvostek's signs*, page 150.)

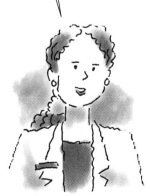

Patients receiving massive blood transfusions are at risk for hypocalcemia.

Checking for Trousseau's and Chvostek's signs

Testing for Trousseau's and Chvostek's signs can aid in the diagnosis of tetany and hypocalcemia. Here's how to check for these important signs.

Trousseau's sign

To check for Trousseau's sign, apply a blood pressure cuff to the patient's upper arm and inflate it to a pressure 20 mm Hg above the systolic pressure. Trousseau's sign may appear after 1 to 4 minutes. The patient will experience an adducted thumb, flexed wrist and metacarpophalangeal joints, and extended interphalangeal joints (with fingers together)—carpopedal spasm—indicating tetany, a major sign of hypocalcemia.

Chvostek's sign

You can induce Chvostek's sign by tapping the patient's facial nerve adjacent to the ear. A brief contraction of the upper lip, nose, or side of the face indicates Chvostek's sign.

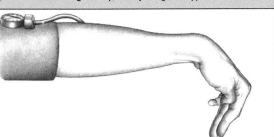

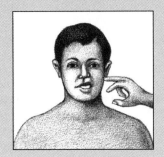

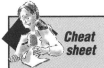

Cheat sheet

Possible indicators of hypocalcemia

- Anxiety
- Confusion
- Decreased cardiac output
- Arrhythmias
- Fractures
- Irritability
- Muscle cramps
- Paresthesia of the face, fingers, or toes
- Positive Chvostek's or Trousseau's signs
- Prolonged ST segment
- Lengthened QT interval
- Tetany
- Tremors
- Twitching

More signs

Fractures may occur more easily in a patient who is hypocalcemic for an extended period. The patient may also have brittle nails or dry skin and hair.

Other signs of hypocalcemia include:
- diarrhea
- hyperactive deep tendon reflexes
- diminished response to digoxin
- decreased cardiac output and subsequent arrhythmias
- prolonged ST segment on the electrocardiogram (ECG)
- lengthened QT interval on the ECG, which places the patient at risk for a form of ventricular tachycardia called "torsades de pointes."

What tests show

The following test results can help doctors diagnose hypocalcemia as well as determine the severity of the deficiency:
- total serum calcium level less than 8.9 mg/dl

- an ionized calcium level below 4.5 mg/dl
- characteristic ECG changes.

How hypocalcemia is treated

Treatment for hypocalcemia focuses on correcting the imbalance as quickly and as safely as possible. The underlying cause should be addressed to prevent recurrence.

Acute hypocalcemia requires immediate correction by administering either I.V. calcium gluconate or I.V. calcium chloride. Although calcium chloride contains three times as much available calcium as calcium gluconate, the latter is more commonly used. Magnesium replacement may also be needed, because hypocalcemia doesn't respond to calcium therapy alone. (See *Administering I.V. calcium safely*, page 152.)

Chronic hypocalcemia requires vitamin D supplements to facilitate GI absorption of calcium. Oral calcium supplements also help increase calcium levels.

The patient's diet should also be adjusted to allow for an adequate intake of calcium, vitamin D, and protein. In cases where the patient also has a high phosphorus level, aluminum hydroxide antacids may be given to bind with excess phosphorus. (See *When treatment doesn't work*.)

How you intervene

If your patient is at increased risk for hypocalcemia, assess him carefully, especially if he has had parathyroid or thyroid surgery or has received massive blood transfusions. If your patient is a breast-feeding mother, assess her for adequate vitamin D intake and exposure to sunlight.

When assessing a patient you suspect has hypocalcemia, obtain a complete medical history. Note if the patient has ever had neck surgery. Hypoparathyroidism may develop immediately or several years after neck surgery. Ask a patient who has chronic hypocalcemia if he has a history of fractures. Obtain a list of medications the patient is taking; the list may help you determine the underlying cause of hypocalcemia. Make sure you also assess the effects of symptoms on the patient's ability to perform activities of daily living.

Calcium by the bed

If your patient is recovering from parathyroid or thyroid surgery, keep calcium gluconate at the bedside. A handy supply of the drug

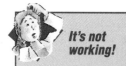

It's not working!

When treatment doesn't work

If treatment for hypocalcemia doesn't seem to be working, then:
- check the magnesium level. A low magnesium level must be corrected before I.V. calcium will increase serum calcium levels.
- check the phosphate level. If the phosphate level is too high, calcium won't be absorbed. Reduce the phosphate level first.
- mix I.V. calcium in dextrose solutions only. Normal saline may cause calcium to be excreted.

Administering I.V. calcium safely

Be prepared to administer parenteral calcium to a patient who has symptomatic hypocalcemia. Always clarify whether the doctor orders calcium gluconate or calcium chloride. Doses vary according to the specific drug. Note the type and dosage of each calcium preparation carefully, and follow these steps when administering it.

Preparing
Dilute the prescribed I.V. calcium preparation in dextrose 5% in water. Never dilute calcium in solutions containing bicarbonate because precipitation will occur. Avoid giving the patient calcium diluted in normal saline solution because the sodium chloride will increase renal calcium loss.

Administering
Always administer I.V. calcium slowly, according to the doctor's order or established protocol. Never give it rapidly because it may result in syncope, hypotension, and cardiac arrhythmias. Initially, calcium may be given as a slow I.V. bolus. If hypocalcemia persists, the initial bolus may be followed by a slow I.V. drip using an infusion pump.

Monitoring
Overcorrection may lead to hypercalcemia. Watch for signs and symptoms of hypercalcemia, including anorexia, nausea, vomiting, lethargy, and confusion. Institute cardiac monitoring, and observe the patient for cardiac arrhythmias, especially if the patient is receiving digoxin. Observe the I.V. site for signs of infiltration; calcium can cause tissue sloughing and necrosis. Closely monitor serum calcium levels.

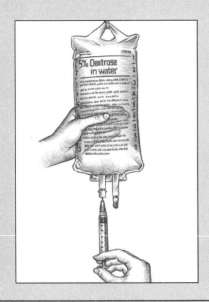 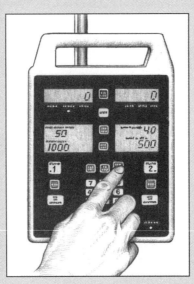 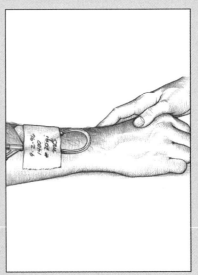

ensures a quick response to signs of a sudden drop in calcium levels. If the patient develops hypocalcemia, here's what you can do.

Monitor

• Monitor vital signs, and assess the patient frequently. Monitor respiratory status, including rate, depth, and rhythm. Watch for stridor, dyspnea, and crowing.

Teaching points

Teaching about hypocalcemia

When teaching about hypocalcemia, cover these topics and then evaluate the patient's learning:
- description of hypocalcemia, its causes, and treatment
- importance of a high-calcium diet
- sources of calcium in diet
- avoidance of long-term laxative use
- medications
- importance of exercise
- warning signs and symptoms and when to report them
- need to report pain during I.V. infusion of calcium
- possible use of female hormones in patients with osteoporosis.

- If the patient shows overt signs of hypocalcemia, keep a tracheotomy tray and a handheld resuscitation bag at the bedside in case laryngospasm occurs.
- Place your patient on a cardiac monitor, and evaluate him for changes in heart rate and rhythm. Notify the doctor if the patient develops arrhythmias, such as ventricular tachycardia or heart block.
- Check the patient for Chvostek's sign or Trousseau's sign. (See *Teaching about hypocalcemia.*)

Maintain and administer

- Monitor a patient receiving I.V. calcium for arrhythmias, especially if he's also taking digoxin. Calcium and digoxin have similar effects on the heart.
- Insert and maintain a patent I.V. line for calcium therapy.
- Administer I.V. calcium replacement therapy carefully. Ensure the patency of the I.V. line because infiltration can cause tissue necrosis and sloughing.
- Administer oral replacements as ordered. Give calcium supplements 1 to 1½ hours after meals. If GI upset occurs, give the supplement with milk.

Follow-up

- Monitor pertinent laboratory test results, including not only calcium levels but also albumin levels and those of other electrolytes such as magnesium. Remember to check the ionized calcium level after every 4 units of blood transfused.

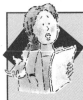

Chart smart

Documenting hypocalcemia

Here's a list of key points to document when caring for a patient with hypocalcemia:
- vital signs, including cardiac rhythm
- intake and output
- seizure activity
- safety measures
- assessments, interventions, and the patient's response
- patency and appearance of I.V. site, before and after calcium infusion
- pertinent laboratory results, including calcium levels
- time that you notified the doctor
- patient teaching.

- Encourage the older patient to take a calcium supplement as ordered and to exercise as much as he can tolerate to prevent calcium loss from bones.
- Take precautions for seizures such as padding bed side rails.
- Reorient a confused patient. Provide a calm, quiet environment.
- Document all care given to the patient and all observations made. (See *Documenting hypocalcemia*.)

Hypercalcemia

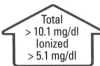

Total
> 10.1 mg/dl
Ionized
> 5.1 mg/dl

Hypercalcemia occurs when the serum calcium level rises above 10.1 mg/dl, the ionized serum calcium level rises above 5.1 mg/dl, and the rate of calcium entry into extracellular fluid exceeds the rate of calcium excretion by the kidneys.

How it happens

Any situation that causes an increase in the total serum or ionized calcium level can lead to hypercalcemia. The condition is usually caused by an increase in the resorption of calcium from bone. Hyperparathyroidism and cancer are the two major causes of hypercalcemia.

> ### Drugs associated with hypercalcemia
>
> Here's a list of medications that can cause hypercalcemia:
> - antacids that contain calcium
> - calcium preparations (oral or I.V.)
> - lithium
> - thiazide diuretics
> - vitamin A
> - vitamin D.

Blame the other hyper

With hyperparathyroidism, the most common cause of hypercalcemia, the body excretes more PTH than normal, which greatly strengthens the effects of the hormone. Calcium resorption from bone and reabsorption from the kidneys are also increased, as is calcium absorption from the intestines.

Malignant invasion

Cancer, the second most common cause of hypercalcemia, causes bone destruction as malignant cells invade the bones and may cause the release of a substance similar to PTH. That hormone causes an increase in serum calcium levels.

When that happens, the kidneys can become overwhelmed and unable to excrete all that excess calcium, which in turn keeps calcium levels elevated. A patient who has squamous cell carcinoma of the lung is especially prone to hypercalcemia, as is a patient with myeloma or breast cancer.

Other causes

Hypercalcemia can also be caused by an increase in the absorption of calcium in the GI tract or by a decrease in the excretion of calcium by the kidneys. These mechanisms may occur alone or in combination.

Hyperthyroidism can cause an increase in calcium release as more calcium is resorbed from bone. Multiple fractures or prolonged immobilization can also cause an increase in calcium release from bone.

Hypophosphatemia and acidosis (which increases calcium ionization) are linked with hypercalcemia. (See *Drugs associated with hypercalcemia*.) Certain medications are also associated with the condition. For instance, abusing antacids that contain calcium, receiving an overdose of calcium (from calcium medications given during cardiopulmonary resuscitation, for example),

> When serum calcium levels increase, I'm overwhelmed and unable to excrete the excess calcium. Oh woe is me!

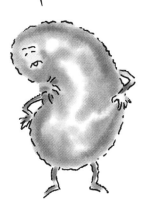

or ingesting excessive amounts of vitamin D can prompt an increase in serum calcium levels.

Vitamin A overdose can lead to increased bone resorption of calcium. Use of lithium or thiazide diuretics can decrease calcium excretion by the kidneys. Milk-alkali syndrome, a condition in which calcium and alkali are combined, also raises calcium levels.

What to look for

Signs and symptoms of hypercalcemia are intensified if the condition develops acutely. Symptoms are also more severe if calcium levels are greater than 15 mg/dl.

Many symptoms stem from the effects of excess calcium in the cells, which causes a decrease in cell membrane excitability, especially in the tissues of the skeletal muscle, the heart muscle, and the nervous system.

The patient with hypercalcemia may complain of fatigue or exhibit confusion or personality changes. Lethargy can progress to coma in severe cases.

Affecting the muscles

As calcium levels rise, the patient develops muscle weakness, hyporeflexia, and decreased muscle tone. Hypercalcemia may lead to hypertension.

Because heart muscle and the cardiac conduction system are affected by hypercalcemia, arrhythmias, such as bradycardia, can lead to cardiac arrest. ECG tests may reveal a shortened QT interval and a shortened ST segment. Also look for digoxin toxicity if the patient is receiving digoxin.

Affecting other systems

Hypercalcemia can also lead to GI symptoms, which are commonly the first indicators that the patient notices. The patient may experience anorexia, nausea, or vomiting. Bowel sounds are decreased. Constipation can occur because of calcium's effect on smooth muscle and subsequent decrease in GI motility. Abdominal pain and paralytic ileus may result.

As the kidneys work overtime to remove excess calcium, renal problems may develop. The patient may experience polyuria and subsequent dehydration. Hypercalcemia can also cause kidney stones and other calcifications. Renal failure may be the end result. Also, the patient may develop pathologic fractures and bone pain. (See *Danger signs of hypercalcemia*.)

Cheat sheet

Signs and symptoms of hypercalcemia

Signs and symptoms of hypercalcemia include:
- abdominal pain and constipation
- anorexia
- behavioral changes, including confusion
- bone pain
- characteristic ECG changes
- decreased DTRs
- extreme thirst
- hypertension
- lethargy
- muscle weakness
- nausea
- polyuria
- vomiting.

What tests show

If you suspect that your patient has hypercalcemia, look for:
- serum calcium level above 10.1 mg/dl
- ionized calcium level above 5.1 mg/dl
- digoxin toxicity (if your patient is taking digoxin)
- X-rays revealing pathologic fractures
- characteristic ECG changes.

How hypercalcemia is treated

If hypercalcemia produces no symptoms, treatment may consist only of managing the underlying cause. Dietary intake of calcium may be reduced and medications or infusions containing calcium stopped. Treatment for asymptomatic hypercalcemia also includes measures to increase the excretion of calcium and to decrease bone resorption of it.

Hydrate!

You can help increase excretion of calcium by hydrating the patient, which encourages diuresis. Normal saline solution is typically used for hydration in these cases. The sodium in the solution inhibits renal tubular reabsorption of calcium.

Loop diuretics, such as furosemide (Lasix) and ethacrynic acid (Edecrin), also promote calcium excretion. Thiazide diuretics aren't used for hypercalcemia because they inhibit calcium excretion.

For patients with life-threatening hypercalcemia, measures to increase calcium excretion may include hemodialysis or peritoneal dialysis with a solution that contains little or no calcium.

Back to the bones

Measures to inhibit bone resorption of calcium may also be used to help reduce calcium levels in extracellular fluids. Corticosteroids administered I.V. and then orally can block bone resorption and decrease calcium absorption from the GI tract.

Etidronate disodium, commonly used to treat hypercalcemia, inhibits the action of osteoclasts in bone, thereby reducing bone resorption. This medication takes full effect in 2 to 3 days. Pamidronate disodium, which is similar to etidronate disodium, can also be used to inhibit bone resorption. Mithramycin, a chemotherapeutic drug, can decrease bone resorption of calcium and is used mostly when the hypercalcemia is due to cancer. Calcitonin inhibits bone resorption as well, but its effects are short lived. (See *When treatment doesn't work*.)

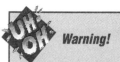

Warning!

Danger signs of hypercalcemia

Watch for these danger signs of hypercalcemia:
- arrhythmias such as bradycardia
- cardiac arrest
- coma
- paralytic ileus
- stupor.

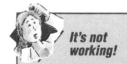

It's not working!

When treatment doesn't work

If your patient doesn't seem to be responding to treatment for hypercalcemia, make sure he isn't still taking vitamin D supplements.

Keep in mind that calcitonin may be given to decrease calcium levels rapidly, but the effects are only temporary.

How you intervene

Make sure you monitor patients at risk for hypercalcemia, such as those who have cancer or parathyroid disorders, are immobile, or are receiving a calcium supplement. For a patient who develops hypercalcemia, you'll want to take the following actions.

Monitor

- Monitor vital signs and assess the patient frequently.
- Watch the patient for arrhythmias. Assess neurologic and neuro-muscular function and report any changes.
- Monitor the patient's fluid intake and output.
- Monitor serum electrolyte levels, especially calcium, to determine the effectiveness of treatment and to detect new imbalances that might result from therapy.

Maintain and administer

- Insert and maintain I.V. access. Normal saline solution is usually administered at a rate of 200 to 500 ml/hour. Monitor the patient for signs of pulmonary edema, such as crackles and dyspnea.
- If administering a diuretic, make sure the patient is properly hydrated first so he doesn't experience volume depletion.
- Encourage the patient to drink 3 to 4 qt (3 to 4 L) of fluid daily, unless contraindicated, to stimulate calcium excretion from the

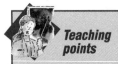

Teaching points

Teaching about hypercalcemia

When teaching about hypercalcemia, cover these topics and then evaluate the patient's learning:
- description of hyper-calcemia, its causes, and treatment
- risk factors
- importance of in-creased fluid intake
- dietary guidelines for a low-calcium diet
- prescribed medica-tions, including possible adverse effects
- warning signs and symptoms
- avoidance of supple-ments and antacids that contain calcium.

Chart smart

Documenting hypercalcemia

Here's a list of key points to document when caring for a patient with hypercalcemia:
- assessments, including neurologic examination and level of con-sciousness
- vital signs, including cardiac rhythm
- intake and output
- interventions, including I.V. therapy, and the patient's response
- signs and symptoms
- safety measures taken
- patient teaching done and the patient's response
- notification of the doctor
- pertinent laboratory results, including calcium levels.

kidneys and to decrease the risk of calculi formation. (See *Teaching about hypercalcemia.*)
• Strain the urine for calculi. Also check for flank pain, which can indicate the presence of renal calculi.
• If the patient is receiving digoxin, watch for signs and symptoms of a toxic reaction, such as anorexia, nausea, vomiting, or an irregular heart rate.
• Get the patient up and moving around as soon as possible to prevent bones from releasing calcium.
• Handle a patient who has chronic hypercalcemia gently to prevent pathologic fractures. Reposition bedridden patients frequently. Perform active or passive range-of-motion exercises to prevent complications from immobility.
• Provide a safe environment. Keep side rails raised as needed, keep the bed in its lowest position, keep the wheels locked, and make sure the patient's belongings and call button are within reach. If the patient is confused, reorient him.
• Offer emotional support to the patient and his family throughout treatment. Overt signs of hypercalcemia can be emotionally distressing for all involved.
• Chart all care given and the patient's response. (See *Documenting hypercalcemia.*)

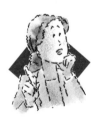

Quick quiz

1. Albumin affects calcium levels by:
    A. blocking phosphorus absorption, which prevents calcium excretion.
    B. binding with calcium, which makes the calcium ineffective.
    C. inhibiting magnesium uptake, which prevents calcium absorption.

Answer: B. Albumin binds with calcium and renders it ineffective.

2. The most common cause of hypocalcemia involves a dysfunction of:
    A. antidiuretic hormone.
    B. growth hormone.
    C. parathyroid hormone (PTH).

Answer: C. PTH promotes reabsorption of calcium from the bone to the serum. When secretion of PTH is decreased, hypocalcemia results.

3.   If your patient is hypercalcemic, you would expect to:
   A.   administer I.V. sodium bicarbonate.
   B.   administer vitamin D.
   C.   hydrate the patient.

Answer: C. Hydrating a patient with oral or I.V. fluids will increase the urine excretion of calcium and help lower serum calcium levels.

4.   Hypercalcemia would be most likely to develop in:
   A.   a 60-year-old man who has squamous cell carcinoma of the lung.
   B.   an 80-year-old woman who has heart failure and is taking furosemide (Lasix).
   C.   a 25-year-old trauma patient who has received massive blood transfusions.

Answer: A. Squamous cell carcinoma of the lung can lead to hypercalcemia.

5.   You're told during shift report that your patient has a positive Chvostek's sign. You would expect his laboratory tests results to reveal:
   A.   total serum calcium level below 8.9 mEq/L.
   B.   total serum calcium level above 10.1 mEq/L.
   C.   ionized calcium level above 5.1 mg/dl.

Answer: A. Chvostek's sign, along with Trousseau's sign, is associated with hypocalcemia. Only a total serum calcium level below 8.9 mEq/L indicates that condition.

Scoring

☆☆☆   If you answered all five questions correctly, we're impressed! We wonder, have you been hanging out in Professor Chvostek's lab?

☆☆   If you answered three or four correctly, oh my! Have you been reading Professor Trousseau's diary, by chance?

☆   If you answered fewer than three correctly, that's fine. We have a great seat for you at the Chvostek-Trousseau lecture series!

When phosphorus tips the balance

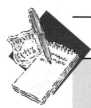

Just the facts

This chapter describes how to recognize and correct phosphorus imbalances. In this chapter, you'll learn:

♦ what role phosphorus plays in the body

♦ how the body regulates phosphorus

♦ what hypophosphatemia and hyperphosphatemia are and how to manage them.

A look at phosphorus

Phosphorus is the primary anion, or negatively charged ion, found in the intracellular fluid. It's contained in the body as phosphate. (The two words — *phosphorus* and *phosphate* — are commonly used interchangeably.) About 85% of phosphorus exists in bone and teeth, combined in a 1:2 ratio with calcium. About 14% is in soft tissue, and less than 1% is in extracellular fluid.

What it does

An essential element of all body tissues, phosphorus is vital to various body functions. It plays a crucial role in cell membrane integrity (phospholipids make up the cell membranes), muscle function, neurologic function, and the metabolism of carbohydrate, fat, and protein. Phosphorus is a primary ingredient in 2,3-diphosphoglycerate (2,3-DPG), a compound in red blood cells (RBCs) that facilitates oxygen delivery from RBCs to the tissues.

Phosphorus is also involved in the buffering of acids and bases. It promotes energy transfer to cells through the formation of energy-storing substances such as adenosine triphosphate (ATP). It's also important for white blood cell (WBC) phagocytosis and for platelet function. Finally, along with calcium, phosphorus is an essential component of bones and teeth.

Serum levels don't tell the whole story

Normal serum phosphorus levels in adults range from 2.5 to 4.5 mg/dl (or 1.8 to 2.6 mEq/L). In comparison, the normal phosphorus level in the cells is 100 mEq/L. Because phosphorus is located primarily within the cells, serum levels may not always reflect the total amount of phosphorus in the body.

Keeping levels regulated

The total amount of phosphorus in the body is related to dietary intake, hormonal regulation, kidney excretion, and transcellular shifts. For adults, the range for the recommended daily requirement of phosphorus is 800 to 1,200 mg. Phosphorus is readily absorbed through the GI tract, and the amount absorbed is proportional to the amount ingested. (See *Dietary sources of phosphorus.*)

Most ingested phosphorus is absorbed through the jejunum. The kidneys excrete about 90% of phosphorus as they regulate serum levels. (The GI tract excretes the rest.) If dietary intake of phosphorus increases, the kidneys increase excretion to maintain normal levels of phosphorus. A low-phosphorus diet causes the kidneys to reabsorb more phosphorus in the proximal tubules in order to conserve it.

Calcium and PTH

The parathyroid gland controls hormonal regulation of phosphorus levels by affecting the activity of parathyroid hormone (PTH). (See *PTH and phosphorus.*) Changes in calcium levels, rather than changes in phosphorus levels, affect the release of PTH. You may recall that phosphorus balance is closely related to that of calcium.

Normally, calcium and phosphorus have an inverse relationship: If one is elevated, the other is decreased. When the serum calcium level is low, the phosphorus level is high. PTH is released, causing an increase in calcium and phosphorus resorption from bone and raising both the calcium and phosphorus levels. Phosphorus absorption from the intestines is also increased. (Activated vitamin D—calcitriol—also enhances its absorption in the intestines.)

PTH then acts on the kidneys to increase excretion of phosphorus. The renal effect of PTH outweighs its other effects on the serum phosphorus level, particularly that of returning the phos-

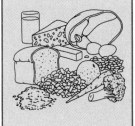

Dietary sources of phosphorus

Major dietary sources of phosphorus include:
- cheese
- dried beans
- eggs
- fish
- milk products
- nuts and seeds
- organ meats (such as brain and liver)
- poultry
- whole grains.

PTH and phosphorus

This illustration shows how parathyroid hormone (PTH) affects serum phosphorus (P) levels—by increasing phosphorus release from bone, increasing phosphorus absorption from the intestines, and decreasing phosphorus reabsorption in the renal tubules.

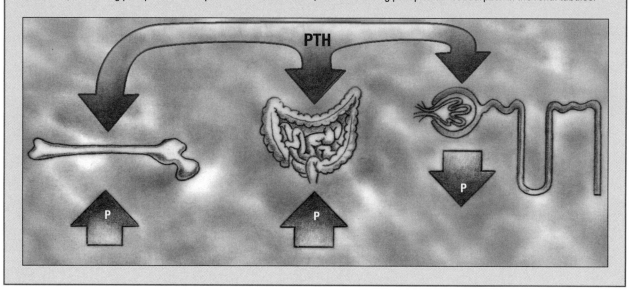

phorus level to normal. Reduced PTH levels allow for phosphorus reabsorption by the kidneys. As a result, serum levels rise.

Shifts affect serum levels

Certain conditions cause phosphorus to move, or shift, in and out of cells. Insulin moves not only glucose but also phosphorus into the cell. Alkalosis results in the same kind of phosphorus shift. Those shifts affect serum phosphorus levels. (See *The elderly at risk*, page 164.)

Hypophosphatemia

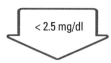

< 2.5 mg/dl

Hypophosphatemia occurs when the serum phosphorus level falls below 2.5 mg/dl (or 1.8 mEq/L). Although this condition generally indicates a deficiency of phosphorus, it can occur under various circumstances when total body phosphorus stores are normal. Severe hypophosphatemia occurs when serum phosphorus levels are less than 1 mg/dl and the body can't support its energy needs. The condition may lead to organ failure.

How it happens

Three underlying mechanisms can lead to hypophosphatemia: a shift of phosphorus from extracellular fluid to intracellular fluid, a decrease in intestinal absorption of phosphorus, and an increased loss of phosphorus through the kidneys. Some causes of hypophosphatemia may involve more than one mechanism.

Several factors may cause phosphorus to shift from extracellular fluid into the cell. Here are the most common causes.

Hyperventilation

Respiratory alkalosis can stem from a number of conditions that produce hyperventilation, including sepsis, alcohol withdrawal, heat stroke, and acute salicylate poisoning. Although the mechanism that prompts respiratory alkalosis to induce hypophosphatemia is unknown, the response is a shift of phosphorus into the cells and a resulting decrease in serum phosphorus levels.

Insulin drives it into the cell

Hyperglycemia, an elevated serum glucose level, causes the release of insulin, which transports glucose and phosphorus into the cells. The same effect may occur in a diabetic patient who's receiving insulin or in a significantly malnourished patient; at particular risk for malnourishment are those who are elderly, debilitated, or alcoholic and those who have anorexia nervosa.

After initiation of enteral or parenteral feeding, and when phosphorus supplementation is insufficient, phosphorus shifts into the cells. This shift is called "refeeding syndrome" and usually occurs 3 or more days after feedings begin. Patients recovering from hypothermia can also develop hypophosphatemia as phosphorus moves into the cells.

Absorption problems

Malabsorption syndromes, starvation, and prolonged or excessive use of phosphorus-binding antacids are among the many causes of impaired intestinal absorption of phosphorus. Because vitamin D contributes to intestinal absorption of phosphorus, inadequate vitamin D intake or synthesis can inhibit phosphorus absorption. Diarrhea or laxative abuse can also result in increased GI loss of phosphorus.

Don't forget the kidneys

Diuretic use is the most common cause of phosphorus loss through the kidneys. Thiazides, loop diuretics, and acetazolamide are the diuretics that most commonly cause hypophosphatemia. (See *Drugs associated with hypophosphatemia.*) The second

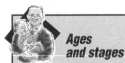

Ages and stages

The elderly at risk

Elderly patients are at risk for altered electrolyte levels for two main reasons. First, they have a lower ratio of lean body weight to total body weight, which places them at risk for water deficit. Second, their thirst response is diminished and their renal function decreased, which makes maintaining electrolyte balance more difficult. Age-related renal changes include changes in renal blood flow and glomerular filtration rate.

An elderly patient's medication can also alter his electrolyte levels by affecting the absorption of phosphate. Therefore, ask him if he uses over-the-counter medications, such as antacids, laxatives, herbs, and teas.

Drugs associated with hypophosphatemia

The following drugs are commonly associated with hypophosphatemia:
- acetazolamide, thiazide diuretics (chlorothiazide and hydrochlorothiazide), loop diuretics (bumetanide and furosemide), and other diuretics
- antacids, such as aluminum carbonate, aluminum hydroxide, calcium carbonate, and magnesium oxide
- insulin
- laxatives.

most common cause is diabetic ketoacidosis (DKA) in diabetic patients who have poorly controlled blood glucose levels. In DKA, an osmotic diuresis is induced from high glucose levels. This results in a significant loss of phosphorus from the kidneys. Ethanol affects phosphorus reabsorption in the kidney so that more phosphorus is excreted in the urine.

A buildup of PTH, which occurs with hyperparathyroidism and hypocalcemia, also leads to hypophosphatemia. Finally, hypophosphatemia occurs in patients who have extensive burns. Although the mechanism is unclear, the condition is suspected to occur in response to the extensive diuresis of salt and water that typically occurs during the first 2 to 4 days after a burn injury. Respiratory alkalosis and carbohydrate administration may also play a role here.

The characteristics of hypophosphatemia are apparent in many organ systems.

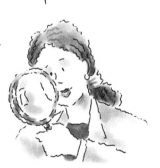

What to look for

The characteristics of hypophosphatemia are apparent in many organ systems. Signs and symptoms may develop acutely due to rapid decreases in phosphorus or gradually as the result of slow, continual decreases in phosphorus.

Hypophosphatemia affects the musculoskeletal, central nervous, cardiac, and hematologic systems. Because phosphorus is required to make high-energy ATP, many of the signs and symptoms of hypophosphatemia are related to low energy stores.

Getting weak

With hypophosphatemia, muscle weakness, malaise, and anorexia occur. The patient may experience a weakened hand grasp, slurred speech, or dysphagia. He also may develop myalgia (tenderness or pain in the muscles).

Respiratory failure may result from weakened respiratory muscles and poor contractility of the diaphragm. Respirations may appear shallow and ineffective. In later stages, the patient may be cyanotic. *Keep in mind that it may be difficult to wean a mechanically ventilated patient with hypophosphatemia from the ventilator.*

With severe hypophosphatemia, rhabdomyolysis (skeletal muscle destruction) can occur with altered muscle cell activity. Muscle enzymes such as creatine kinase are released from the cells into the extracellular fluid. Loss of bone density, osteomalacia (softening of the bones), and bone pain may also occur with prolonged hypophosphatemia. Fractures can result.

Neuroeffects

Without enough phosphorus, the body can't make enough ATP, a cornerstone of energy metabolism. As a result, central nervous system cells can malfunction, causing paresthesia, irritability, apprehension, and confusion. The neurologic effects of hypophosphatemia may progress to seizures and coma.

Weak heartbeats

The heart's contractility is decreased due to low energy stores of ATP. As a result, the patient may develop hypotension and a low cardiac output. Severe hypophosphatemia may lead to cardiomyopathy, which can be reversed with treatment.

Oxygen delivery drop-off

A drop in production of 2,3-DPG causes a decrease in oxygen delivery to tissues. Because hemoglobin has a stronger affinity for oxygen than for other gases, oxygen is less likely to be given up to the tissues as it circulates through the body. As a result, less oxygen is delivered to the myocardium, which can cause chest pain.

Hypophosphatemia may also cause hemolytic anemia because of changes in the structure and function of RBCs.

Patients with hypophosphatemia are more susceptible to infection because of the effect of low levels of ATP in WBCs. Lack of ATP results in a decreased functioning of leukocytes. Chronic hypophosphatemia also affects platelet function, resulting in bruising and bleeding, particularly mild GI bleeding.

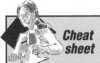

Cheat sheet

Signs and symptoms of severe hypophosphatemia

- Hypotension
- Decreased cardiac output
- Cardiomyopathy
- Rhabdomyolysis
- Cyanosis
- Respiratory failure

What tests show

The following diagnostic test results may indicate hypophosphatemia or a related condition:
- serum phosphorus level of less than 2.5mg/dl (or 1.8 mEq/L)
- elevated creatine kinase level if rhabdomyolysis is present
- X-ray studies that reveal the skeletal changes typical of osteomalacia or bone fractures.

How hypophosphatemia is treated

Treatment varies with the severity and cause of the condition. It includes treating the underlying cause and correcting the imbalance with phosphorus replacement and a high-phosphorus diet. The route of replacement therapy depends on the severity of the imbalance.

For mild to moderate...

Treatment for mild-to-moderate hypophosphatemia includes a diet high in phosphorus-rich foods, such as eggs, nuts, whole grains, meat, fish, poultry, and milk products. However, if calcium is contraindicated or the patient can't tolerate milk, oral phosphorus supplements are indicated. Oral supplements include Neutra-Phos and Neutra-Phos-K and can be used for moderate hypophosphatemia. Dosage limitations are related to the adverse effects, most notably nausea and diarrhea. (See *When dietary changes aren't working*.)

For more severe...

For patients with severe hypophosphatemia or a nonfunctioning GI tract, I.V. phosphorus replacement is the recommended choice. Two preparations are used: I.V. potassium phosphate and I.V. sodium phosphate. Dosage is guided by the patient's response to treatment and serum phosphorus levels.

Potassium phosphate should be administered slowly (no more than 10 mEq/hour). Adverse effects of I.V. replacement for hypophosphatemia include hyperphosphatemia and hypocalcemia.

How you intervene

If your patient is beginning total parenteral nutrition or is otherwise at risk for developing hypophosphatemia, monitor him for signs and symptoms of this imbalance. If the patient has already developed hypophosphatemia, your nursing care should focus on careful monitoring, safety measures, and interventions to restore normal serum phosphorus levels. (See *Teaching about hypophosphatemia*, page 168.) Alert the doctor to any changes in the patient's condition and take these other actions.

Assess and monitor

- Monitor vital signs. Remember that hypophosphatemia can lead to respiratory failure, low cardiac output, confusion, seizures, or coma.
- Assess the patient's level of consciousness and neurologic status each time you check his vital signs. Document your observa-

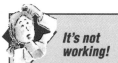

It's not working!

When dietary changes aren't working

If your patient's phosphorus-rich diet hasn't raised serum phosphorus levels as you had hoped, it's time to ask the following questions.
- Is a GI problem making phosphorus digestion difficult?
- Is your patient using a phosphate-binding antacid?
- Is your patient abusing alcohol?
- Is your patient using a thiazide diuretic?
- Is your patient complying with the treatment regimen for diabetes?

tions and the patient's neurologic status on a flow sheet so changes can be noted immediately, even on other shifts. (See *Documenting hypophosphatemia.*)

• Monitor the rate and depth of respirations, especially if the patient has severe hypophosphatemia. Report signs and symptoms of hypoxia, such as confusion, restlessness, increased respiratory rate and, in later stages, cyanosis. If possible, take steps to prevent hyperventilation, because it worsens respiratory alkalosis and can lower phosphorus levels. Follow arterial blood gas results and pulse oximetry levels to monitor the effectiveness of ventilation. Wean patients from the ventilator slowly.

• Monitor the patient for evidence of heart failure related to reduced myocardial functioning. Such evidence includes crackles, shortness of breath, decreased blood pressure, and elevated heart rate.

• Monitor the patient's temperature at least every 4 hours. Check WBC counts. Follow strict sterile technique in changing dressings. Report signs of infection.

• Assess the patient frequently for evidence of decreasing muscle strength, such as weak hand grasps or slurred speech, and document your findings regularly.

Chart smart

Documenting hypophosphatemia

When caring for a patient with hypophosphatemia, make sure you document:
• vital signs
• neurologic status, including level of consciousness, restlessness, apprehension
• muscle strength
• respiratory assessment
• serum electrolyte levels and other pertinent laboratory data
• notification of the doctor
• I.V. therapy, including condition of I.V. site, medication, dose, patient's response
• seizures, if any
• your interventions and the patient's response
• safety measures to protect patient
• patient teaching.

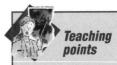

Teaching points

Teaching about hypophosphatemia

When teaching about hypophosphatemia, cover these topics and then evaluate the patient's learning:
• description of hypophosphatemia and its risk factors, prevention, and treatment
• medications ordered
• need to consult with a dietitian
• need for a high-phosphorus diet
• avoidance of antacids that contain phosphorus
• warning signs and symptoms and when to report them
• need to maintain follow-up appointments.

Assess, administer, and maintain

- Administer prescribed phosphorus supplements. Keep in mind that oral supplements may cause diarrhea. To improve their taste, mix them with juice.
- Insert an I.V. line, as ordered, and keep it patent. Infuse phosphorus solutions slowly, using an infusion device to control the rate. During infusions, watch for signs of hypocalcemia, hyperphosphatemia, and I.V. infiltration. Potassium phosphate can cause tissue sloughing and necrosis.
- Administer an analgesic, if ordered.
- Make sure the patient maintains bed rest, if ordered, for his own safety. Keep the bed in its lowest position, with the wheels locked and the side rails raised. If the patient is at risk for seizures, pad the side rails and keep an artificial airway at the patient's bedside.

Follow up

- Orient the patient as needed. Keep clocks, calendars, and familiar personal objects within his sight.
- Inform the patient and his family that confusion caused by a low phosphorus level is only temporary and will most likely decrease with therapy.
- Record the patient's fluid intake and output.
- Carefully monitor serum electrolyte levels, especially calcium and phosphorus levels as well as other pertinent laboratory test results. Report abnormalities.
- Assist patient with ambulation and activities of daily living, if needed, and keep essential objects near the patient to prevent accidents.

Hyperphosphatemia

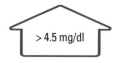
> 4.5 mg/dl

Hyperphosphatemia occurs when the serum phosphorus levels exceed 4.5 mg/dl (or 2.6 mEq/L) and usually reflects the kidneys' inability to excrete excess phosphorus. The condition commonly occurs along with an increased release of phosphorus from damaged cells. Severe hyperphosphatemia occurs when the serum phosphorus levels reach 6 mg/dl or higher.

How it happens

Hyperphosphatemia results from a number of underlying mechanisms, including impaired renal excretion of phosphorus, a shift of phosphorus from the intracellular fluid to the extracellular fluid, and an increase in dietary intake of phosphorus.

Kidney filter fails

Hyperphosphatemia most commonly results from renal failure due to the kidneys' inability to excrete excess phosphorus.

When the glomerular filtration rate begins to drop below 30 ml/minute, the kidneys can't filter excess phosphorus adequately. Because the kidneys are responsible for most of the excretion of phosphorus, their inability to filter phosphorus leads to an elevated serum phosphorus level.

Hypoparathyroidism

A risk after thyroid or parathyroid surgery, hypoparathyroidism impairs synthesis of parathyroid hormone. When less PTH is synthesized, less phosphorus is excreted from the kidneys. The result? Elevated serum phosphorus levels.

Puttin' on the transcellular shift

Several conditions can cause phosphorus to shift from the intracellular fluid to the extracellular fluid. Acid-base imbalances, such as respiratory acidosis and DKA, are common examples. Anything that causes cellular destruction can also result in a transcellular shift of phosphorus.

Destruction of cells can trigger the release of intracellular phosphorus into the extracellular fluid, causing serum phosphorus levels to rise. Chemotherapy, for example, causes significant cell destruction, as do muscle necrosis and rhabdomyolysis, conditions that can stem from infection, heat stroke, and trauma.

Increased intake of phosphorus

Excessive intake of phosphorus can result from overadministration of phosphorus supplements or of laxatives or enemas that contain phosphorus (such as Fleet enemas).

Excessive intake of vitamin D can result in increased absorption of phosphorus and lead to an elevated serum phosphorus level. (See *Drugs associated with hyperphosphatemia* and *Cow's milk and hyperphosphatemia*.) Poor renal function increases the risk of hyperphosphatemia because of the increased intake of phosphorus.

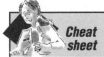

Cheat sheet

Signs and symptoms of hyperphosphatemia

- Anorexia
- Chvostek's or Trousseau's sign
- Conjunctivitis, visual impairment
- Decreased mental status
- Hyperreflexia
- Hypocalcemic ECG changes
- Muscle weakness, cramps, spasm
- Nausea and vomiting
- Papular eruptions
- Paresthesia
- Tetany

What to look for

Hyperphosphatemia causes few clinical problems by itself. However, phosphorus and calcium levels have an inverse relationship: If one is high, the other is low. Because of this seesaw relationship, hyperphosphatemia may lead to hypocalcemia, which can be life-threatening.

Drugs associated with hyperphosphatemia

The following drugs may cause hyperphosphatemia:
• enemas such as Fleet enemas
• laxatives containing phosphorus or phosphate
• oral phosphorus supplements (Neutra-Phos)
• parenteral phosphorus supplements (sodium phosphate, potassium phosphate)
• vitamin D supplements.

Ages and stages

Cow's milk and hyperphosphatemia

Infants fed cow's milk are predisposed to hyperphosphatemia because cow's milk contains more phosphorus than breast milk.

Muscles and nerves

The patient may develop paresthesia in the fingertips and around the mouth, which may increase in severity and spread proximally along the limbs and to the face. Muscle spasm, cramps, pain, and weakness may also occur and may be severe enough to prevent the patient from performing normal activities. The patient may also exhibit hyperreflexia and positive Chvostek's and Trousseau's signs.

Neurologic signs and symptoms include decreased mental status and seizures. Electrocardiogram (ECG) changes include a prolonged QT interval and ST segment. The patient may experience anorexia, nausea, and vomiting. Bone development may also be affected.

Calcification cues

When phosphorus levels rise, phosphorus binds with calcium, forming an insoluble compound called calcium phosphate. Organ dysfunction can result when calcium phosphate precipitates, or is deposited, in the heart, lungs, kidneys, corneas, or other soft tissues. This process, called calcification, usually occurs as a result of chronically elevated phosphorus levels. (See *A look at calcification*, page 172.)

With calcification, the patient may experience arrhythmias, an irregular heart rate, and decreased urine output. Corneal haziness, conjunctivitis, and impaired vision may occur, and papular eruptions may develop on the skin.

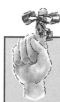

Memory jogger

To help you remember some of the signs and symptoms of hyperphosphatemia, think of the word CHEMO. (Keep in mind that chemotherapy can lead to hyperphosphatemia.)

Cardiac irregularities

Hyperreflexia

Eating poorly

Muscle weakness

Oliguria

What tests show

The following findings may indicate hyperphosphatemia or a related condition such as hypocalcemia:
• serum phosphorus level above 4.5 mg/dl (or 2.6 mEq/L)
• serum calcium level below 8.9 mg/dl

• X-ray studies that may reveal skeletal changes due to osteodystrophy (defective bone development) in chronic hyperphosphatemia

• increased blood urea nitrogen (BUN) and creatinine levels, which reflect worsening renal function

• ECG changes characteristic of hypocalcemia.

How hyperphosphatemia is treated

An elevated serum phosphorus level may be treated with drugs and other therapeutic measures. The treatment is aimed at correcting the underlying disorder, if one exists.

Now I get it!

A look at calcification

When serum phosphorus levels are high, phosphorus binds with calcium to form an insoluble compound called calcium phosphate. The compound is deposited in the heart, lungs, kidneys, eyes, skin, and other soft tissues, where it interferes with normal organ and tissue function. This illustration shows some of the effects of this calcification.

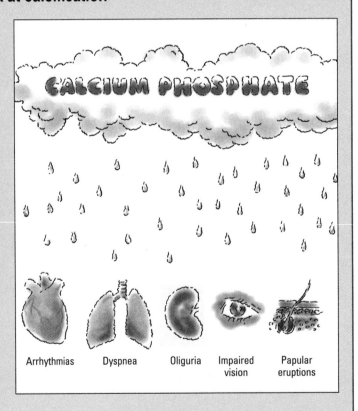

CALCIUM PHOSPHATE

Arrhythmias   Dyspnea   Oliguria   Impaired vision   Papular eruptions

Try a low-phosphorus diet

If a patient's elevated serum phosphorus level is due to excessive phosphorus intake, the condition may be easily remedied by reducing phosphorus intake. Therapeutic measures include reducing dietary intake of phosphorus and eliminating the use of phosphorus-based laxatives and enemas. (See *When dietary changes aren't enough.*)

Decreasing absorption

Drug therapy may help decrease absorption of phosphorus in the GI system. Drug therapy may include aluminum, magnesium, or calcium gel or phosphate-binding antacids. For patients with underlying renal insufficiency or renal failure, use of magnesium antacids may result in hypermagnesemia and should be avoided.

Keep in mind that a mildly elevated phosphorus level may benefit a patient with renal failure. High phosphorus levels allow more oxygen to move from the RBCs to tissues, which can help prevent hypoxemia and limit the effects of chronic anemia on oxygen delivery.

Treat what's underneath

Treatment for the underlying cause of respiratory acidosis or DKA can lower serum phosphorus levels. In a diabetic patient, the administration of insulin causes phosphorus to shift back into the cell, which can result in a decrease in serum phosphorus levels.

When the situation worsens

For patients with severe hyperphosphatemia, I.V. saline solution may be given to promote renal excretion of phosphorus. However, this treatment requires that the patient has functional kidneys and can tolerate the increased load of sodium and fluid.

As a final therapeutic intervention, hemodialysis or peritoneal dialysis may be initiated if the patient has chronic renal failure or an extreme case of acute hyperphosphatemia with symptomatic hypocalcemia.

How you intervene

Identify patients at risk for hyperphosphatemia, and monitor them carefully. Use care when administering phosphorus in I.V. infusions, enemas, and laxatives because the extra phosphorus may cause hyperphosphatemia. If your patient has already developed hyperphosphatemia, your nursing care should focus on careful monitoring, safety measures, and interventions to restore normal

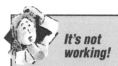

It's not working!

When dietary changes aren't enough

If your patient's low-phosphorus diet hasn't changed his serum phosphorus level, it's time to ask the following questions.

• Is the patient taking the medication (phosphorus-binding antacids) as directed?
• Is the patient continuing to use laxatives or enemas that contain phosphate?
• Are the patient's kidneys functioning?
• Has the underlying cause of hyperphosphatemia been corrected?

Teaching points

Teaching about hyperphosphatemia

Before your patient heads home, cover these topics with him and evaluate his learning:
- causes and treatment
- prescribed medications
- avoidance of preparations that contain phosphorus
- avoidance of high-phosphorus foods
- warning signs and symptoms
- referrals to dietitian and social services, if indicated.

Chart smart

Documenting hyperphosphatemia

When caring for a patient with hyperphosphatemia, make sure you document the following:
- all assessment findings
- intake and output
- I.V. therapy and medications given
- muscle spasms, cramps, pain, strength
- paresthesia in the fingertips and around the mouth
- visual disturbances
- safety measures to protect patient
- notification of the doctor
- your interventions, including patient teaching and the patient's response.

serum phosphorus levels. Follow these steps to provide care for the patient.

• Monitor vital signs, keeping in mind the signs and symptoms of hypocalcemia. If you note any signs or symptoms of worsening hypocalcemia, such as paresthesia in the fingers or around the mouth, hyperactive reflexes, or muscle cramps, notify the doctor promptly. (See *Teaching about hyperphosphatemia.*) Also notify the doctor if you detect signs or symptoms of calcification, including oliguria, visual impairment, conjunctivitis, irregular heart rate or palpitations, and papular eruptions.

• Monitor fluid intake and output. If urine output falls below 30 ml/hour, notify the doctor immediately. Decreased urine output can seriously affect renal clearance of excess serum phosphorus.

• Carefully monitor serum electrolyte levels, especially calcium and phosphorus. Report changes immediately. Also monitor blood urea nitrogen (BUN) and serum creatinine levels, because hyperphosphatemia can impair renal tubules when calcification occurs.

• Keep a flow sheet of daily laboratory test results for a patient at risk. Include BUN and serum phosphorus, calcium, and creatinine levels as well as fluid intake and output. Keep the flow sheet on a clipboard so changes can be detected immediately. (See *Documenting hyperphosphatemia.*)

Administer and follow up

• Administer prescribed medications, monitor their effectiveness, and assess the patient for possible adverse reactions. Give antacids with meals to increase their effectiveness in binding phosphorus.

• Prepare the patient for possible dialysis if hyperphosphatemia is severe.

• If a patient's condition results from chronic renal failure or if his treatment includes a low-phosphorus diet, consult a dietitian to assist the patient in complying with dietary restrictions.

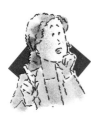

Quick quiz

1. If your patient has hyperphosphatemia, he may also have the secondary electrolyte disturbance:
    A.   hypermagnesemia.
    B.   hypocalcemia.
    C.   hypernatremia.
Answer: B. Phosphorus and calcium have an inverse relationship: If the serum phosphorus levels are increased, then the serum calcium levels are decreased.

2. For a patient with hyperphosphatemia and renal failure, avoid giving the phosphate-binding antacid:
    A.   aluminum hydroxide.
    B.   calcium carbonate.
    C.   magnesium oxide.
Answer: C. Administering an antacid that contains magnesium to a patient with renal failure can result in hypermagnesemia.

3. Many of the signs and symptoms of hypophosphatemia are related to:
    A.   low energy stores.
    B.   hypercalcemia.
    C.   extensive diuresis.
Answer: A. The body needs phosphorus to make adenosine triphosphate, which provides all the cells—especially muscles—with energy.

4. The binding of phosphorus and calcium in a patient with hyperphosphatemia can lead to:
    A.   increased calcium release by the kidneys.
    B.   widespread calcification of tissues.
    C.   decreased calcium uptake by the pituitary gland.
Answer: B. Hyperphosphatemia results in hypocalcemia. The calcium and phosphorus bind together and are deposited in the tissues, resulting in calcification.

5.   You're advised that your alcoholic patient will be receiving his first infusion of total parenteral nutrition (TPN) tonight. Before hanging the first solution, you'll want to make sure:
    A.   patient's serum phosphorus level is normal.
    B.   patient isn't allergic to phosphorus.
    C.   patient's urine output is greater than 30 ml/hour.

Answer: A. A low serum phosphorus level can drop even more if a patient receives TPN. The high glucose load causes phosphorus to shift into the cells.

6.   Your patient's ability to be weaned from mechanical ventilation would be most likely affected by a serum phosphorus level:
    A.   higher than 8 mg/dl.
    B.   between 2 and 4 mg/dl.
    C.   lower than 1 mg/dl.

Answer: C. Severe hypophosphatemia can lead to respiratory muscle weakness and impaired contractility of the diaphragm, which compromises the patient's ability to breathe spontaneously.

Scoring

☆☆☆   If you answered all six questions correctly, wow! You're phospho-fabulous!

☆☆   If you answered four or five correctly, way to go! How about a lovely plate of baked halibut?

☆   If you answered fewer than four correctly, that's OK. Here's a delicious egg-and-cheese sandwich. Enjoy!

When chloride tips the balance

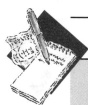

Just the facts

This chapter discusses how to care for patients who have either a chloride deficit or excess. In this chapter, you'll learn:

♦ why chloride is important in the body

♦ how chloride and sodium are related

♦ how the body regulates the chloride level

♦ how to recognize and treat high and low chloride levels.

A look at chloride

Chloride is the most abundant anion (negatively charged ion) in extracellular fluid. It moves in and out of the cells with sodium and potassium and combines with major cations (positively charged ions) to form sodium chloride, hydrochloric acid, potassium chloride, calcium chloride, and other important compounds. High levels of chloride are found in cerebrospinal fluid (CSF), but the anion can also be found in bile and in gastric and pancreatic juices.

What it does

Because of its negative charge, chloride travels with positively charged sodium and helps maintain serum osmolality and water balance. Chloride and sodium also work together to form CSF. The choroid plexus, a tangled mass of tiny blood vessels inside the ventricles of the brain, depends on these two electrolytes to attract water and to form the fluid component of CSF.

In the stomach, chloride is secreted by the gastric mucosa as hydrochloric acid, providing the acid medium conducive to digestion and enzyme activation. Chloride helps maintain acid-base balance and assists in carbon dioxide transport in the red blood cells.

On the level

Serum chloride levels normally range between 96 and 106 mEq/L. By comparison, the chloride level inside a cell is 4 mEq/L. Chloride levels remain relatively stable with age. Because chloride balance is closely associated with sodium balance, the levels of both electrolytes usually change in direct proportion to one another. (See *Chloride levels.*)

Chloride control

Chloride regulation depends on intake and excretion of chloride and reabsorption of chloride ions in the kidneys. The daily chloride requirement for adults is 750 mg. Most diets provide sufficient chloride in the form of salt (usually as sodium chloride) in the same foods that contain sodium. (See *Dietary sources of chloride.*)

Most chloride is absorbed in the intestines with only a small portion lost in the feces. Chloride is produced mainly in the stomach as hydrochloric acid, so chloride levels can be influenced by GI disorders.

Linked electrolytes

Because chloride and sodium are closely linked, a change in one electrolyte level causes a comparable change in the other. Chloride levels can also be indirectly affected by aldosterone secretion, which causes the renal tubules to reabsorb sodium. As positively charged sodium ions are reabsorbed, negatively charged chloride ions are passively reabsorbed because of their electrical attraction to sodium.

Acids and bases

Regulation of chloride levels also involves acid-base balance. Chloride is reabsorbed and excreted in direct opposition to bicarbonate. When chloride levels change, the body attempts to keep its positive-negative balance by making corresponding changes in the levels of bicarbonate (another negatively charged ion) in the kidneys. (Remember, bicarbonate is alkaline.)

When chloride levels decrease, the kidneys retain bicarbonate and bicarbonate levels increase. When chloride levels increase, the kidneys excrete bicarbonate and bicarbonate levels decrease. Therefore, changes in chloride and bicarbonate levels can lead to acidosis or alkalosis. (See *Chloride and bicarbonate.*)

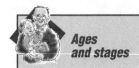

Ages and stages

Chloride levels

Patients between ages 60 and 90 have chloride levels between 98 and 107 mEq/L; patients age 90 and older, between 98 and 111 mEq/L.

Dietary sources of chloride

Dietary sources of chloride include:
- fruits
- vegetables
- table salt
- salty foods
- processed meats
- canned vegetables.

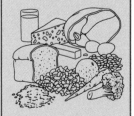

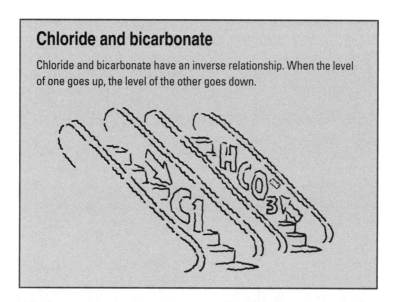

Chloride and bicarbonate

Chloride and bicarbonate have an inverse relationship. When the level of one goes up, the level of the other goes down.

Hypochloremia

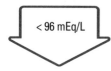

< 96 mEq/L

Hypochloremia is a deficiency of chloride in extracellular fluid. The condition occurs when serum chloride levels fall below 96 mEq/L. When serum chloride levels drop, levels of sodium, potassium, calcium, and other electrolytes may be affected. If much more chloride than sodium is lost, hypochloremic alkalosis may occur.

How it happens

Serum chloride levels drop when chloride intake or absorption decreases or when chloride losses increase. Losses may occur through the skin (chloride is found in sweat), the GI tract, or the kidneys. Changes in sodium levels or acid-base balance also alter chloride levels.

Down with intake

Reduced chloride intake may occur in infants being fed chloride-deficient formula and in people on salt-restricted diets. Patients dependent on I.V. fluids are also at risk if the fluids lack chloride (for example, a dextrose solution without electrolytes).

Excessive chloride losses can occur with prolonged vomiting, diarrhea, severe diaphoresis, gastric surgery, nasogastric (NG) suctioning, and other GI tube drainage. Severe vomiting can cause a loss of hydrochloric acid from the stomach, an acid deficit in the

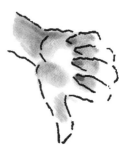

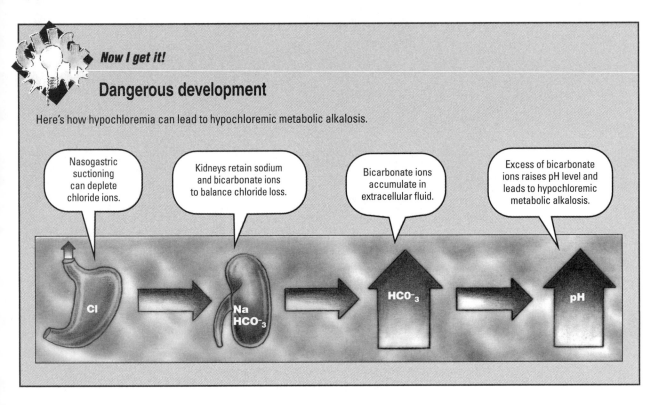

Now I get it!

Dangerous development

Here's how hypochloremia can lead to hypochloremic metabolic alkalosis.

Nasogastric suctioning can deplete chloride ions.

Kidneys retain sodium and bicarbonate ions to balance chloride loss.

Bicarbonate ions accumulate in extracellular fluid.

Excess of bicarbonate ions raises pH level and leads to hypochloremic metabolic alkalosis.

Cl

Na
HCO⁻₃

HCO⁻₃

pH

body, and subsequent metabolic alkalosis. Patients with cystic fibrosis can also lose more chloride than normal. Any prolonged and untreated hypochloremic state can result in a state of hypochloremic alkalosis. (See *Dangerous development.*)

People at risk for hypochloremia include children with prolonged vomiting from pyloric obstruction and those with draining fistulas and ileostomies that can cause a loss of chloride from the GI tract. Diuretics, such as furosemide (Lasix), ethacrynic acid (Edecrin), and hydrochlorothiazide can also cause an excessive loss of chloride from the kidneys. (See *Drug culprits.*)

Wait, there's more

Other causes of hypochloremia include sodium and potassium deficiency or metabolic alkalosis; conditions that affect acid-base or electrolyte balance, such as untreated diabetic ketoacidosis and Addison's disease; and rapid removal of ascitic fluid (which contains sodium) during paracentesis. Also, patients who have heart failure may develop hypochloremia because serum chloride levels are diluted by excess fluid in the body.

Drug culprits

Drugs commonly associated with hypochloremia include the following types of diuretics:
• loop (such as furosemide)
• osmotic (such as mannitol)
• thiazide (such as hydrochlorothiazide).

What to look for

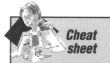

Patients who have hypochloremia may have signs and symptoms of acid-base and electrolyte imbalances. You may notice signs of hyponatremia, hypokalemia, or metabolic alkalosis. Alkalosis results in a high pH and, to compensate, respirations become slow and shallow as the body tries to retain carbon dioxide and restore the pH level to normal.

The nerves also become more excitable, so look for tetany, hyperactive deep tendon reflexes, and muscle hypertonicity. (See *Danger signs of hypochloremia.*) The patient may have muscle cramps, twitching, and weakness and be agitated or irritable. If hypochloremia goes unrecognized, it can become life-threatening. As the chloride imbalance worsens (along with other imbalances), the patient may suffer arrhythmias, seizures, coma, or respiratory arrest.

> ### Cheat sheet
>
> ## Possible indicators of hypochloremia
>
> - Hyperactive DTRs
> - Muscle hypertonicity
> - Signs and symptoms of acid-base and electrolyte imbalances
> - Tetany

What tests show

The following diagnostic test results are associated with hypochloremia:
- serum chloride level below 96 mEq/L
- serum sodium level below 135 mEq/L (indicates hyponatremia)
- serum pH greater than 7.45 and serum bicarbonate level greater than 26 mEq/L (indicates metabolic alkalosis).

How hypochloremia is treated

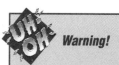

Treatment for hypochloremia focuses on correcting the underlying cause, such as low dietary chloride intake, prolonged vomiting, or gastric suctioning. Chloride may be replaced through fluid administration or drug therapy. The patient also may require treatment for associated metabolic alkalosis or electrolyte imbalances such as hypokalemia.

Chloride may be given orally; for example, in a salty broth. If the patient can't take oral supplements, he may receive medications or normal saline solution I.V. To avoid hypernatremia (high sodium level) or to treat hypokalemia, potassium chloride may be administered I.V.

Check out underlying causes

Treatment for associated metabolic alkalosis usually addresses the underlying causes. The underlying cause of diaphoresis, vomiting or other GI losses, or renal losses should be investigated. Rarely, metabolic alkalosis may be treated by administering am-

> ### Warning!
>
> ## Danger signs of hypochloremia
>
> Suspect that your patient with hypochloremia is really in trouble if he has any of these late-developing danger signs:
> - seizures and coma
> - arrhythmias
> - respiratory arrest.

monium chloride, an acidifying agent that's used when alkalosis is caused by chloride loss. Drug dosage depends on the severity of the alkalosis. The effects of ammonium chloride last only 3 days. After that, the kidneys begin to excrete the extra acid. (See *When treatment isn't working.*)

How you intervene

Be sure to monitor patients at risk for hypochloremia, such as those receiving diuretic therapy or NG suctioning. When caring for a patient with hypochloremia, you'll also want to take these nursing actions.

Monitor

• Monitor level of consciousness (LOC), muscle strength, and movement. Notify the doctor if the patient's condition worsens.
• Monitor vital signs, especially respiratory rate and pattern, and observe for worsening respiratory function. Also monitor cardiac rhythm because hypokalemia may be present with hypochloremia. Have emergency equipment handy in case the patient's condition deteriorates.
• Monitor and record serum electrolyte levels, especially chloride, sodium, potassium, and bicarbonate. Also assess arterial blood gas (ABG) results for acid-base imbalance.

Administer and maintain

• If the patient is alert and can swallow without difficulty, offer foods high in chloride, such as tomato juice or salty broth. Don't let the patient fill up on plain drinking water. (See *Teaching about hypochloremia.*)
• Insert an I.V. line, as ordered, and keep it patent. Administer chloride and potassium replacements as ordered.
• If administering ammonium chloride, assess the patient for pain at the infusion site and adjust the rate, if needed. This drug is metabolized by the liver, so don't give it to patients with severe hepatic disease.
• Use normal saline solution, not tap water, to flush the patient's NG tube.
• Accurately measure and record intake and output, including the volume of vomitus and gastric contents from suction and other GI drainage tubes.
• Provide a safe environment. Help the patient ambulate, and keep his personal items and call button within reach. Institute seizure precautions, as needed.
• Provide a quiet environment, explain interventions, and reorient the patient, as needed.

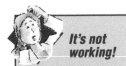

It's not working!

When treatment isn't working

If treatment for hypochloremia doesn't seem to be working, make sure the patient isn't drinking large amounts of water, which can cause him to excrete large amounts of chloride. Review the causes of hypochloremia to identify new or coexisting conditions that might be causing chloride loss.

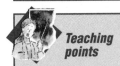

Teaching points

Teaching about hypochloremia

When teaching about hypochloremia, cover these topics and then evaluate the patient's learning:
• signs and symptoms, complications, and risk factors for hypochloremia
• warning signs to report to the doctor
• dietary supplements
• medications if prescribed.

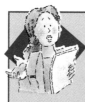

Chart smart

Documenting hypochloremia

If your patient has hypochloremia, make sure your documentation includes:
- vital signs, including cardiac rhythm
- intake and output
- serum electrolyte levels and arterial blood gas results
- your assessment, including level of consciousness, seizure activity,
and respiratory status
- time of notification of the doctor
- I.V. therapy, along with other interventions, and the patient's response
- safety measures implemented
- teaching done and the patient's response.

- Document all care and the patient's response. (See *Documenting hypochloremia.*)

Hyperchloremia

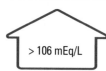

> 106 mEq/L

Hyperchloremia, an excess of chloride in extracellular fluid, occurs when serum chloride levels exceed 106 mEq/L. This condition is associated with other acid-base imbalances and rarely occurs alone.

How it happens

Because chloride regulation and sodium regulation are closely related, hyperchloremia may also be associated with hypernatremia.
Chloride and bicarbonate have an inverse relationship, so an excess of chloride ions may be linked to a decrease in bicarbonate.
Excess serum chloride results from increased chloride intake or
absorption, from acidosis, or from chloride retention by the kidneys.

Up with intake and absorption

Increased intake of chloride as sodium chloride can cause hyperchloremia, especially if water is lost from the body at the same
time. That water loss raises the chloride level even more. In-

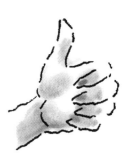

creased chloride absorption by the bowel can occur in patients who have had anastomoses joining the ureter and intestines.

Conditions that alter electrolyte and acid-base balance and cause metabolic acidosis include dehydration, renal tubular acidosis, renal failure, respiratory alkalosis, salicylate toxicity, hyperparathyroidism, hyperaldosteronism, and hypernatremia.

Drug-related retention

Several medications can also contribute to hyperchloremia. For example, direct ingestion of ammonium chloride or other drugs that contain chloride or cause chloride retention can lead to hyperchloremia. Ion exchange resins that contain sodium, such as Kayexalate, can cause chloride to be exchanged for potassium in the bowel. When chloride follows sodium into the bloodstream, serum chloride levels rise. Carbonic anhydrase inhibitors, such as acetazolamide, also promote chloride retention in the body. (See *Drug offenders.*)

> ### Drug offenders
>
> These drugs can cause hyperchloremia:
> - acetazolamide
> - ammonium chloride
> - phenylbutazone
> - sodium polystyrene sulfonate (Kayexalate)
> - salicylates (overdose)
> - triamterene.

What to look for

Hyperchloremia rarely produces signs and symptoms on its own. Instead, the major signs and symptoms are essentially those of metabolic acidosis, including tachypnea, lethargy, weakness, diminished cognitive ability, and deep, rapid respirations (Kussmaul's respirations).

Left untreated, acidosis can lead to arrhythmias, decreased cardiac output, a further decrease in the patient's LOC, and even coma. Metabolic acidosis related to a high chloride level is called "hyperchloremic metabolic acidosis." (See *Anion gap and metabolic acidosis.*)

If a patient has an increased serum chloride level, his serum sodium level is probably high as well, which can lead to fluid retention. He also may be agitated and have dyspnea, tachycardia, hypertension, or pitting edema—signs of hypernatremia and hypervolemia.

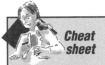

Cheat sheet

Signs and symptoms of hyperchloremia

- Those associated with metabolic acidosis (it rarely produces signs and symptoms on its own)

Severe signs of metabolic acidosis
- Arrhythmias
- Decreased cardiac output
- Decreased LOC that may progress to coma

What tests show

The following diagnostic test results typically occur in hyperchloremia:
- serum chloride level greater than 106 mEq/L
- serum sodium level greater than 145 mEq/L
- serum pH level less than 7.35, a serum bicarbonate level less than 22 mEq/L, and a normal anion gap (8 to 14 mEq/L). These findings suggest metabolic acidosis.

Now I get it!

Anion gap and metabolic acidosis

Hyperchloremia increases the likelihood that a patient will develop hyperchloremic metabolic acidosis. The illustration below shows the relationship between chloride and bicarbonate in the development of that form of acidosis.

How it happens

A normal anion gap in a patient with metabolic acidosis indicates that the acidosis is most likely caused by a loss of bicarbonate ions by the kidneys or the GI tract. In such cases, a corresponding increase in chloride ions also occurs.

Acidosis can also result from an accumulation of chloride ions in the form of acidifying salts. A corresponding decrease in bicarbonate ions occurs at the same time. In this illustration, the chloride level is high (> 106 mEq/L) and the bicarbonate level is low (< 22 mEq/L).

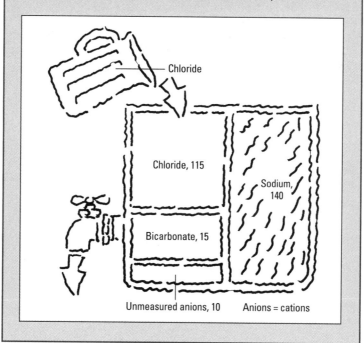

How hyperchloremia is treated

Treatments for hyperchloremia include correcting the underlying cause as well as restoring fluid, electrolyte, and acid-base balance. (See *Diuretics to the rescue.*) Dehydrated patients may receive fluids to dilute the chloride and speed renal excretion of chloride ions. Sodium and chloride intake also may be restricted.

If the patient's liver function is adequate, he may receive an infusion of lactated Ringer's solution to convert lactate to bicarbonate in the liver and to increase the base bicarbonate level and correct acidosis. In severe hyperchloremia, I.V. sodium bicarbonate may be administered to raise serum bicarbonate levels. Because bicarbonate and chloride compete for sodium, I.V. sodium bicarbonate therapy can lead to renal excretion of chloride ions and correction of acidosis.

How you intervene

Try to prevent hyperchloremia by monitoring high-risk patients. If your patient develops a chloride imbalance:
• Monitor vital signs, including cardiac rhythm.
• If the patient is confused, reorient him as needed, and provide a safe, quiet environment to prevent injury. Teach the patient's family to do the same. (See *Teaching about hyperchloremia.*)
• Continually assess the patient, paying particular attention to the neurologic, cardiac, and respiratory examinations. Report changes to the doctor immediately.

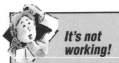

It's not working!

Diuretics to the rescue

If the patient doesn't seem to respond to therapy, the doctor may order diuretics to eliminate chloride. Although other electrolytes will be lost, the chloride level should decrease.

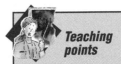

Teaching points

Teaching about hyperchloremia

Make sure you cover the following topics about hyperchloremia and that you evaluate your patient's learning:
• signs and symptoms, complications, and risk factors of hyperchloremia
• what symptoms to report to the doctor
• dietary restrictions if ordered
• medications if prescribed.
• importance of replenishing lost fluids during hot weather.

Chart smart

Documenting hyperchloremia

Your documentation for a patient with hyperchloremia should include:
• vital signs, including cardiac rhythm
• level of consciousness, muscle strength, and activity level
• serum electrolyte and arterial blood gas levels
• fluid intake and output
• safety precautions taken
• your assessment and interventions—and the patient's responses
• patient teaching.

• Look for changes in the respiratory pattern that may indicate a worsening of the acid-base imbalance.
• Insert an I.V. and maintain its patency. Administer I.V. fluids and medications as ordered. Watch for signs of fluid overload.
• Evaluate muscle strength and adjust activity level accordingly.
• If the patient is receiving high doses of sodium bicarbonate, watch for signs and symptoms of overcompensation, such as metabolic alkalosis, which may cause central and peripheral nervous system overstimulation. Also watch for signs of hypokalemia as potassium is forced into the cells.
• Restrict fluids, sodium, and chloride, if ordered.
• Monitor and record serum electrolyte levels and ABG results.
• Monitor and record fluid intake and output.(See *Documenting hyperchloremia.*)

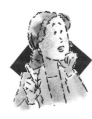

Quick quiz

1. Chloride is largely produced by the:
   A.   brain.
   B.   kidneys.
   C.   stomach.

Answer: C. The chloride ion is largely produced by gastric mucosa and occurs in the form of hydrochloric acid.

2. If the level of bicarbonate ions increases, the level of chloride ions:
   A.   increases.
   B.   decreases.
   C.   stays the same.

Answer: B. The relationship between chloride ions and bicarbonate ions is inversely proportional. If one level rises, the other level drops.

3. If your postoperative patient has a chloride imbalance, you would also expect to see a change in the electrolyte:
   A.   calcium.
   B.   potassium.
   C.   sodium.

Answer: C. Sodium and chloride move together through the body, so an imbalance in one may cause an imbalance in the other.

4.   For a patient who has a low serum chloride level, you would expect the patient to have the acid-base imbalance:

    A.   respiratory acidosis.

    B.   metabolic acidosis.

    C.   metabolic alkalosis.

Answer: C. A drop in chloride ions causes the body to retain bicarbonate, a base, and results in hypochloremic metabolic alkalosis.

5.   Deep, rapid breathing may indicate a:

    A.   serum chloride level greater than 106 mEq/L.

    B.   serum chloride less than 96 mEq/L.

    C.   pH greater than 7.45.

Answer: A. Deep, rapid breathing, or Kussmaul's respirations, is the body's attempt to blow off excess acid in the form of carbon dioxide. When this occurs, suspect metabolic acidosis, a condition associated with a serum chloride level greater than 106 mEq/L.

Scoring

☆☆☆   If you answered all five questions correctly, incredible! You're hereby named Most Exalted Keeper of the Chloride Key!

☆☆   If you answered three or four correctly, super! You're hereby named Royal High Assistant to the Most Exalted Keeper of the Chloride Key!

☆   If you answered fewer than three correctly, that's OK. You're hereby named Notable Grand Associate to the Royal High Assistant to the Most Exalted Keeper of the Chloride Key.

When acids and bases tip the balance

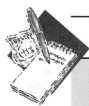

Just the facts

This chapter explains the basics — and more — of acidosis and alkalosis. In this chapter, you'll learn:

♦ how the body compensates for acid-base imbalances

♦ what conditions may trigger them

♦ how to differentiate among the four respiratory and metabolic acid-base imbalances

♦ how to care for the patient with an acid-base imbalance.

A look at acid-base imbalances

The body constantly works to maintain the balance between acids and bases. Without that balance, the cells can't function properly. Acid-base balance depends on the regulation of free hydrogen ions. The concentration of hydrogen ions in body fluids determines the extent of acidity or alkalinity, both of which are measured in pH. (For more information about pH, see chapter 3, Balancing acids and bases.)

When acid-base values stray

Blood gas measurements remain the major diagnostic tool for evaluating acid-base states. An arterial blood gas (ABG) analysis includes the following tests: pH, which measures the hydrogen ion (H+) concentration and is an indication of the blood's acidity or alkalinity; partial pressure of arterial carbon dioxide ($Paco_2$), which reflects the adequacy of ventilation by the lungs; and bicarbonate level (HCO_3^-), which reflects the activity of the kidneys in retaining or excreting bicarbonate. (See *The ABC's of ABG*.)

The ABC's of ABG

Use these three main values when analyzing arterial blood gas (ABG):

pH	7.35 to 7.45
$Paco_2$	35 to 45 mm Hg
HCO_3^-	22 to 26 mEq/L

Normal fix-me-ups

Most of the time, the body's compensatory mechanisms restore acid-base balance — or at least prevent the life-threatening consequences of an imbalance. Those compensatory mechanisms include chemical buffers, certain respiratory reactions, and certain kidney reactions.

For example, the body compensates for a primary respiratory disturbance such as respiratory acidosis by inducing metabolic alkalosis. Unfortunately, not all attempts to compensate are equal. The respiratory system is efficient and can compensate for metabolic disturbances quickly, whereas the metabolic system, working through the kidneys, can take hours or days to compensate for an imbalance. This chapter takes a closer look at each of the four major acid-base imbalances.

Respiratory acidosis

A compromise in any of the three essential parts of breathing — ventilation, perfusion, or diffusion — may result in respiratory acidosis. This acid-base disturbance is characterized by alveolar hypoventilation, meaning that the patient's pulmonary system is unable to rid the body of enough carbon dioxide (CO_2) to maintain a healthy pH balance.

The lack of efficient CO_2 release leads to hypercapnia, in which the $Paco_2$ is greater than 45 mm Hg. The condition can be acute, resulting from sudden failure in ventilation, or chronic, resulting from chronic pulmonary disease.

In acute respiratory acidosis, the pH drops below normal (lower than 7.35). In chronic respiratory acidosis, commonly due to chronic obstructive pulmonary disease (COPD), the pH stays within normal limits (7.35 to 7.45) because the kidneys have had time to compensate for the imbalance. (More on that complex phenomenon later.)

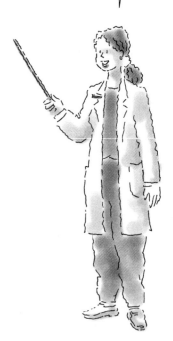

A compromise in any of the three essential parts of breathing may result in respiratory acidosis.

How it happens

When a patient hypoventilates, CO_2 builds up in the bloodstream and the pH drops below normal — respiratory acidosis. The kidneys try to compensate for a drop in pH by conserving bicarbonate (base) ions, or generating them in the kidney, which in turn raises the pH. (See *What happens in respiratory acidosis.*)

Now I get it!

What happens in respiratory acidosis

This series of illustrations shows at the cellular level how respiratory acidosis develops.

Step 1

When pulmonary ventilation decreases, retained carbon dioxide (CO_2) combines with water (H_2O) to form carbonic acid (H_2CO_3) in larger-than-normal amounts. The carbonic acid dissociates to release free hydrogen ions (H) and bicarbonate ions (HCO_3^-). The excessive carbonic acid causes a drop in pH. *Look for a Paco$_2$ level above 45 mm Hg and a pH level below 7.35.*

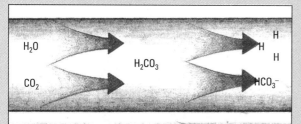

Step 2

As the pH level falls, 2,3-diphosphoglycerate (2,3-DPG) increases in the red blood cells and causes a change in hemoglobin (Hb) that makes the hemoglobin release oxygen (O_2). The altered hemoglobin, now strongly alkaline, picks up hydrogen ions and CO_2, thus eliminating some of the free hydrogen ions and excess CO_2. *Look for decreased arterial oxygen saturation.*

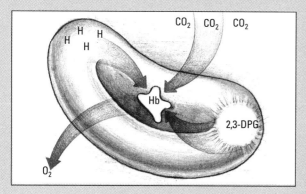

Step 3

Whenever Paco$_2$ increases, CO_2 builds up in all tissues and fluids, including cerebrospinal fluid and the respiratory center in the medulla. The CO_2 reacts with water to form carbonic acid, which then breaks into free hydrogen ions and bicarbonate ions. The increased amount of CO_2 and free hydrogen ions stimulate the respiratory center to increase the respiratory rate. An increased respiratory rate expels more CO_2 and helps to reduce the CO_2 level in the blood and other tissues. *Look for rapid, shallow respirations and a decreasing Paco$_2$.*

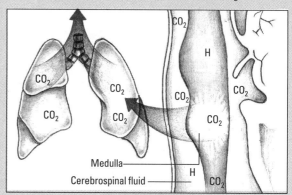

Medulla
Cerebrospinal fluid

Step 4

Eventually, CO_2 and hydrogen ions cause cerebral blood vessels to dilate, which increases blood flow to the brain. That increased flow can cause cerebral edema and depress central nervous system activity. *Look for headache, confusion, lethargy, nausea, or vomiting.*

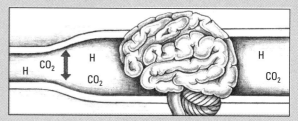

(continued)

What happens in respiratory acidosis (continued)

Step 5
As respiratory mechanisms fail, the increasing $Paco_2$ stimulates the kidneys to conserve bicarbonate and sodium ions and to excrete hydrogen ions, some in the form of ammonium (NH_4). The additional bicarbonate and sodium combine to form extra sodium bicarbonate ($NaHCO_3$), which is then able to buffer more free hydrogen ions. *Look for increased acid content in the urine, increasing serum pH and bicarbonate levels, and shallow, depressed respirations.*

Step 6
As the concentration of hydrogen ions overwhelms the body's compensatory mechanisms, the hydrogen ions move into the cells, and potassium ions move out. A concurrent lack of oxygen causes an increase in the anaerobic production of lactic acid, which further skews the acid-base balance and critically depresses neurologic and cardiac functions. *Look for hyperkalemia, arrhythmias, increased $Paco_2$, decreased Pao_2, decreased pH, and decreased level of consciousness.*

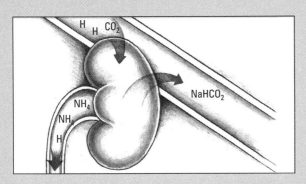

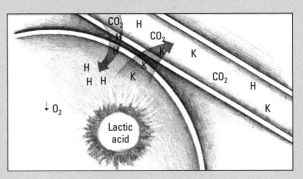

Respiratory acidosis can result from neuromuscular problems, depression of the respiratory center in the brain, lung disease, or an airway obstruction.

Respirations lack drive

In certain neuromuscular diseases—such as Guillain-Barré syndrome, myasthenia gravis, and poliomyelitis—the respiratory muscles fail to respond properly to the respiratory drive, resulting in respiratory acidosis. Diaphragmatic paralysis, which commonly occurs with spinal cord injury, works the same way to cause respiratory acidosis.

Hypoventilation from central nervous system (CNS) trauma or brain lesions—such as tumors, vascular disorders, or infections—may impair the patient's ventilatory drive. Obesity (as in pickwickian syndrome) or primary hypoventilation (as in Ondine's curse) may contribute to this imbalance as well. Also, certain drugs—including anesthetics, hypnotics, narcotics, and sedatives—can depress the respiratory center of the brain, leading to hypercapnia. (See *Drugs associated with respiratory acidosis*.)

Drugs associated with respiratory acidosis

The following drugs are associated with respiratory acidosis:
• anesthetics
• hypnotics
• narcotics
• sedatives.

Pulmonary problems pose risk

Lung diseases that decrease the amount of pulmonary surface area available for gas exchange can prompt respiratory acidosis. Less surface area decreases the amount of gas exchange that can occur, thus impeding CO_2 exchange. Examples of pulmonary problems that can decrease surface area include respiratory infections, COPD, acute asthma attacks, chronic bronchitis, late stages of adult respiratory distress syndrome, pulmonary edema, conditions in which there's increased dead space in the lungs (hypoventilation), and physiologic or anatomic shunts.

Chest-wall trauma (leading to pneumothorax or flail chest) can also cause respiratory acidosis. The ventilatory drive remains intact, but the chest-wall mechanics of the collapsed lung don't allow for sufficient alveolar ventilation to meet the body's needs. Chest-wall mechanics can also be impeded as a result of the rib cage distortion caused by fibrothorax or kyphoscoliosis.

Danger! Obstruction!

Respiratory acidosis can also be caused by airway obstruction, which leads to carbon dioxide retention in the lungs. Airway obstruction can occur as a result of retained secretions, tumors, anaphylaxis, laryngeal spasm, or lung diseases that interfere with alveolar ventilation. *Keep in mind that children are prone to airway obstruction, as are elderly patients and debilitated patients, who may not be able to effectively clear secretions.* (See *Infants and acidosis.*)

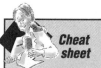

Cheat sheet

Causes of respiratory acidosis

• Hypoventilation from CNS trauma or tumor that depresses respiratory center
• Neuromuscular diseases that affect respiratory drive
• Lung diseases that decrease amount of surface area available for gas exchange
• Airway obstruction
• Chest-wall trauma
• Certain drugs that depress respiratory center primary hypoventilation

Ages and stages

Infants and acidosis

Infants commonly have problems with acid-base imbalances, particularly acidosis. Because of their low residual lung volume, any alteration in their respiration can rapidly and dramatically change their partial pressure of arterial carbon dioxide, leading to acidosis.

Infants also have a high metabolic rate, which yields large amounts of metabolic wastes and acids that must be excreted by the kidneys. This, along with their immature buffer system, leaves infants prone to acidosis.

Who's at risk

Treatments can induce respiratory acidosis. For instance, mechanical ventilation that underventilates a patient can cause CO_2 retention. A postoperative patient is at risk for respiratory acidosis if fear of pain prevents him from participating in pulmonary hygiene measures, such as coughing and deep breathing. Also, analgesics or sedatives can depress the medulla, which is responsible for controlling respirations. Depressing the medulla can lead to inadequate ventilation and subsequent respiratory acidosis.

What to look for

Signs and symptoms of respiratory acidosis depend on the cause of the condition. The patient may complain of a headache because carbon dioxide dilates cerebral blood vessels. (See *Signs and symptoms of respiratory acidosis.*)

CNS depression may result in an altered level of consciousness (LOC), ranging from restlessness, confusion, and apprehension to somnolence and coma. If the acidosis remains untreated, a fine flapping tremor and depressed reflexes may develop. The patient may also report nausea and vomiting, and the skin may be warm and flushed.

Most patients with respiratory acidosis have rapid, shallow respirations. They will be dyspneic and possibly diaphoretic. Auscultation will reveal diminished or absent breath sounds over the affected area. However, if acidosis stems from CNS trauma or lesions or drug overdose, the respiratory rate will be greatly decreased.

In a patient with acidosis, hyperkalemia, *and* hypoxemia, you may note tachycardia and ventricular arrhythmias. Cyanosis is a late sign of the condition. Resulting myocardial depression may lead to shock and, ultimately, cardiac arrest.

What tests show

Several test results may help confirm diagnosis of respiratory acidosis and guide treatment:
• ABG analysis is the key test for detecting respiratory acidosis. Typically, the pH is below 7.35, and the $Paco_2$ is above 45 mm Hg. The HCO_3^- level varies, depending on how long the acidosis has been present. In a patient with acute respiratory acidosis, the HCO_3^- level may be normal; in a patient with chronic respiratory acidosis, it may be above 26 mEq/L. (See *ABG results in respiratory acidosis.*)

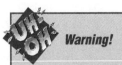

Warning!

Signs and symptoms of respiratory acidosis

The following assessment findings commonly occur in patients with respiratory acidosis:
• apprehension
• confusion
• decreased deep-tendon reflexes
• diaphoresis
• dyspnea, with rapid, shallow respirations
• nausea or vomiting
• restlessness
• tachycardia
• tremors
• warm, flushed skin.

ABG results in respiratory acidosis

This chart shows typical arterial blood gas (ABG) findings in uncompensated and compensated respiratory acidosis.

	Uncompensated	Compensated
pH	< 7.35	Normal
$Paco_2$ (mm Hg)	> 45	> 45
HCO_3^- (mEq/L)	Normal	> 26

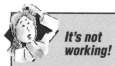

It's not working!

When hypoventilation can't be corrected

If hypoventilation can't be corrected, expect your patient to have an artificial airway inserted and to be placed on mechanical ventilation. Be aware that bronchoscopy may be needed to remove retained secretions.

• Chest X-rays can help pinpoint causes, such as COPD, pneumonia, pneumothorax, and pulmonary edema.
• Serum electrolyte levels with potassium greater than 5 mEq/L typically indicate hyperkalemia. In acidosis, potassium leaves the cell, so expect the serum level to be elevated.
• Drug screening may confirm a suspected overdose.

How respiratory acidosis is treated

Treatment of respiratory acidosis focuses on improving ventilation and lowering the $Paco_2$ level. If respiratory acidosis stems from nonpulmonary conditions, such as neuromuscular disorders or a drug overdose, treatment goals involve correcting the underlying cause.

Treatment for respiratory acidosis with a pulmonary cause includes:
• a bronchodilator to open constricted airways
• supplemental oxygen as needed
• drug therapy to treat hyperkalemia
• an antibiotic to treat infection
• chest physiotherapy to remove secretions from the lungs
• removal of a foreign body from the patient's airway, if needed.
(See *When hypoventilation can't be corrected.*)

How you intervene

If your patient develops respiratory acidosis, maintain a patent airway. Help remove any foreign bodies from the airway and establish an artificial airway. Provide adequate humidification to ensure moist secretions. Additional measures include the following.

Assess and monitor

- Monitor vital signs, and assess cardiac rhythm. Respiratory acidosis can cause tachycardia, alterations in respiratory rate and rhythm, hypotension, and arrhythmias.
- Continue to assess respiratory patterns, and report changes quickly. Prepare for mechanical ventilation, if indicated.
- Monitor the patient's neurologic status, and report significant changes. Also monitor the patient's cardiac function, because respiratory acidosis may progress to shock and cardiac arrest.
- Report any variations in ABG, pulse oximetry, or serum electrolyte levels.

Maintain

- Give medications, such as an antibiotic or a bronchodilator, as prescribed. (See *Teaching about respiratory acidosis*.)
- Administer oxygen as ordered. Generally, lower concentrations of oxygen are given to patients with COPD. The medulla of a patient with COPD is accustomed to high CO_2 levels. A lack of oxygen, called the "hypoxic drive," stimulates those patients to breathe. Too much oxygen diminishes that drive and depresses respiratory efforts.
- Perform tracheal suctioning, incentive spirometry, postural drainage, and coughing and deep breathing, as indicated.
- Make sure the patient takes in enough fluids, both oral and I.V., and maintain accurate intake and output records. (See *Documenting respiratory acidosis*.)

Chart smart

Documenting respiratory acidosis

When providing nursing care for a patient with respiratory acidosis, document:
- vital signs and cardiac rhythm
- intake and output
- your assessment and interventions, and the patient's response
- notification of doctor
- patient teaching
- medications administered, oxygen therapy, and ventilator settings
- character of pulmonary secretions
- serum electrolyte levels and arterial blood gas results.

Teaching points

Teaching about respiratory acidosis

Make sure you cover these topics with your patient, and then evaluate his learning:
- description of the condition and how to prevent it
- reasons for repeated arterial blood gas analyses
- deep-breathing exercises
- prescribed medications
- home oxygen therapy, if indicated
- warning signs and symptoms and when to report them
- proper technique for using bronchodilators, if appropriate
- need for frequent rest
- need for increased caloric intake, if appropriate.

- Provide reassurance to the patient and family.
- Keep in mind that any sedatives you give to the patient can decrease his respiratory rate.
- Institute safety measures as needed to protect a confused patient.

Questions to consider

As you reevaluate your patient's condition, consider the following questions:
- Have the patient's respiratory rate and LOC returned to normal?
- Does auscultation of the patient's chest reveal reduced adventitious breath sounds?
- Have all tachycardias or ventricular arrhythmias been stabilized?
- Have the patient's cyanosis and dyspnea diminished?
- Have the patient's ABG results and serum electrolyte levels returned to normal?
- Do chest X-rays show improvement in the condition of the patient's lungs?

Respiratory alkalosis

Respiratory alkalosis, which is the opposite of respiratory acidosis, results from alveolar hyperventilation and hypocapnia. In respiratory alkalosis, the pH is greater than 7.45 and the $Paco_2$ is less than 35 mm Hg. The condition may be acute, resulting from a sudden increase in ventilation, or chronic, which may be difficult to identify because of renal compensation.

How it happens

Any clinical condition that increases the respiratory rate or depth can cause the lungs to eliminate, or blow off, CO_2. Because CO_2 is an acid, eliminating it causes a decrease in $Paco_2$ along with an increase in pH—alkalosis.

Hyperventilation (gasp!)

The most common cause of acute respiratory alkalosis is hyperventilation stemming from anxiety. Pain, which also causes an increased respiratory rate, can have the same effect. Hyperventilation is an early sign of salicylate intoxication and also occurs with the use of nicotine and xanthines such as aminophylline. (See *Drugs associated with respiratory alkalosis.*)

Drugs associated with respiratory alkalosis

The following drugs are associated with respiratory alkalosis:
- catecholamines
- nicotine
- salicylates
- xanthines such as aminophylline.

Hypermetabolic states—such as fever, liver failure, and sepsis (especially gram-negative sepsis)—can lead to respiratory alkalosis. Certain drugs can also stimulate an increase in respiratory drive.

Conditions that affect the respiratory control center in the medulla are also a danger. For example, the higher progesterone levels of pregnancy may stimulate this center, while stroke or trauma may injure it, both resulting in respiratory alkalosis.

Hypoxia (pant!)

Acute hypoxia secondary to high altitude, pulmonary disease, severe anemia, pulmonary embolus, or hypotension can cause respiratory alkalosis. Such conditions may overstimulate the respiratory center and make the patient breathe faster and deeper. Overventilation during mechanical ventilation causes the lungs to blow off more CO_2, resulting in respiratory alkalosis.

What to look for

An increase in the rate and depth of respirations is a primary sign of respiratory alkalosis. It's also common for the patient to have tachycardia. The patient may appear anxious and restless as well as complain of muscle weakness or difficulty breathing. (See *What happens in respiratory alkalosis.*)

In extreme alkalosis, confusion or syncope may occur. Because of the lack of CO_2 in the blood and its effect on cerebral blood flow and the respiratory center, you may see alternating periods of apnea and hyperventilation. The patient may complain of tingling in the fingers and toes.

You may see electrocardiogram (ECG) changes, including a prolonged PR interval, a flattened T wave, a prominent U wave, and a depressed ST segment. (For more information, see Chapter 6, When potassium tips the balance.)

Symptoms worsen as calcium levels drop because of vasoconstriction of peripheral and cerebral vessels resulting from hypoxia. You may see hyperreflexia, carpopedal spasm, tetany, arrhythmias, a progressive decrease in the patient's LOC, seizures, or coma. (See *Signs and symptoms of respiratory alkalosis*, page 201.)

What tests show

Several diagnostic test results may be helpful in detecting and treating respiratory alkalosis.

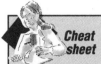

Cheat sheet

Causes of respiratory alkalosis

- Any condition that increases respiratory rate and depth
- Hyperventilation
- Hypercapnia
- Hypermetabolic states
- Liver failure
- Certain drugs
- Conditions that affect brain's respiratory control center
- Acute hypoxia secondary to high altitude, pulmonary disease, severe anemia, pulmonary embolus, and hypotension.

Now I get it!

What happens in respiratory alkalosis

This series of illustrations shows at the cellular level how respiratory alkalosis develops.

Step 1

When pulmonary ventilation increases above the amount needed to maintain normal carbon dioxide (CO_2) levels, excessive amounts of CO_2 are exhaled. This causes hypocapnia (a fall in $Paco_2$), which leads to a reduction in carbonic acid (H_2CO_3) production, a loss of hydrogen ions (H) and bicarbonate ions (HCO_3^-), and a subsequent rise in pH. *Look for a pH level above 7.45, a $Paco_2$ level below 35 mm Hg, and a bicarbonate level below 22 mEq/L.*

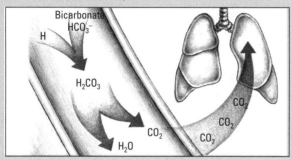

Step 2

In defense against the rising pH, hydrogen ions are pulled out of the cells and into the blood in exchange for potassium ions (K). The hydrogen ions entering the blood combine with bicarbonate ions to form carbonic acid, which lowers the pH. *Look for a further decrease in bicarbonate levels, a fall in pH, and a fall in serum potassium levels (hypokalemia).*

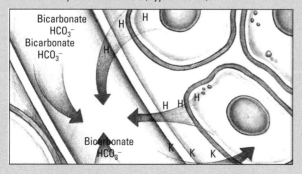

Step 3

Hypocapnia stimulates the carotid and aortic bodies and the medulla, which causes an increase in heart rate without an increase in blood pressure. *Look for angina, electrocardiogram changes, restlessness, and anxiety.*

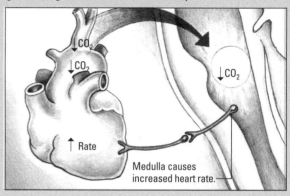

Medulla causes increased heart rate.

Step 4

Simultaneously, hypocapnia produces cerebral vasoconstriction, which prompts a reduction in cerebral blood flow. Hypocapnia also overexcites the medulla, pons, and other parts of the autonomic nervous system. *Look for increasing anxiety, diaphoresis, dyspnea, alternating periods of apnea and hyperventilation, dizziness, and tingling in the fingers or toes.*

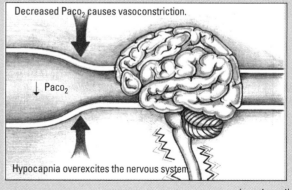

Decreased $Paco_2$ causes vasoconstriction.

$\downarrow Paco_2$

Hypocapnia overexcites the nervous system.

(continued)

What happens in respiratory alkalosis *(continued)*

Step 5
When hypocapnia lasts more than 6 hours, the kidneys increase secretion of bicarbonate and reduce excretion of hydrogen. Periods of apnea may result if the pH remains high and the $Paco_2$ remains low. *Look for slowing of the respiratory rate, hypoventilation, and Cheyne-Stokes respirations.*

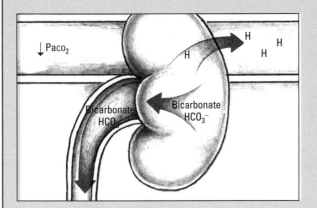

Step 6
Continued low $Paco_2$ increases cerebral and peripheral hypoxia from vasoconstriction. Severe alkalosis inhibits calcium (Ca) ionization, which in turn causes increased nerve excitability and muscle contractions. Eventually, the alkalosis overwhelms the central nervous system and the heart. *Look for decreasing level of consciousness, hyperreflexia, carpopedal spasm, tetany, arrhythmias, seizures, and coma.*

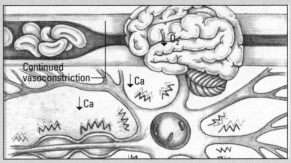

- ABG analysis is the key diagnostic test for identifying respiratory alkalosis. Typically, the pH is above 7.45, and the $Paco_2$ level is below 35 mm Hg. The HCO_3^- level may be normal (22 to 26 mEq/L) when the alkalosis is acute, but usually falls below 22 mEq/L when chronic. (See *ABG results in respiratory alkalosis.*)
- Serum electrolyte levels may point to a metabolic disorder that could be causing compensatory respiratory alkalosis. Hypokalemia may be evident (decreased LOC). The ionized serum calcium level may be decreased in those with severe respiratory alkalosis.
- ECG findings may indicate arrhythmias or the changes associated with hypokalemia or hypocalcemia.
- Toxicology screening may reveal salicylate poisoning.

How respiratory alkalosis is treated

Treatment focuses on correcting the underlying disorder, which may require removing the causative agent, such as a salicylate or other drug, or taking steps to reduce fever and eliminate the source of sepsis.

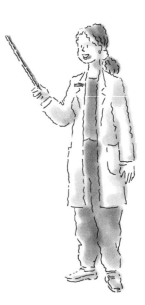

ABG results in respiratory alkalosis

This chart shows typical arterial blood gas (ABG) findings in uncompensated and compensated respiratory alkalosis.

	Uncompensated	Compensated
pH	> 7.45	Normal
$Paco_2$ (mm Hg)	< 35	< 35
HCO_3^- (mEq/L)	Normal	< 22

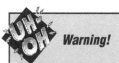

Warning!

Signs and symptoms of respiratory alkalosis

The following assessment findings commonly occur in patients with respiratory alkalosis:
• anxiety
• diaphoresis
• dyspnea, increased respiratory rate and depth
• electrocardiogram changes
• hyperreflexia
• paresthesia
• restlessness
• tachycardia
• tetany.

If acute hypoxemia is the cause, oxygen therapy is initiated. If anxiety is the cause, the patient may receive a sedative or an anxiolytic.

Hyperventilation can be counteracted by having the patient breathe into a paper bag, which forces the patient to breathe exhaled CO_2, thereby raising the CO_2 level. If a patient's respiratory alkalosis is iatrogenic, mechanical ventilator settings may be adjusted by decreasing the tidal volume or the number of breaths per minute.

How you intervene

• Monitor patients at risk for developing respiratory alkalosis. Allay anxiety whenever possible to prevent hyperventilation. Recommend activities that promote relaxation. Help the patient breath into a paper bag, if indicated.
• Monitor vital signs. Report changes in neurologic, neuromuscular, or cardiovascular functioning.
• Monitor ABG and serum electrolyte levels, and immediately report any variations. *Remember that twitching and cardiac arrhythmias may be associated with alkalosis and electrolyte imbalances.*
• If the patient is receiving mechanical ventilation, check ventilator settings frequently. Monitor ABG levels after making changes in settings.
• Provide undisturbed rest periods after the patient's respiratory rate returns to normal; hyperventilation may result in severe fatigue.
• Stay with the patient during periods of extreme stress and anxiety. Offer reassurance, and maintain a

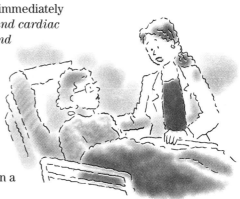

calm, quiet environment. (See *Teaching about respiratory alkalosis.*)
• Institute safety measures and seizure precautions as needed. Document all care. (See *Documenting respiratory alkalosis.*)

Metabolic acidosis

Metabolic acidosis is characterized by a pH below 7.35 and an HCO_3^- level below 22 mEq/L. This disorder depresses the CNS. Left untreated, it may lead to ventricular arrhythmias, coma, and cardiac arrest.

How it happens

The underlying mechanisms in metabolic acidosis are a loss of HCO_3^- from extracellular fluid, an accumulation of metabolic acids, or a combination of the two. If the patient's anion gap (measurement of the difference between the amount of sodium and the amount of bicarbonate in the blood) is greater than 14 mEq/L, then the acidosis is due to an accumulation of metabolic acids (unmeasured anions).

If the metabolic acidosis is associated with a normal anion gap (8 to 14 mEq/L), loss of HCO_3^- may be the cause. (See *What happens in metabolic acidosis.*)

Gain acids, lose bases

Metabolic acidosis is characterized by a gain in acids or a loss of bases from the plasma. The condition may be related to an over-

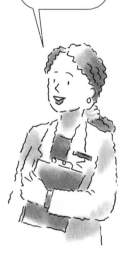

Document all care.

Now I get it!

What happens in metabolic acidosis

This series of illustrations shows at the cellular level how metabolic acidosis develops.

Step 1

As hydrogen ions (H) start to accumulate in the body, chemical buffers (plasma bicarbonate and proteins) in the cells and extra-cellular fluid bind with them. *No signs are detectable at this stage.*

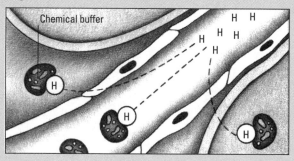

Step 2

Excess hydrogen ions that the buffers can't bind with decrease the pH and stimulate chemoreceptors in the medulla to increase the respiratory rate. The increased respiratory rate lowers the $Paco_2$, which allows more hydrogen ions to bind with bicarbonate ions (HCO_3^-). Respiratory compensation occurs within minutes but isn't sufficient to correct the imbalance. *Look for a pH level below 7.35, a bicarbonate level below 22 mEq/L, a decreasing $Paco_2$ level, and rapid, deeper respirations.*

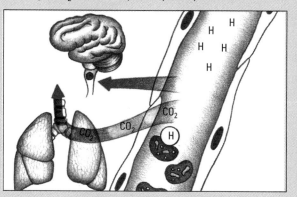

Step 3

Healthy kidneys try to compensate for acidosis by secreting excess hydrogen ions into the renal tubules. Those ions are buffered by phosphate or ammonia and then are excreted into the urine in the form of a weak acid. *Look for acidic urine.*

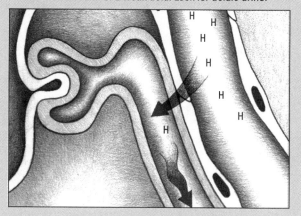

Step 4

Each time a hydrogen ion is secreted into the renal tubules, a sodium ion (Na) and a bicarbonate ion are absorbed from the tubules and returned to the blood. *Look for pH and bicarbonate levels that return slowly to normal.*

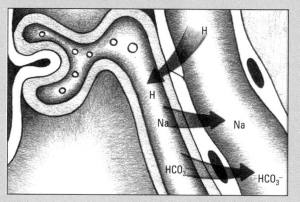

(continued)

What happens in metabolic acidosis *(continued)*

Step 5

Excess hydrogen ions in the extracellular fluid diffuse into cells. To maintain the balance of the charge across the membrane, the cells release potassium ions into the blood. *Look for signs and symptoms of hyperkalemia, including colic and diarrhea, weakness or flaccid paralysis, tingling and numbness in the extremities, bradycardia, a tall T wave, a prolonged PR interval, and a wide QRS complex.*

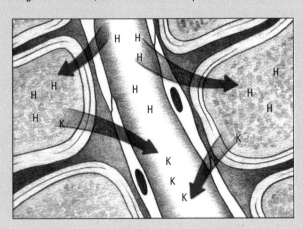

Step 6

Excess hydrogen ions alter the normal balance of potassium, sodium, and calcium ions (Ca), leading to reduced excitability of nerve cells. *Look for signs and symptoms of progressive central nervous system depression, including lethargy, dull headache, confusion, stupor, and coma.*

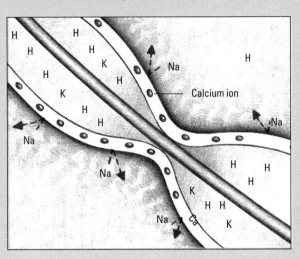

production of ketone bodies. Fatty acids are converted to ketone bodies when glucose supplies have been used and the body draws on fat stores for energy. Conditions that cause an overproduction of ketone bodies include diabetes mellitus, chronic alcoholism, severe malnutrition or starvation, poor dietary intake of carbohydrates, hyperthyroidism, and severe infection with accompanying fever.

Lactic acidosis can cause or worsen metabolic acidosis and can occur secondarily to shock, heart failure, pulmonary disease, hepatic disorders, seizures, or strenuous exercise.

Kidney culprit

Metabolic acidosis can also stem from a decreased ability of the kidneys to excrete acids, as occurs in renal insufficiency or renal failure with acute tubular necrosis.

Gut reactions

Metabolic acidosis also occurs with excessive GI losses from diarrhea, intestinal malabsorption, a draining fistula of the pancreas or liver, or a urinary diversion to the ileum. Other causes include hyperaldosteronism and use of a potassium-sparing diuretic such as acetazolamide, which inhibits the secretion of acid.

Poison pills

At particular risk for metabolic acidosis are patients with poisoning or a toxic reaction to a drug, which can occur following inhalation of toluene or ingestion of a salicylate (such as aspirin or an aspirin-containing medication), methanol, ethylene glycol, paraldehyde, hydrochloric acid, or ammonium chloride.

What to look for

Metabolic acidosis typically produces respiratory, neurologic, and cardiac signs and symptoms. As acid builds up in the bloodstream, the lungs compensate by blowing off CO_2.

Hyperventilation, especially increased depth of respirations, is the first clue to metabolic acidosis. Called Kussmaul's respirations, the breathing is rapid and deep. A diabetic who experiences Kussmaul's respirations may have a fruity odor to his breath. The odor stems from catabolism of fats and excretion of acetone through the lungs.

Depressed CNS

As the pH drops, the CNS is further depressed, as is myocardial function. Cardiac output and blood pressure drop, and arrhythmias may occur if the patient also has hyperkalemia.

Initially, the skin is warm and dry as a result of peripheral vasodilation, but as shock develops, the skin becomes cold and clammy. The patient may complain of weakness and a dull headache as the cerebral vessels dilate.

The patient's LOC may deteriorate from confusion to stupor and coma. A neuromuscular examination may show diminished muscle tone and deep tendon reflexes. Metabolic acidosis also has an effect on the GI system, causing anorexia, nausea, and vomiting. (See *Signs and symptoms of metabolic acidosis*.)

What tests show

Several test results may be helpful in diagnosing and treating metabolic acidosis.
• ABG analysis is the key diagnostic test for detecting metabolic acidosis. Typically, the pH is below 7.35. The $Paco_2$ may be less

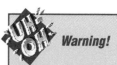

Warning!

Signs and symptoms of metabolic acidosis

The following assessment findings commonly occur in patients with metabolic acidosis:
• confusion
• decreased deep-tendon reflexes
• dull headache
• hyperkalemic signs and symptoms, including abdominal cramping, diarrhea, muscle weakness, and electrocardiogram changes
• hypotension
• Kussmaul's respirations
• lethargy
• warm, dry skin.

ABG results in metabolic acidosis

This chart shows typical arterial blood gas (ABG) findings in uncompensated and compensated metabolic acidosis.

	Uncompensated	Compensated
pH	< 7.35	Normal
$Paco_2$ (mm Hg)	Normal	< 35
HCO_3^- (mEq/L)	< 22	< 22

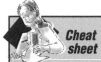

Cheat sheet

Causes of metabolic acidosis

- Loss of bicarbonate (base)
- Accumulation of metabolic acids (acid)
- Overproduction of ketone bodies
- Decreased ability of kidneys to excrete acids
- Excessive GI losses from diarrhea, intestinal malabsorption, or urinary diversion to the ileum
- Hyperaldosteronism
- Use of potassium-sparing diuretics
- Poisoning or toxic drug reaction

than 35 mm Hg, indicating compensatory attempts by the lungs to rid the body of excess CO_2. (See *ABG results in metabolic acidosis.*)

- Serum potassium levels are usually elevated as hydrogen ions move into the cells and potassium moves out to maintain electroneutrality.
- Blood glucose and serum ketone levels rise in patients with diabetic ketoacidosis (DKA).
- Plasma lactate levels rise in patients with lactic acidosis. (See *A look at lactic acidosis.*)
- The anion gap is increased—this measurement is calculated by subtracting the amount of negative ion (chloride plus bicarbonate) from the amount of the positive ion (sodium). Sometimes the amount of potassium ion is added to the amount of positive ion, but the amount of potassium ion is usually so small that the calculation doesn't change. The normal anion gap is 8 to 14 mEq/L.
- ECG changes associated with hyperkalemia—such as tall T waves, prolonged PR intervals, and wide QRS complexes— may be found.

How metabolic acidosis is treated

Treatment aims to correct the acidosis as quickly as possible by addressing both the symptoms and the underlying cause. Respiratory compensation is usually the first line of therapy, including mechanical ventilation, if needed.

Adjust the potassium

For diabetics, expect to administer rapid-acting insulin to reverse DKA and drive potassium back into the cell. For any patient with

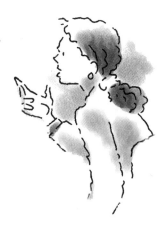

A look at lactic acidosis

Lactate, produced as a result of carbohydrate metabolism, is metabolized by the liver. The normal lactate level is 0.93 to 1.65 mEq/L. With tissue hypoxia, however, cells are forced to switch to anaerobic metabolism and more lactate is produced. When lactate accumulates in the body faster than it can be metabolized, lactic acidosis occurs. It can happen any time the demand for oxygen in the body is greater than its availability.

The causes of lactic acidosis include septic shock, cardiac arrest, pulmonary disease, seizures, and strenuous exercise.

The latter two cause transient lactic acidosis. Hepatic disorders can also cause lactic acidosis, because the liver isn't able to metabolize lactate.

Treatment
Treatment focuses on eliminating the underlying cause. If the pH is under 7.1, sodium bicarbonate may be given. Use caution when administering sodium bicarbonate, however, because it may cause alkalosis.

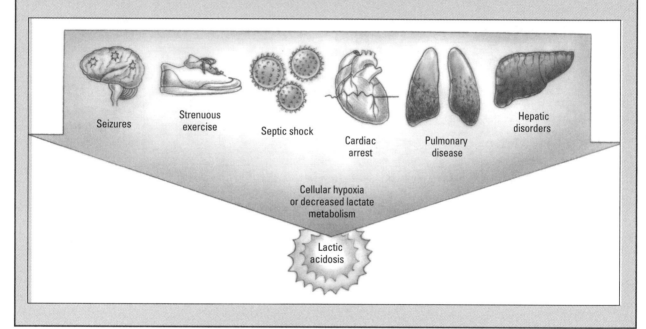

Seizures

Strenuous exercise

Septic shock

Cardiac arrest

Pulmonary disease

Hepatic disorders

Cellular hypoxia or decreased lactate metabolism

Lactic acidosis

metabolic acidosis, monitor serum potassium levels. Even though high serum levels exist initially, serum potassium levels will drop as the acidosis is corrected and may result in hypokalemia. Any other electrolyte imbalances are evaluated and corrected.

Replace the bicarbonate

Sodium bicarbonate is administered I.V. to neutralize blood acidity in patients with a pH lower than 7.1 and bicarbonate loss. Fluids are replaced parenterally as required. Dialysis may be initiated in patients with renal failure or a toxic reaction to a drug. Such patients may receive an antibiotic to treat sources of infection or an antidiarrheal to treat diarrhea-induced bicarbonate loss.

Be on the alert

Watch for worsening of CNS status or deteriorating laboratory and ABG test results. Ventilatory support may be needed, so prepare for intubation. Dialysis may be needed for patients with renal failure, especially when complicated by diabetes. Maintain a patent I.V. line to administer emergency drugs, and flush the line with normal saline solution before and after administering sodium bicarbonate because the bicarbonate may inactivate or cause precipitation of many drugs. (See *Acidosis and dopamine*.)

How you intervene

If your patient is at risk for metabolic acidosis, careful monitoring can help prevent it from developing. If your patient has metabolic acidosis, nursing care includes immediate emergency interventions and long-term treatment of the condition and its underlying causes. Observe the following guidelines:

Assess and monitor

- Monitor vital signs, and assess cardiac rhythm.
- Prepare for mechanical ventilation or dialysis as required.
- Monitor the patient's neurologic status closely because changes can occur rapidly. Notify the doctor of any changes in the patient's condition.
- Insert an I.V. line, as ordered, and maintain patent I.V. access. Have a large-bore catheter in place for emergency situations. Administer I.V. fluid, a vasopressor, an antibiotic, and other medications, as prescribed.
- Administer sodium bicarbonate as ordered. Remember to flush the I.V. line with normal saline solution before and after giving bicarbonate because the chemical can inactivate many drugs or cause them to precipitate. Be aware that too much bicarbonate can cause metabolic alkalosis and pulmonary edema.
- Position the patient to promote chest expansion and facilitate breathing. If the patient is stuporous, turn him frequently. (See *Teaching about metabolic acidosis*.)
- Take steps to help eliminate the underlying cause. For example, administer insulin and I.V. fluids as prescribed to reverse DKA.
- Watch for any secondary changes, such as declining blood pressure, that hypovolemia may cause.

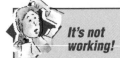

It's not working!

Acidosis and dopamine

If you're administering dopamine to a patient and it isn't raising his blood pressure as you expected, investigate your patient's pH. A pH level below 7.1 (as can happen in severe metabolic acidosis) causes resistance to vasopressor therapy. Correct the pH level, and the dopamine may prove to be more effective.

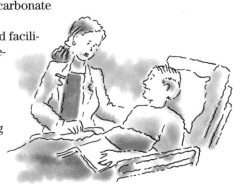

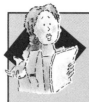

Chart smart

Documenting metabolic acidosis

When caring for a patient with metabolic acidosis, document the following information:
• assessment findings, including results of neurologic examination
• intake and output
• notification of doctor
• patient teaching
• prescribed medications and I.V. therapy, and patient's response
• safety measures implemented
• serum electrolyte levels and arterial blood gas results
• ventilator or dialysis data
• vital signs and cardiac rhythm.

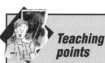

Teaching points

Teaching about metabolic acidosis

Make sure you cover these topics with your patient, and then evaluate his learning:
• basics of the condition and its treatment
• testing of blood glucose levels, if indicated
• need for strict adherence to antidiabetic therapy, if appropriate
• avoidance of alcohol
• warning signs and symptoms and when to report them
• prescribed medications
• avoidance of ingestion of toxic substances.

• Monitor the patient's renal function by recording intake and output. (See *Documenting metabolic acidosis.*)
• Watch for changes in the serum electrolyte levels, and monitor ABG results throughout treatment to check for overcorrection.
• Orient the patient as needed. If he's confused, take steps to ensure his safety, such as keeping the bed in the lowest position.
• Investigate reasons for the patient's ingestion of toxic substances.

Questions to consider

Physical examination and further diagnostic tests may provide additional information about your patient's metabolic acidosis. As you reevaluate the patient's condition, consider the following questions:
• Has the patient's LOC returned to normal?
• Have his vital signs stabilized?
• Have his ABG results, blood glucose levels, and serum electrolyte levels improved?
• Is his cardiac output normal?
• Has he regained a normal sinus rhythm (or his previously stable underlying rhythm)?
• Is he ventilating adequately?

Metabolic alkalosis

Metabolic alkalosis is characterized by a blood pH above 7.45 and is accompanied by an HCO_3^- level above 26 mEq/L. In acute metabolic alkalosis, the HCO_3^- level may be as high as 50 mEq/L. With early diagnosis and prompt treatment, the prognosis for effective treatment is good. Left untreated, metabolic alkalosis can result in coma, arrhythmias, and death.

How it happens

In metabolic alkalosis, the underlying mechanisms include a loss of hydrogen ions (acid), a gain in HCO_3^-, or both. $Paco_2$ greater than 45 mm Hg (possibly as high as 60 mm Hg) indicates that the lungs are compensating for the alkalosis. Renal compensation is more effective, but slower as well. Metabolic alkalosis is commonly associated with hypokalemia, particularly from the use of thiazides, furosemide, ethacrynic acid, and other diuretics that deplete potassium stores. In hypokalemia, the kidneys conserve potassium. At the same time, the kidneys also increase the excretion of hydrogen ions, which prompts alkalosis from the loss of acid. Metabolic alkalosis may also occur with hypochloremia and hypocalcemia. (See *What happens in metabolic alkalosis.*)

GI problems

Metabolic alkalosis can result from many causes, the most common of which is excessive acid loss from the GI tract. Vomiting causes loss of hydrochloric acid from the stomach. Children who have pyloric stenosis can develop this disorder. Alkalosis also results from nasogastric (NG) suctioning, presenting a risk for surgical patients and patients with GI disorders.

Diuretic risks

Diuretic therapy presents another risk of metabolic alkalosis. Thiazide and loop diuretics can lead to a loss of hydrogen, potassium, and chloride ion from the kidneys. Hypokalemia causes hydrogen ion excretion from the kidneys as they try to conserve potassium. Potassium moves out of the cell as hydrogen moves in, resulting in alkalosis.

With the fluid loss of diuresis, the kidneys attempt to conserve sodium and water. For sodium to be reabsorbed, hydrogen ions must be excreted. In a process known as contraction alkalosis, bicarbonate is reabsorbed and metabolic alkalosis results.

Now I get it!

What happens in metabolic alkalosis

This series of illustrations shows at the cellular level how metabolic alkalosis develops.

Step 1

As bicarbonate ions (HCO_3^-) start to accumulate in the body, chemical buffers (in extracellular fluid and cells) bind with the ions. *No signs are detectable at this stage.*

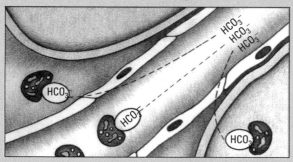

Step 2

Excess bicarbonate ions that don't bind with chemical buffers elevate serum pH levels, which in turn depress chemoreceptors in the medulla. Depression of those chemoreceptors causes a decrease in respiratory rate, which increases the $Paco_2$. The additional CO_2 combines with water to form carbonic acid (H_2CO_3). *Note:* Lowered oxygen levels limit respiratory compensation. *Look for a serum pH level above 7.45, a bicarbonate level above 26 mEq/L, a rising $Paco_2$, and slow, shallow respirations.*

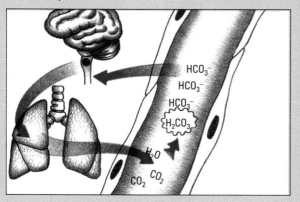

Step 3

When the bicarbonate level exceeds 28 mEq/L, the renal glomeruli can no longer reabsorb excess bicarbonate. That excess bicarbonate is excreted in the urine; hydrogen ions are retained. *Look for alkaline urine and pH and bicarbonate levels that return slowly to normal.*

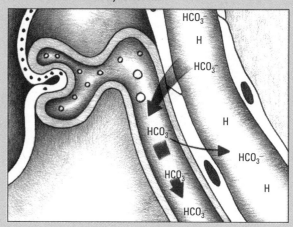

Step 4

To maintain electrochemical balance, the kidneys excrete excess sodium ions (Na), water, and bicarbonate. *Look for polyuria initially, then signs and symptoms of hypovolemia, including thirst and dry mucous membranes.*

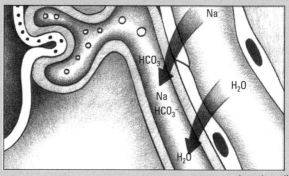

(continued)

What happens in metabolic alkalosis *(continued)*

Step 5

Lowered hydrogen ion levels in the extracellular fluid cause the ions to diffuse out of the cells. To maintain the balance of charge across the cell membrane, extracellular potassium ions (K) move into the cells. *Look for signs and symptoms of hypokalemia, including anorexia, muscle weakness, loss of reflexes, and others.*

Step 6

As hydrogen ion levels decline, calcium (Ca) ionization decreases. That decrease in ionization makes nerve cells more permeable to sodium ions. Sodium ions moving into nerve cells stimulate neural impulses and produce overexcitability of the peripheral and central nervous systems. *Look for tetany, belligerence, irritability, disorientation, and seizures.*

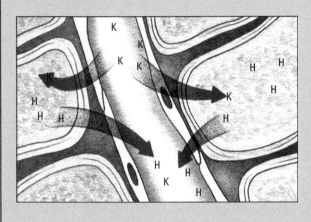

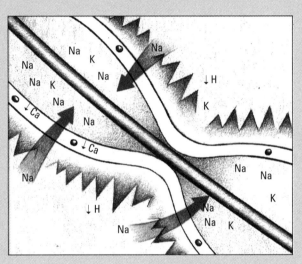

More metabolic mishaps

Cushing's disease can lead to metabolic alkalosis by causing retention of sodium and chloride and urinary loss of potassium and hydrogen. Rebound alkalosis following correction of organic acidosis, such as after cardiac arrest and administration of sodium bicarbonate, can also cause metabolic alkalosis. Posthypercapnic alkalosis occurs when chronic CO_2 retention is corrected by mechanical ventilation and the kidneys haven't yet corrected the chronically high HCO_3^- levels.

Metabolic alkalosis can also result from kidney disease, such as renal artery stenosis, or from multiple transfusions. Certain drugs, such as corticosteroids and antacids that contain sodium bicarbonate, can also lead to metabolic alkalosis. (See *Drugs associated with metabolic alkalosis.*)

What to look for

Initially, your patient may have slow, shallow respirations as hypoventilation, a compensatory mechanism, occurs. However, this mechanism is limited because hypoxemia soon develops, which stimulates ventilation. The signs and symptoms of metabolic alkalosis are commonly associated with an underlying condition. The resulting hypokalemic or hypocalcemic ECG changes may be seen, as well as hypotension.

It hits the neuro system

Metabolic alkalosis results in neuromuscular excitability, which causes muscle twitching, weakness, and tetany. Reflexes are hyperactive. The patient may experience numbness and tingling of the fingers, toes, and mouth area. Neurologic symptoms include apathy and confusion. Seizures, stupor, and coma may result.

Keep track of these tracts

If hypokalemia affects the GI tract, the patient will probably experience anorexia, nausea, and vomiting. If it affects the genitourinary (GU) tract—that is, if the kidneys are affected—polyuria may result. If left untreated, metabolic alkalosis can result in arrhythmias and death. (See *Signs and symptoms of metabolic alkalosis*, page 214.)

What tests show

The following tests may be helpful in the diagnosis and treatment of metabolic alkalosis.
- ABG analysis may reveal a blood pH above 7.45 and an HCO_3^- level above 26 mEq/L. If the underlying cause is excessive acid loss, the HCO_3^- level may be normal. The $Paco_2$ level may be above 45 mm Hg, indicating respiratory compensation. (See *ABG results in metabolic alkalosis*, page 214.)
- Serum electrolyte levels usually indicate low potassium, calcium, and chloride levels. HCO_3^- levels are elevated.
- ECG changes may occur, such as a low T wave that merges with the P wave.

How metabolic alkalosis is treated

Treatment aims to correct the acid-base imbalance.
- I.V. administration of ammonium chloride is rarely done but may be necessary in severe cases.

Drugs associated with metabolic alkalosis

The following drugs are commonly associated with metabolic alkalosis:
- antacids (sodium bicarbonate, calcium carbonate)
- corticosteroids
- thiazide and loop diuretics.

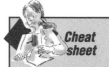

Cheat sheet

Causes of metabolic alkalosis

- Excessive acid loss from the GI tract
- Diuretic therapy (from hydrogen, potassium, and chloride loss from the kidneys)
- Cushing's disease (from retention of sodium and chloride and excretion of potassium and hydrogen)

ABG results in metabolic alkalosis

This chart shows typical arterial blood gas (ABG) findings in uncompensated and compensated metabolic alkalosis.

	Uncompensated	Compensated
pH	> 7.45	Normal
$Paco_2$ (mm Hg)	Normal	> 45
HCO_3^- (mEq/L)	> 26	> 26

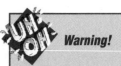

Warning!

Signs and symptoms of metabolic alkalosis

The following assessment findings commonly occur in patients with metabolic alkalosis:
• anorexia
• apathy
• confusion
• cyanosis
• hypotension
• loss of reflexes
• muscle twitching
• nausea
• paresthesia
• polyuria
• vomiting
• weakness.

• Thiazide diuretics and NG suctioning are discontinued. An antiemetic may be administered to treat underlying nausea and vomiting.
• Acetazolamide (Diamox) may be added to increase renal excretion of HCO_3^-.

How you intervene

If your patient is at risk for metabolic alkalosis, careful monitoring can help prevent its development. If your patient has metabolic alkalosis, follow these guidelines:
• Monitor vital signs, including cardiac rhythm and respiratory pattern.
• Assess the patient's LOC when taking his health history or by talking with him while you're performing the physical examination. For instance, apathy and confusion may be evident in a patient's conversation.
• Administer oxygen, as ordered, to treat hypoxemia.
• Institute seizure precautions when needed, and explain them to the patient and his family. (See *Teaching about metabolic alkalosis.*)
• Maintain patent I.V. access as ordered.
• Administer diluted potassium solutions with an infusion device.
• Monitor intake and output. (See *Documenting metabolic alkalosis.*)
• Infuse 0.9% ammonium chloride no faster than 1 L over 4 hours. Faster administration may cause hemolysis of red blood cells. Don't administer the drug to a patient who has hepatic or renal disease.

Assess the patient's level of consciousness.

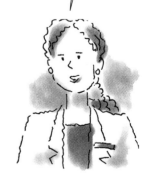

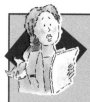

Chart smart

Documenting metabolic alkalosis

When providing nursing care to a patient with metabolic alkalosis, document:
- vital signs
- I.V. therapy
- interventions and the patient's response
- medications
- intake and output
- oxygen therapy
- notification of doctor
- safety measures
- serum electrolyte levels and arterial blood gas results.

Teaching points

Teaching about metabolic alkalosis

Make sure you cover these topics with your patient, and then evaluate his learning of:
- basics of the condition and its treatment
- need to avoid overuse of alkaline agents and diuretics
- prescribed medications, especially adverse effects of potassium-wasting diuretics or potassium chloride supplements
- warning signs and symptoms and when to report them.

- Irrigate an NG tube with normal saline solution instead of tap water, to prevent loss of gastric electrolytes.
- Assess laboratory test results, such as ABG and serum electrolyte levels. Notify the doctor of any changes.
- Watch closely for signs of muscle weakness, tetany, or decreased activity.

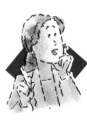

Quick quiz

1. The body compensates for chronic respiratory alkalosis by developing:
- A. metabolic alkalosis.
- B. respiratory acidosis.
- C. metabolic acidosis.

Answer: C. When hypocapnia lasts more than 6 hours, the kidneys compensate by increasing excretion of HCO_3^- and reducing excretion of hydrogen ions. Hydrogen ions return to the blood to decrease the pH, causing chemoreceptors in the medulla to decrease the respiratory rate.

2. You're taking care of a patient with obesity-hypoventilation syndrome. You expect to see signs of chronic respiratory acidosis in the patient's ABG results. Which of the following compensatory mechanisms do you look for?

    A.   Respiratory alkalosis
    B.   Metabolic acidosis
    C.   Metabolic alkalosis

Answer: C. As respiratory mechanisms fail, the body compensates by using the increased $Paco_2$ to excrete hydrogen and to stimulate the kidneys to retain HCO_3^- and sodium ions. As a result, more sodium bicarbonate is available to buffer free hydrogen ions (metabolic alkalosis). Ammonium ions are also excreted to remove hydrogen.

3. If your patient's NG tube is attached to suction, you know the patient may develop metabolic alkalosis. The body compensates for metabolic alkalosis by developing which of the following?

    A.   Respiratory alkalosis
    B.   Respiratory acidosis
    C.   Metabolic acidosis

Answer: B. Excess unbound HCO_3^- elevates blood pH, which depresses the chemoreceptors in the medulla, decreasing respirations and increasing blood CO_2 levels (respiratory acidosis). CO_2 combines with water to form H_2CO_3.

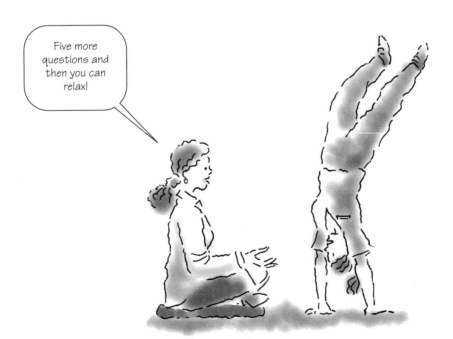

4. When assessing a patient with DKA, you detect Kussmaul's respirations. You realize the body is compensating for primary metabolic acidosis with:

    A.   respiratory alkalosis.

    B.   respiratory acidosis.

    C.   metabolic alkalosis.

Answer: A. Excess hydrogen that can't be buffered reduces blood pH and stimulates chemoreceptors in the medulla, which in turn increases the respiratory rate (leading to respiratory alkalosis). This mechanism lowers CO_2 levels and allows more hydrogen to bind with HCO_3^-.

5. In a patient with COPD, which of the following is the primary imbalance?

    A.   Respiratory alkalosis

    B.   Respiratory acidosis

    C.   Metabolic alkalosis

Answer: B. COPD results in destruction of the alveoli, thereby decreasing the surface area of the lungs available for gas exchange. With alveolar ventilation decreased, the $Paco_2$ increases. The CO_2 combines with H_2O to form excessive amounts of H_2CO_3. The H_2CO_3 dissociates to release free hydrogen and bicarbonate ions, thereby decreasing the pH (respiratory acidosis).

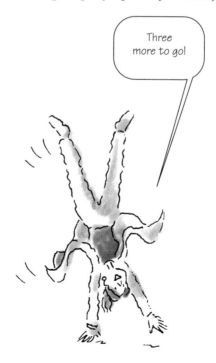

6.   Your bedridden patient has these ABG results: pH, 7.5; $Paco_2$, 26 mm Hg; HCO_3^-, 24 mEq/L. He's dyspneic and he has a swollen right calf. The patient most likely is suffering from:

    A.   a pulmonary embolus.

    B.   heart failure.

    C.   dehydration.

Answer: A. Unexplained respiratory alkalosis may mean a pulmonary embolus (in this case, most likely a thrombus in the leg as a result of immobility).

7.   If administering dopamine to a patient with hypotension proves ineffective, how should you proceed?

    A.   Change to dobutamine.

    B.   Investigate the patient's pH.

    C.   Check the patient's serum potassium level.

Answer: B. If you're administering dopamine to a patient and it isn't elevating his blood pressure as you expected, you should investigate the patient's pH. A pH level below 7.1 causes resistance to vasopressor therapy.

8.   Before and after you administer sodium bicarbonate, you should flush the I.V. line with:

    A.   heparin.

    B.   sterile water.

    C.   normal saline solution.

Answer: C. You should flush the I.V. line with normal saline solution before and after giving bicarbonate.

Scoring

☆☆☆   If you answered all eight questions correctly, *wow!* Test the pH of the nearest pool, and jump in for a refreshing swim!

☆☆   If you answered five to seven correctly, excellent! You're just about ready to do your first solo balancing act!

☆   If you answered fewer than five correctly, take heart. You're still a boffo buffer in our book. (*Buffer*, get it? For chemical buffers? Oh well, can't win 'em all.)

Part III

Disorders that cause imbalances

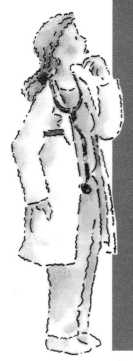

Heart failure

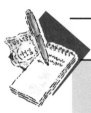

Just the facts

This chapter explains the basics about this disorder and its effects on fluid, electrolyte, and acid-base balance. In this chapter, you'll learn:

♦ what heart failure is and how it happens

♦ which imbalances can occur as a result of heart failure or its treatment

♦ how to effectively care for patients with heart failure

♦ how to chart the care you give to patients with heart failure.

A look at heart failure

Heart failure is a clinical syndrome of myocardial dysfunction that causes diminished cardiac output. From the subtle loss of normal ventricular function to the presence of symptoms that no longer respond to medical therapy, heart failure occurs when the heart can't pump enough blood to meet the body's metabolic needs. How the ventricles function depends on the interaction among the four factors that regulate the cardiac output:
- preload (volume)
- afterload (pressure)
- contractility (squeeze)
- heart rate.

Cycle survey

It's important to remember that two periods—diastole and systole—make up the normal cardiac cycle. Diastole is the portion of the cycle during which the heart is at rest, filling the ventricles with blood. Systole is the portion of the cycle during which the ventricles contract, ejecting their volume of blood.

Chain reaction

When any of the four interrelated factors are altered, cardiac output may be altered. For example, when the preload (volume) delivered to the ventricles during diastole is inadequate, cardiac output may be compromised, and heart failure may result. Further, when the afterload (pressure) against which the ventricles must contract is elevated during systole, cardiac output may be compromised and heart failure may result.

Heart failure may result when the balance of these four interrelated factors is altered during either diastole or systole. When heart failure is due to inadequate filling of the ventricles, the syndrome is described as diastolic heart failure; when it's due to inadequate contraction, systolic heart failure. This ventricular dysfunction may occur in either the left or right ventricle.

How it happens

Normally, the pumping actions of the right and left sides of the heart complement each other, producing a synchronized and continuous blood flow. With an underlying disorder, though, one side may fail while the other continues to function normally for some time. Because of the prolonged strain, the functioning side eventually fails, resulting in total heart failure.

First, the left side

Usually, the heart's left side fails first. Left-sided heart failure typically leads to and is the main cause of right-sided heart failure.

Here's what happens: Diminished left ventricular function allows blood to pool in the ventricle and atrium and eventually to back up into the pulmonary veins and capillaries. (See *Left-sided heart failure.*)

As the pulmonary circulation becomes engorged, rising capillary pressure pushes sodium and water into the interstitial space, causing pulmonary edema. The right ventricle becomes stressed because it's pumping against greater pulmonary vascular resistance and left ventricular pressure.

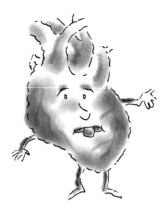

Then, the right side

As the right ventricle starts to fail, symptoms worsen. Blood pools in the right ventricle and the right atrium. The backed-up blood causes pressure and congestion in the venae cavae and systemic circulation. (See *Right-sided heart failure,* page 224.)

Blood also distends the visceral veins, especially the hepatic vein. As the liver and spleen become engorged, their function is impaired. Rising capillary pressure forces excess fluid from the

Now I get it!

Left-sided heart failure

This illustration shows what happens when left-sided heart failure develops. The left side of the heart normally receives oxygenated blood returning from the lungs and then pumps blood through the aorta to all tissues. Left-sided heart failure causes blood to back up into the lungs, which results in such respiratory symptoms as tachypnea and shortness of breath.

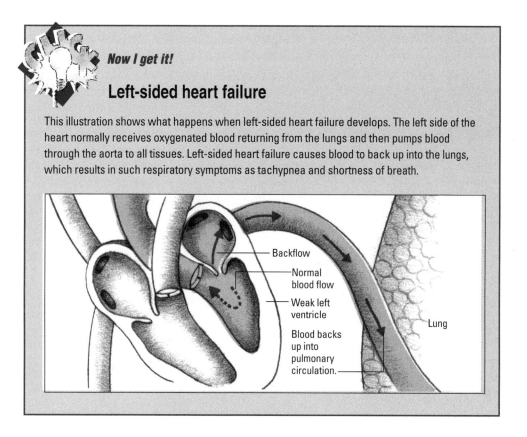

capillaries into the interstitial space. This causes tissue edema, especially in the lower extremities and abdomen.

Compensatory responses

When the heart begins to fail, the body responds with three compensatory mechanisms to maintain blood flow to the tissues. These mechanisms include sympathetic nervous system activation, increased preload, and hypertrophy of the cardiac cells. Initially, the compensatory mechanisms serve to increase the cardiac output. However, these mechanisms will eventually contribute to heart failure.

The sympathetic nervous system

Diminished cardiac output activates the sympathetic nervous system, causing an increased heart rate and increased contractility. This initially increases the cardiac output. However, both increased heart rate and increased contractility increase the heart's

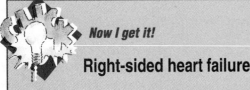

Now I get it!

Right-sided heart failure

This illustration shows what happens when right-sided heart failure develops. The right side of the heart normally receives deoxygenated blood returning from the tissues and then pumps that blood through the pulmonary artery into the lungs. Right-sided heart failure causes blood to back up past the vena cava and into the systemic circulation. This, in turn, causes enlargement of the abdominal organs and tissue edema.

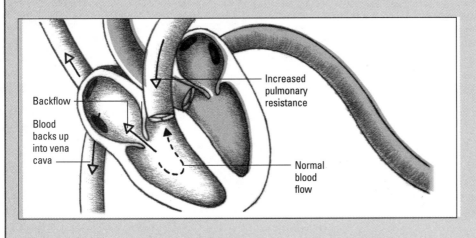

demand for oxygen, thereby increasing the work that the heart must do to meet this demand. (Over time, this contributes to heart failure, rather than compensating for it.)

With increased demand, blood then shunts away from areas of low priority (such as the skin and kidneys) to areas of high priority (such as the heart and brain).

Pulmonary congestion, a complication of heart failure, can lead to pulmonary edema, a life-threatening condition. Decreased perfusion to major organs, particularly the brain and kidneys, may cause these organs to fail, necessitating dialysis for kidney failure. The patient's LOC may decrease, possibly leading to coma. Myocardial infarction (MI) may occur because myocardial oxygen demands can't be sufficiently met.

Increased preload

When blood is shunted away from areas of low priority, the kidneys, sensing a reduced renal blood flow, activate the renin-angiotensin-aldosterone system. This results in sodium and water retention, which increases blood volume (preload). Again, initially this serves to increase the cardiac output. However, over time, the heart can't pump this increased volume effectively, and heart failure is facilitated rather than compensated.

Cardiac hypertrophy

When the heart is under strain, it responds by increasing its muscle mass, a condition called cardiac hypertrophy. As the cardiac wall thickens, the heart's demand for blood and oxygen grows. The patient's heart may be unable to meet this demand, further compromising the condition.

When pressure inside the chambers (usually the left ventricle) rises for a sustained period, the heart compensates by stretching, a condition called cardiac dilation. Eventually, stretched muscle fibers become overstrained, reducing the heart's ability to pump.

Imbalances caused by heart failure

Several imbalances may result from the heart's failure to pump blood and perfuse tissues adequately. Imbalances may also result from stimulation of the renin-angiotensin-aldosterone system or from certain treatments such as diuretic therapy. Fluid, electrolyte, and acid-base imbalances associated with heart failure include:
- hypervolemia and hypovolemia
- hyperkalemia and hypokalemia
- hypochloremia, hypomagnesemia, hyponatremia
- metabolic acidosis and alkalosis
- respiratory acidosis and alkalosis.

Problems with volume

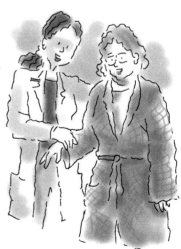

Hypervolemia—the most common fluid imbalance associated with heart failure—results from the heart's failure to propel blood forward, consequent vascular pooling, and sodium and water reabsorption triggered by the renin-angiotensin-aldosterone system. Excess extracellular fluid volume commonly causes peripheral edema.

Hypovolemia is usually associated with overly aggressive diuretic therapy and can be especially dangerous in older adult patients because it causes confusion and hypotension.

Hyponatremia

Hyponatremia may result from sodium loss due to diuretic abuse. In some cases, it may result from a dilutional effect that occurs when water reabsorption is greater than sodium reabsorption.

Other electrolyte imbalances

In patients with heart failure, prolonged use of diuretic without adequate potassium replacement can cause hypokalemia. Hypomagnesemia may accompany hypokalemia, particularly if the patient is receiving a diuretic. Many diuretics cause the kidneys to excrete magnesium.

Hyperkalemia may occur from the use of a potassium-sparing diuretic. Hypochloremia results from excessive diuretic therapy.

Lactic acid on the rise

When cells don't receive enough oxygen, they produce more lactic acid. Poor tissue perfusion in the patient with heart failure allows lactic acid to accumulate, which in turn leads to metabolic acidosis. Metabolic alkalosis may be caused by excessive diuretic use, which causes bicarbonate retention.

In the early stages of heart failure, as the respiratory rate increases, more carbon dioxide (CO_2) is blown off from the lungs, which raises the pH and leads to respiratory alkalosis. As heart failure progresses, gas exchange is further impaired. CO_2 accumulates, resulting in respiratory acidosis.

What causes heart failure

A wide range of pathophysiologic processes can cause heart failure, including conditions that directly damage the heart, such as MI, myocarditis, myocardial fibrosis, and ventricular aneurysm. The damage from these disorders causes a subsequent decrease in the contractility of the heart.

Ventricular overload can also cause heart failure. This overload may be caused by increased blood volume in the heart (called increased preload) as a result of aortic insufficiency or a ventricular septal defect. Systemic or pulmonary hypertension or an elevation in pressure against which the heart must pump (called increased afterload) as a result of aortic or pulmonic stenosis may also cause this overload.

Restricted ventricular diastolic filling, characterized by the presence of so little blood that the ventricle can't pump it effectively, can also cause heart failure. Such diastolic filling is triggered by constrictive pericarditis or cardiomyopathy, tachyarrhythmias, cardiac tamponade, or mitral or aortic stenosis and usually occurs in older patients.

Increasing the risk

Certain conditions can predispose a person to heart failure, especially if he has an underlying disease. Such conditions include:
• anemia, which causes the heart rate to speed up to maintain tissue oxygenation
• pregnancy and thyrotoxicosis, which increase the demand for cardiac output
• infections, which increase metabolic demands and further burden the heart
• increased physical activity, emotional stress, greater sodium or water intake, or failure to comply with the prescribed treatment regimen for underlying heart disease
• pulmonary embolism, which elevates pulmonary arterial pressures and can cause right-sided heart failure.

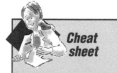

Cheat sheet

Causes of heart failure

• Myocardial infarction
• Myocardial fibrosis
• Ventricular aneurysm
• Ventricular overload
• Restricted ventricular diastolic filling

What to look for

Signs and symptoms of heart failure vary according to the site of the failure and the stage of the disease. Expect to encounter a combination of the following findings.

Left-sided heart failure

If your patient has left-sided heart failure and tissue hypoxia, then he'll probably complain of fatigue, weakness, orthopnea, and exertional dyspnea. The patient may also report paroxysmal nocturnal dyspnea.

He may use two or three pillows to elevate his head to sleep, or he may have to sleep sitting up in a chair. Shortness of breath may awaken him shortly after he falls asleep, forcing him to quickly sit upright to catch his breath. He may have dyspnea, coughing, and wheezing even when he sits up. Tachypnea may occur, and you may note crackles on inspiration. Coughing may progress to the point where the patient produces pink, frothy sputum as he develops pulmonary edema.

The patient may be tachycardic. Auscultation of heart sounds may reveal third and fourth heart sounds as the myocardium becomes less compliant. Hypoxia and hypercapnia can affect the central nervous system, causing restlessness, confusion, and a progressive decrease in the patient's level of consciousness. Later, with continued decrease in cardiac output, the kidneys may be affected, and oliguria may develop.

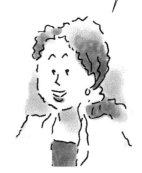

Expect a combination of findings.

Right-sided heart failure

Inspection of a patient with right-sided heart failure may reveal venous engorgement. When the patient sits upright, his neck veins may appear distended, feel rigid, and exhibit exaggerated pulsations. Edema may develop, and the patient may report a weight gain. Nail beds may appear cyanotic. Anorexia and nausea may occur. The liver may be enlarged and slightly tender. This condition may progress to congestive hepatomegaly, ascites, and jaundice.

Advanced heart failure

In a patient with advanced heart failure, pulse pressure may be diminished, reflecting reduced stroke volume. Occasionally, diastolic pressure rises from generalized vasoconstriction. The skin feels cool and clammy. Progression of heart failure may lead to palpitations, chest tightness, and arrhythmias. Cardiac arrest may occur. (See *Recognizing advanced heart failure.*)

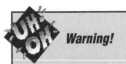

Warning!

Recognizing advanced heart failure

The following assessment findings commonly occur in patients with heart failure:
- cool and clammy skin
- diminished pulse pressure
- elevated diastolic pressure
- chest tightness
- arrhythmias
- cardiac arrest (may occur).

What tests show

Because the causes of heart failure are so varied, several tests may help confirm the diagnosis.
- Electrocardiograms can detect arrhythmias.
- Chest X-rays show edema, effusion, and congestion.
- Echocardiograms reveal enlarged heart chambers and changes in ventricular function.
- Hemodynamic pressure readings reveal increased central venous pressure and pulmonary artery wedge pressure.

How heart failure is treated

Heart failure is a medical emergency. Relieving dyspnea and improving arterial oxygenation are the immediate therapeutic goals. Secondary goals include minimizing or eliminating the underlying cause, reducing sodium and water retention, optimizing cardiac preload and afterload, and enhancing myocardial contractility.

Diuretics: First-line treatment

One or more drugs—such as a diuretic, a vasodilator, or an inotropic agent—are usually needed to manage heart failure. Diuretic therapy, the starting point of this treatment, increases sodium and water elimination by the kidneys. By reducing fluid overload, diuretics decrease total blood volume and relieve circulatory congestion. *For most diuretics to work effectively, the patient must control his sodium intake.*

Diuretics include thiazide diuretics and loop diuretics, such as furosemide and bumetanide. Because thiazide and loop diuretics work at different sites in the nephron, they produce a synergistic effect when given in combination. Potassium-sparing diuretics, such as spironolactone and triamterene, may be used.

Any patient who takes a diuretic should be carefully monitored, because it can disturb the electrolyte balance and lead to metabolic alkalosis, metabolic acidosis, or other complications.

Reducing preload and afterload

Vasodilators can reduce preload or afterload by decreasing arterial and venous vasoconstriction. Reducing preload and afterload helps increase stroke volume and cardiac output.

Angiotensin-converting enzyme (ACE) inhibitors such as captopril decrease both afterload and preload. Because ACE inhibitors prevent potassium loss, hyperkalemia may develop in patients who are also taking a potassium-sparing diuretic. For this reason, diuretic therapy should be discontinued when ACE inhibitor therapy begins.

Nitrates, primarily vasodilators, also dilate arterial smooth muscle at higher doses. Most heart failure patients tolerate nitrates well. Nitrates are available in several forms. I.V., oral, and topical ointment or patches are considered the most useful for heart failure therapy.

Beta-adrenergic blockers such as carvedilol decrease afterload through their vasodilating action. Specifically, they cause peripheral vasodilation, decreasing systemic pressure directly and cardiac workload indirectly. In addition, beta-adrenergic blocker therapy enhances longevity.

Inotropic drugs such as digoxin increase contractility in the failing heart muscle. They also slow conduction through the atrioventricular node. Other drugs—such as dopamine, dobutamine, milrinone, and inamrinone—may be indicated for patients with acute heart failure to increase myocardial contractility and cardiac output. Hydralazine and nitroprusside may also be used to treat heart failure.

Morphine is commonly used in heart failure patients with acute pulmonary edema. Besides reducing anxiety, it decreases preload and afterload by dilating veins.

Urgency may call for surgery

Patients with severe heart failure may require surgery. In cardiomyoplasty, a muscle is wrapped around the failing heart to boost its pumping action. In a left ventriculectomy, a section of

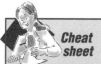

Cheat sheet

Signs and symptoms of heart failure

Left-sided heart failure
• Coughing and pink, frothy sputum
• Exertional dyspnea
• Fatigue
• Oliguria
• Orthopnea
• Pulmonary edema
• Tachycardia
• Tachypnea
• Third and fourth heart sounds
• Weakness

Right-sided heart failure
• Anorexia and nausea
• Arrhythmias
• Cardiac arrest
• Chest tightness
• Cool, clammy skin
• Cyanotic nail beds
• Neck vein distention and rigidity
• Palpitations
• Venous engorgement

nonviable myocardium is removed to reduce ventricular size, which allows the heart to pump more effectively. To help the ventricles propel blood through the vascular system, an intra-aortic balloon counterpulsation or other ventricular assist devices may be implanted. Heart transplant is reserved when there are no other options.

How you intervene

To properly care for a patient with heart failure, you'll need to perform a number of specific nursing interventions, including the following.

Assess, monitor, and administer

• Assess the patient's mental status, and report changes in vital signs or mental status immediately.
• Assess the patient for signs and symptoms of impending cardiac failure, such as fatigue, restlessness, hypotension, rapid respiratory rate, dyspnea, coughing, decreased urine output, liver enlargement, and a rapid, thready pulse.
• Assess the patient for edema. Note the amount and location of the edema and the degree of pitting, if present. (See *Documenting heart failure*.)
• Monitor sodium and fluid intake as prescribed. Hyponatremia and fluid volume deficit can stimulate the renin-angiotensin-aldosterone system and exacerbate heart failure. Usually, mild sodium restriction—whereby the patient uses no added salt—is prescribed.
• Check patient's weight and fluid intake and output daily for significant changes to determine if the patient is in a state of fluid overload. If the patient's weight has increased by two or more pounds over 24 hours, additional diuretic therapy is needed. (See *Teaching about heart failure*.)
• Monitor vital signs, including blood pressure, pulse, respirations, and heart and breath sounds for abnormalities that might indicate a fluid excess or deficit.
• Monitor serum electrolyte levels—especially sodium and potassium—for changes that may indicate an imbalance. Remember that hypokalemia can lead to digoxin toxicity. Monitor arterial blood gas results to assess adequacy of ventilation.
• Maintain continuous cardiac monitoring during acute and advanced stages of disease to identify arrhythmias promptly.
• Administer prescribed medications—such as digoxin, diuretics, ACE inhibitors, and potassium supplements—to support cardiac function and minimize symptoms.

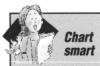

Documenting heart failure

When caring for a patient with heart failure, document:
• condition of skin
• daily weight, intake, and output
• mental status
• notification of doctor
• patient teaching
• tolerance of activity
• positioning of patient and response
• prescribed medications
• edema
• safety measures implemented
• diet restrictions
• vital signs.

Teaching points

Teaching about heart failure

Make sure you cover these topics with your patient, and then evaluate his learning:
• basics of the condition and its treatment
• need for adequate rest
• proper skin care
• prescribed medications
• dietary restrictions
• need to reduce stress and anxiety level
• need for regular exercise
• need for daily weights
• warning signs and symptoms and when to report them
• importance of follow-up.

• Administer oral potassium supplements in orange juice or with meals to promote absorption and prevent gastric irritation.

Provide comfort measures

• Place the patient in Fowler's position, and give supplemental oxygen as ordered to help him breathe more easily.
• Encourage independent activities of daily living as tolerated, though bed rest may be required for some patients. Reposition the patient as needed every 1 to 2 hours. Edematous skin is prone to breakdown.
• Instruct the patient and his family to notify the staff of any changes in the patient's condition, such as increased shortness of breath, chest pain, or dizziness.
• Instruct the patient to call the doctor if his pulse rate is irregular, if it measures fewer than 60 beats/minute, or if he experiences dizziness, blurred vision, shortness of breath, a persistent dry cough, palpitations, increased fatigue, nocturnal dyspnea that comes and goes, swollen ankles, or decreased urine output.

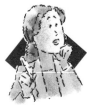

Quick quiz

1. When assessing a patient with left-sided heart failure, you would expect to detect:

    A.   distended neck veins.
    B.   edema of lower extremities.
    C.   dyspnea on exertion.

Answer: C. Diminished left ventricular function allows blood to pool in the ventricle and atrium and eventually to back up into the pulmonary veins and capillaries. As the pulmonary circulation becomes engorged, rising capillary pressure pushes sodium and water into the interstitial space, causing pulmonary edema. Reasons for seeking care include fatigue, exertional dyspnea, orthopnea, weakness, and paroxysmal nocturnal dyspnea.

2. Which of the following is the most common fluid imbalance associated with heart failure?

    A.   Hypervolemia
    B.   Hypovolemia
    C.   Hyperkalemia

Answer: A. Extracellular fluid volume excess results from the heart's failure to propel blood forward, which causes vascular pooling, and from the sodium and water reabsorption triggered by the renin-angiotensin-aldosterone system.

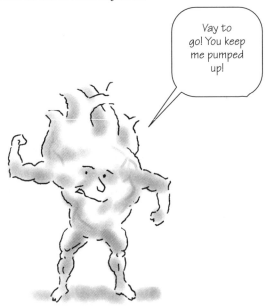

3. Of the following patients admitted to the emergency department, the one *most likely* to develop heart failure is:

    A.   31-year-old woman with pneumonia.

    B.   52-year-old man suffering a heart attack.

    C.   82-year-old woman with chronic dehydration.

Answer: B. The man suffering the heart attack has the greatest risk of developing heart failure from the myocardial damage, which prevents the heart from pumping as effectively as it needs to.

4. Your assessment of a patient reveals an enlarged liver, distended neck veins, and pitting edema of the lower extremities. You suspect that the patient has which of the following conditions?

    A.   Right-sided heart failure

    B.   Left-sided heart failure

    C.   Pulmonary hypertension

Answer: A. These findings indicate that fluid has backed up into the systemic circulation from the right side of the heart.

5. A patient with heart failure is more likely to develop a toxic drug reaction if he has concurrent:

    A.   hyponatremia.

    B.   hyperkalemia.

    C.   hypokalemia.

Answer: C. Hypokalemia, which can occur with diuretic therapy, may lead to digoxin toxicity.

6. The inotropic drug digoxin has which effect on a failing heart muscle?

    A.   Increases contractility

    B.   Decreases afterload

    C.   Decreases both preload and afterload

Answer: A. Inotropic drugs, such as digoxin, increase contractility in the failing heart muscle.

7.   Which drug class given to treat heart failure has been shown to increase longevity?
   A.   ACE inhibitors
   B.   Nitrates
   C.   Beta-adrenergic blockers

Answer: C. Beta-adrenergic blocker therapy enhances longevity.

Scoring

☆☆☆ If you answered all seven questions correctly, we salute your heartfelt effort!

☆☆ If you answered five or six correctly, great! We applaud your boisterous bravado!

☆ If you answered fewer than five correctly, relax. We still commend your veritable valor!

Respiratory failure

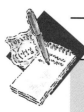

Just the facts

This chapter provides essential information about respiratory failure and its effect on fluid, electrolyte, and acid-base balance. In this chapter, you'll learn:

♦ how respiratory failure occurs

♦ how to recognize the signs and symptoms of respiratory failure

♦ which imbalances occur with respiratory failure and how to manage them.

A look at respiratory failure

When the lungs can't sufficiently maintain arterial oxygenation or eliminate carbon dioxide (CO_2), acute respiratory failure results. Unchecked and untreated, this condition can lead to decreased oxygenation of the body tissues and metabolic acidosis.

In patients with essentially normal lung tissue, respiratory failure usually produces hypercapnia (an above-normal amount of carbon dioxide in the arterial blood) and hypoxemia (a deficiency of oxygen in the arterial blood).

In patients with chronic obstructive pulmonary disease (COPD), however, respiratory failure is signaled only by an acute drop in arterial blood gas (ABG) levels and clinical deterioration. The reason? Patients with COPD consistently have high partial pressure of arterial carbon dioxide ($Paco_2$) levels and low partial pressure of arterial oxygen (Pao_2) levels but are able to compensate and maintain a normal, or near-normal, pH level.

How it happens

In patients with acute respiratory failure, gas exchange is diminished by any combination of the following factors:

- alveolar hypoventilation
- ventilation-perfusion ($\dot{V}/\dot{Q}$) mismatch
- intrapulmonary shunting.

Imbalances associated with respiratory failure include hypervolemia, hypovolemia, hypokalemia, hyperkalemia, respiratory acidosis, respiratory alkalosis, and metabolic acidosis. Let's look at each one individually. (See *What happens in acute respiratory failure.*)

Now I get it!

What happens in acute respiratory failure

Three major malfunctions account for impaired gas exchange and subsequent acute respiratory failure: alveolar hypoventilation, ventilation-perfusion ($\dot{V}/\dot{Q}$) mismatch, and intrapulmonary (right-to-left) shunting.

Alveolar hypoventilation

In alveolar hypoventilation (shown below as the result of airway obstruction), the amount of oxygen brought to the alveoli is diminished, which causes a drop in the partial pressure of arterial oxygen and an increase in alveolar carbon dioxide (CO_2). The accumulation of CO_2 in the alveoli prevents diffusion of adequate amounts of CO_2 from the capillaries, which increases the partial pressure of arterial carbon dioxide.

$\dot{V}/\dot{Q}$ mismatch

$\dot{V}/\dot{Q}$ mismatch, the leading cause of hypoxemia, occurs when insufficient ventilation exists with a normal flow of blood or when, as shown below, normal ventilation exists with an insufficient flow of blood.

Intrapulmonary shunting

Intrapulmonary shunting occurs when blood passes from the right side of the heart to the left side without being oxygenated, as shown below. Shunting can result from untreated ventilation or perfusion mismatches.

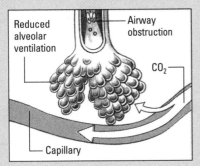

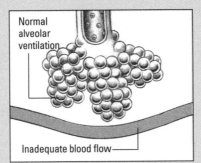

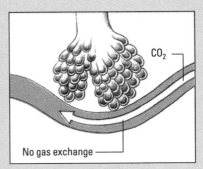

Hypervolemia

Prolonged respiratory treatments, such as nebulizer use, can lead to inhalation and absorption of water vapor. Excessive fluid absorption may also result from increased lung capillary pressure or permeability, which typically occurs in adult respiratory distress syndrome. The excessive fluid absorption may precipitate pulmonary edema.

Hypovolemia

Because the lungs remove water daily through exhalation, an increased respiratory rate can promote excessive loss of water. Excessive loss can also occur with fever or any other condition that increases the metabolic rate and thus the respiratory rate. (See *Causes of respiratory failure.*)

Hypokalemia

If a patient begins to hyperventilate and alkalosis results, hydrogen ions will move out of the cells and potassium ions will move from the blood into the cells. That shift can cause hypokalemia.

Hyperkalemia

In acidosis, excess hydrogen ions move into the cell. Potassium ions then move out of the cell and into the blood to balance the

Causes of respiratory failure

Problems with the brain, lungs, muscles and nerves, or pulmonary circulation can impair gas exchange and cause respiratory failure. Here's a list of conditions that can cause respiratory failure.

Brain	Lungs	Muscles and nerves	Pulmonary circulation
• Anesthesia	• Adult respiratory distress	• Amyotrophic lateral	• Heart failure
• Cerebral hemorrhage	syndrome	sclerosis	• Pulmonary edema
• Cerebral tumor	• Asthma	• Guillain-Barré syndrome	• Pulmonary embolism
• Drug overdose	• Chronic obstructive	• Multiple sclerosis	
• Head trauma	pulmonary disease	• Muscular dystrophy	
• Skull fracture	• Cystic fibrosis	• Myasthenia gravis	
	• Flail chest	• Polio	
	• Massive bilateral	• Spinal cord trauma	
	pneumonia		
	• Sleep apnea		
	• Tracheal obstruction		

positive charges between the two fluid compartments. Hyperkalemia may result.

Respiratory acidosis

Respiratory acidosis, which is due to hypoventilation, results from the inability of the lungs to eliminate sufficient quantities of CO_2. The excess CO_2 combines with water to form carbonic acid. Increased carbonic acid levels result in decreased pH, which contributes to respiratory acidosis.

Respiratory alkalosis

Respiratory alkalosis develops from an excessively rapid respiratory rate, or hyperventilation, and causes excessive carbon dioxide elimination. Loss of carbon dioxide decreases the blood's acid-forming potential and results in respiratory alkalosis.

Metabolic acidosis

Conditions that cause hypoxia cause cells to use anaerobic metabolism. That metabolism creates an increase in the production of lactic acid, which can lead to metabolic acidosis.

What to look for

Hypoxemia and hypercapnia, which are characteristic of acute respiratory failure, stimulate strong compensatory responses from all body systems, especially the respiratory, cardiovascular, and central nervous systems (CNS).

Leading with the lungs

When the body senses hypoxemia or hypercapnia, the respiratory center responds by increasing respiratory depth and then respiratory rate. Signs of labored breathing — flared nostrils, pursed-lip exhalation, and the use of accessory breathing muscles, among others — may signify respiratory failure.

As respiratory failure worsens, muscle retractions between the ribs, above the clavicle, and above the sternum may also occur. The patient is dyspneic and may become cyanotic. Auscultation of the chest reveals diminished or absent breath sounds over the affected area. You may also hear wheezes, crackles, or rhonchi. Respiratory arrest may occur.

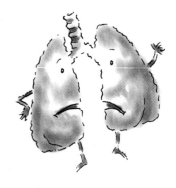

The heart heats up

The sympathetic nervous system usually compensates by increasing the heart rate and constricting blood vessels in an effort to improve cardiac output. The patient's skin may become cool, pale, and clammy. Eventually, as myocardial oxygenation diminishes, cardiac output, blood pressure, and heart rate drop. Arrhythmias develop, and cardiac arrest may occur.

S.O.S. from the CNS

Even a slight disruption in oxygen supply and carbon dioxide elimination can affect brain function and behavior. Hypoxia initially causes anxiety and restlessness, which can progress to marked confusion, agitation, and lethargy. The primary indicator of hypercapnia, headache, occurs as cerebral vessels dilate in an effort to increase the brain's blood supply. If the carbon dioxide level continues to rise, the patient is at risk for seizures and coma. (See *Recognizing worsening respiratory failure*, page 240.)

What tests show

The following diagnostic tests can help in the diagnosis of respiratory failure and can guide its treatment.
• ABG changes indicate respiratory failure. Always compare ABG results with your patient's baseline values. For a patient with previously normal lungs, the pH is usually less than 7.35, the Pao_2 less than 50 mm Hg, and the $Paco_2$ greater than 50 mm Hg. In a patient with COPD, an acute drop in the Pao_2 level of 10 mm Hg or more indicates respiratory failure. *Keep in mind that patients with chronic COPD have a chronically low Pao_2, increased $Paco_2$, increased bicarbonate levels, and normal pH.*
• Chest X-rays may identify an underlying pulmonary condition.
• Electrocardiogram (ECG) changes may show arrhythmias.
• Changes in serum potassium levels may be related to acid-base balance.

How respiratory failure is treated

The underlying cause of respiratory failure must be addressed and the oxygen and carbon dioxide levels improved.

Increase oxygen saturation

Oxygen is given in controlled concentrations, often using a Venturi mask. The goal of oxygen therapy is to prevent oxygen toxicity by administering the lowest dose of oxygen for the shortest period of time, while achieving an oxygen saturation of 90% or more or a Pao_2 level of at least 60 mm Hg.

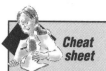

Cheat sheet

Signs and symptoms of respiratory failure

• Increased respiratory depth and rate
• Muscle retraction between the ribs, above the clavicle, and above the sternum
• Increased heart rate, arrhythmias
• Constriction of blood vessels
• Anxiety and restlessness, progressing to confusion, agitation, and lethargy
• Headache
• Acute drop in Pao_2 level of 10 mm Hg or more
• Changes in serum potassium levels

Intubate and ventilate

Intubation and mechanical ventilation are indicated if conservative treatment fails to raise oxygen saturation above 90%. The patient may also be intubated and ventilated if acidemia continues, if he becomes exhausted, or if respiratory arrest occurs. Intubation provides a patent airway. Mechanical ventilation decreases the work of breathing, ventilates the lungs, and improves oxygenation.

Positive end-expiratory pressure (PEEP) therapy may be ordered during mechanical ventilation to improve gas exchange. PEEP maintains positive pressure at the end of expiration, thus preventing the airways and alveoli from collapsing between breaths.

Open the airways

Bronchodilators, especially inhalants, are used to open the airways. If the patient can't inhale effectively or is on a mechanical ventilator, he may receive a bronchodilator via a nebulizer. A corticosteroid, theophylline, and an antibiotic may also be ordered, as may be chest physiotherapy, including postural drainage, chest percussion, and chest vibration. Suctioning may be required to clear the airways. I.V. fluids may be ordered to correct dehydration and to help thin secretions. A diuretic may be used if the patient is experiencing fluid overload.

How you intervene

To care effectively for a patient with respiratory failure, follow these guidelines.

Assess and monitor

- Assess respiratory status; monitor rate, depth, and character of respirations, checking breath sounds for abnormalities.
- Monitor vital signs frequently.
- Monitor the patient's neurologic status; it may become depressed as respiratory failure worsens.
- Ongoing respiratory assessment should include accessory muscle use, changes in breath sounds, ABG analysis, secretion production and clearance, and respiratory rate, depth, and pattern. Notify the doctor if interventions don't improve the patient's condition.
- Monitor fluid status by maintaining accurate fluid intake and output records. Obtain daily weights.
- Evaluate serum electrolyte levels for abnormalities that can occur with acid-base imbalances.

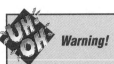

Warning!

Recognizing worsening respiratory failure

The following assessment findings commonly occur in patients with worsening respiratory failure:
- arrhythmias
- bradycardia
- cyanosis
- diminished or absent breath sounds over affected area; may also hear wheezes, crackles, or rhonchi
- dyspnea
- hypotension
- muscle retractions.

- Evaluate ECG results for arrhythmias.
- Monitor oxygen saturation values with a pulse oximeter.
- Monitor ABG levels to assess ventilation.

Maintain and administer

- Intervene as needed to correct underlying respiratory problems and associated alterations in acid-base status.
- Keep a handheld resuscitation bag at the bedside.
- Maintain patent I.V. access as ordered for medication and I.V. fluid administration.
- Administer oxygen as ordered to help maintain adequate oxygenation and to restore the normal respiratory rate.
- Use caution when administering oxygen to a patient with COPD. Increased oxygen levels can depress the breathing stimulus.
- Make sure the ventilator settings are at the ordered parameters.
- Perform chest physiotherapy and postural drainage as needed to promote adequate ventilation.
- If the patient is retaining carbon dioxide, encourage slow deep breaths with pursed lips. Urge him to cough up secretions. If he can't mobilize secretions, suction him when necessary. (See *Teaching about respiratory failure*.)
- Unless the patient is retaining fluid or has heart failure, increase his fluid intake to 2 qt (2 L)/day, to help liquefy secretions.

Provide comfort measures

- Reposition the immobilized patient every 1 to 2 hours.
- Position the patient for optimum lung expansion. Sit the conscious patient upright as tolerated in a supported, forward-leaning position to promote diaphragm movement. Supply an overbed table and pillows for support.
- If the patient isn't on a ventilator, avoid giving him a narcotic or another central nervous system depressant, because either may further suppress respirations.

Provide nutritional support

- Limit carbohydrate intake and increase protein intake, because carbohydrate metabolism causes more carbon dioxide production than protein metabolism.
- Calm and reassure the patient while giving care. Anxiety can raise oxygen demands.
- Pace care activities to maximize the patient's energy level and to provide needed rest. Limit his need to respond verbally. Talking may cause shortness of breath.
- Implement safety measures as needed to protect the patient. Reorient the confused patient.

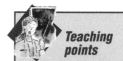

Teaching points

Teaching about respiratory failure

Make sure you cover these points with your patient, and then evaluate his learning:
- basics of the condition and its treatment
- proper pulmonary hygiene and coughing techniques
- need for proper rest
- need to quit smoking, if appropriate
- prescribed medications
- warning signs and symptoms and when to report them
- importance of follow-up appointments
- diet restrictions, if appropriate.

Follow up

• Stress the importance of returning for routine follow-up appointments with the doctor.
• Explain how to recognize signs and symptoms of overexertion, fluid retention, and heart failure. These may include a weight gain of 2 to 3 lb (0.9 to 1.4 kg)/day, edema of the feet or ankles, nausea, loss of appetite, or abdominal tenderness.
• Help the patient develop the knowledge and skills he needs to perform pulmonary hygiene. Encourage adequate hydration to thin secretions — but instruct the patient to notify the doctor of any signs of fluid retention or heart failure.
• Chart all instructions given and care provided. (See *Documenting respiratory failure.*)

Chart smart

Documenting respiratory failure

When caring for a patient with respiratory failure, document:
• breath sounds
• lung secretions
• laboratory results
• breathing exercises and the patient's response
• color and temperature of skin
• daily weights
• intake and output
• measures taken to promote ventilation and the patient's response
• neurologic status
• notification of doctor
• oxygen therapy
• patient teaching
• safety measures.

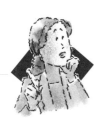

Quick quiz

1. When the body senses hypoxemia or hypercapnia, the brain's respiratory center responds by:
    A.   slowing down the respiratory rate.
    B.   decreasing the heart rate.
    C.   increasing the depth and rate of respirations.

Answer: C. The brain's respiratory center initially causes an increase in respiratory rate. It then causes an increase in respiratory depth in an effort to blow off excess CO_2.

2. Respiratory alkalosis can develop from:
    A.   hyperventilation.
    B.   excessive vomiting.
    C.   prolonged use of antacids.

Answer: A. Respiratory alkalosis develops from an excessively rapid respiratory rate — hyperventilation — which causes excessive CO_2 elimination.

3. Prolonged respiratory treatment, such as nebulizer use, can lead to which of the following conditions?
    A.   Hypovolemia
    B.   Hypervolemia
    C.   Respiratory acidosis

Answer: B. Prolonged respiratory treatments, such as nebulizer use, can lead to the inhalation and absorption of water vapor, which can lead to hypervolemia.

4. The leading cause of hypoxemia is:
    A.   alveolar hypoventilation.
    B.   intrapulmonary shunting.
    C. $\dot{V}/\dot{Q}$ mismatch.

Answer: C. $\dot{V}/\dot{Q}$ mismatch is the leading cause of hypoxemia. It stems from an imbalance in the lungs between ventilation and blood flow.

5. Your patient with respiratory failure has been ordered oxygen by Venturi mask. The goal of oxygen therapy is to achieve a Pa_{O_2} level of at least:
    A.   80 mm Hg.
    B.   60 mm Hg.
    C.   90 mm Hg.

Answer: B. The goal of oxygen therapy is to prevent oxygen toxicity by administering the lowest dose of oxygen for the shortest period of time, while achieving a Pa_{O_2} of at least 60 mm Hg or an oxygen saturation of 90% or more.

6. You're concerned about possible respiratory failure in your newly admitted patient. When administering drug therapy, you should avoid giving him which of the following agents?
    A.   Anticholinergics
    B.   Corticosteroids
    C.   Narcotics

Answer: C. Narcotics depress the respiratory center of the brain and may hasten the development of respiratory failure.

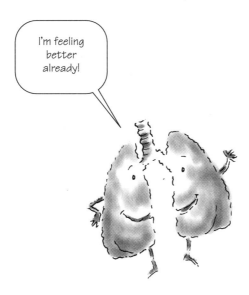

7.   A patient with respiratory failure should limit his intake of:
    A.   protein.
    B.   carbohydrates.
    C.   water.

Answer: B. A patient with respiratory failure should limit carbohydrate intake and increase protein intake because carbohydrate
metabolism causes more carbon dioxide production than protein
metabolism.

Scoring

☆☆☆ If you answered all seven questions correctly, outstanding! You're
an inspiration when it comes to respiration!

☆☆ If you answered five or six correctly, great! Breathe deeply and
appreciate your accomplishment!

☆ If you answered fewer than five correctly, don't worry. Keep your
head up and your heart pumping, there are more chapters to
run through!

Excessive GI fluid loss

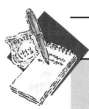

Just the facts

This chapter will guide you through the processes of GI fluid loss and its effect on the patient. In this chapter, you'll learn:

♦ what can cause GI fluid loss

♦ which fluid, electrolyte, and acid-base imbalances occur with excessive GI fluid loss and how to treat them

♦ which signs and symptoms are related to excessive GI fluid loss

♦ what to teach your patient about excessive GI fluid loss.

A look at GI fluid loss

Normally, very little fluid is lost from the GI system. Most of the fluid is reabsorbed in the intestines. However, the potential for significant loss exists because large amounts of fluids — isotonic and hypotonic — pass through the GI system in the course of a day.

Isotonic fluids that may be lost from the GI tract include gastric juices, bile, pancreatic juices, and intestinal secretions. The only hypotonic fluid that may be lost is saliva, which has a lower solute concentration than other GI fluids.

How it happens

Excessive GI fluid loss may come from physical removal of secretions as a result of vomiting, suctioning, or increased or decreased GI tract motility. Excessive fluids can be excreted as waste products or secreted from the intestinal wall into the intestinal lumen, both of which lead to fluid and electrolyte imbalances. (See *Imbalances caused by GI fluid loss*, page 246.)

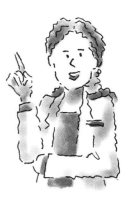

Imbalances caused by GI fluid loss

Excessive GI fluid loss can lead to a number of fluid, electrolyte, and acid-base imbalances. Here's a breakdown of those imbalances.

Fluid imbalances
• *Hypovolemia and dehydration*—Large amounts of fluid can be lost during prolonged, uncorrected vomiting and diarrhea. Hypovolemia can also result if gastric and intestinal suctioning occur without proper monitoring of intake and output to make sure lost fluid and electrolytes are adequately replaced.

Electrolyte imbalances
• *Hypokalemia*—The excessive loss of gastric fluids rich in potassium can lead to hypokalemia.
• *Hypomagnesemia*—Although gastric secretions contain little magnesium, several weeks of vomiting, diarrhea, or gastric suctioning can result in hypomagnesemia. Because hypomagnesemia itself can cause vomiting, the patient's condition may be self-perpetuating.
• *Hyponatremia*—Prolonged vomiting, diarrhea, or gastric or intestinal suctioning can deplete the body's supply of sodium and lead to hyponatremia.
• *Hypochloremia*—Any loss of gastric contents causes the loss of chloride. Prolonged gastric fluid loss can led to hypochloremia.

Acid-base imbalances
• *Metabolic acidosis*—Anything that promotes intestinal fluid loss can result in metabolic acidosis. Intestinal fluid contains large amounts of bicarbonate. With the loss of bicarbonate, pH falls, creating an acidic condition.
• *Metabolic alkalosis*—Loss of gastric fluids from vomiting or the use of drainage tubes in the upper GI tract can lead to metabolic alkalosis. Gastric fluids contain large amounts of acids that, when lost, lead to an increase in pH and alkalosis. Excessive use of antacids can also worsen the imbalance by adding to the alkalotic state.

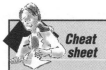

Cheat sheet

Causes of GI fluid loss

• Anorexia nervosa or bulimia
• Antibiotic administration
• Bacterial infection
• Enemas and laxatives
• Enteral tube feedings and ostomies
• Excessive intake of alcoholic substances and illicit drugs
• Hepatitis or pancreatitis
• Increased or decreased GI motility
• Poor absorption or digestion
• Pregnancy
• Pyloric stenosis in young children
• Vomiting or suctioning
• Young age

Osmotic diarrhea may occur in the intestines when a high solute load in the intestinal lumen attracts water into the cavity. Both acids and bases can be lost from the GI tract.

Vomiting and suctioning

Vomiting or mechanical suctioning of stomach contents, as with a nasogastric tube, causes the loss of hydrogen ions and electrolytes, such as chloride, potassium, and sodium. Vomiting also depletes the body's fluid volume supply and causes hypovolemia. Dehydration occurs when more water than electrolytes is lost. *When assessing acid-base balance, remember that the pH of the upper GI tract is low and that vomiting causes the loss of those*

Characteristics and causes of vomiting

Vomiting may lead to serious fluid, electrolyte, and acid-base disturbances and can occur for a variety of reasons. By carefully observing
the characteristics of the vomitus, you may gain clues as to the underlying disorder. Here's what the vomitus may indicate.

Bile-stained (greenish)
Obstruction below the pylorus, as from a duodenal lesion

Bloody
Upper-GI bleeding, as from gastritis or peptic ulcer, if bright or from
gastric or esophageal varices if dark red

Brown with a fecal odor
Intestinal obstruction or infarction

Burning, bitter-tasting
Excessive hydrochloric acid in gastric contents

Coffee-ground consistency
Digested blood from slowly bleeding gastric or duodenal lesions

Undigested food
Gastric outlet obstruction, as from gastric tumor or ulcer

acids and raises the risk of alkalosis. (See *Characteristics and
causes of vomiting.*)

Bowel movements

An increase in the frequency and amount of bowel movements
and a change in the stool toward a watery consistency can cause
excessive fluid loss, resulting in hypovolemia and dehydration.
Besides fluid loss, diarrhea can cause a loss of potassium, magnesium, and sodium. Fluids lost from the lower GI tract carry
a large amount of bicarbonate with them, which lowers the
amount of bicarbonate available to counter the effects of
acids in the body.

Laxatives and enemas

Laxatives and enemas may be used by patients to treat constipation, or they may be given to patients before abdominal
surgery or diagnostic studies to clean the bowel. Excessive
use of laxatives—such as magnesium sulfate, milk of magne-

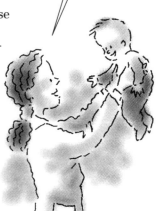

Young children are particularly vulnerable to fluid loss from diarrhea.

sia, and Fleet Phospho-soda—can cause high magnesium (hypermagnesemia) and phosphorus (hyperphosphatemia) levels.

Excessive use of commercially prepared enemas containing sodium and phosphate, such as Fleet enemas, can cause high phosphorus and sodium (hypernatremia) levels if the enemas are absorbed before they can be eliminated. Excessive use of tapwater enemas can cause a decrease in sodium levels because water absorbed by the colon can have a dilutional effect on sodium.

Who's at risk?

Excessive GI fluid loss can result from several conditions, including:

• bacterial infections of the GI tract, which are usually accompanied by vomiting or diarrhea
• antibiotic administration, which removes normal flora and promotes diarrhea
• young age, which makes the person vulnerable to diarrhea, a frequent cause of GI fluid loss in children
• pregnancy, which may be accompanied by vomiting
• pancreatitis or hepatitis, which may be accompanied by vomiting
• pyloric stenosis in young children, which may be accompanied by vomiting.

A delicate balance

Imbalances can also result from fecal impaction, poor absorption of foods, poor digestion, anorexia nervosa, or bulimia as well as excessive intake of alcoholic substances and some illicit drugs. Such disorders as anorexia nervosa and bulimia, which primarily affect young women, typically involve the use of laxatives and vomiting as a means of controlling weight. This can lead to numerous fluid, electrolyte, and acid-base imbalances. (See *Adolescents and GI fluid loss.*) Other disorders that can cause disturbances in fluid, electrolyte, or acid-base balance include the presence of fistulas involving the GI tract, GI bleeding, intestinal obstruction, and paralytic ileus.

The use of enteral tube feedings and ostomies (especially ileostomies) may also lead to imbalances. Enteral tube feedings may cause diarrhea or vomiting, depending on their composition and the patient's condition. Suctioning of gastric secretions through tubes may deplete the body of vital fluids, electrolytes, and acids. Saliva may be lost from the body when it can't be swallowed, as with dysphagia related to extensive head and neck cancer.

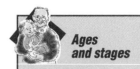

Ages and stages

Adolescents and GI fluid loss

When treating an adolescent, especially a girl, for excessive GI fluid loss, assess for signs and symptoms of anorexia and bulimia. Teeth that appear yellow and worn away and a history of laxative or diet pill use are two obvious signs.

Also, assess the patient for use of alternative diet therapies, particularly pills containing mahuang or ephedrine, which speeds the metabolism by mimicking the effects of adrenaline on the system.

What to look for

With excessive fluid loss, the patient may show signs of hypovolemia. Look for these signs and symptoms:
• The body tries to compensate for hypovolemia by increasing the heart rate. Along with tachycardia, blood pressure falls as intravascular volume is lost.
• The patient's skin may be cool and dry as the body shunts blood flow to major organs. Skin turgor may be decreased or the eyeballs may appear to be sunken, as occurs with dehydration. Urine output decreases as kidneys try to conserve fluid and electrolytes.
• Cardiac arrhythmias may occur from electrolyte imbalances, such as those related to potassium and magnesium. The patient may become weak and confused. Mental status may deteriorate as fluid, electrolyte, and acid-base imbalances progress.
• Respirations may change according to the type of acid-base imbalance the patient develops. For instance, acidosis will cause respirations to be deeper as the patient tries to blow off acid from the lungs.
• The patient will also have signs and symptoms related to the underlying disorder — for instance, pancreatitis. (See *Recognizing excessive GI fluid loss*.)

What tests show

Diagnostic test results related to the fluid, electrolyte, and acid-base imbalances associated with excessive GI fluid loss can help to direct nursing interventions. Such results include:
• changes in arterial blood gas levels related to metabolic acidosis and metabolic alkalosis
• alterations in the levels of certain electrolytes, such as potassium, magnesium, and sodium.
• hematocrit that may be falsely elevated in a volume-depleted patient
• cultures of body fluid samples that may help to identify bacteria responsible for the underlying disorder.

How GI fluid losses are treated

Treatment is aimed at the underlying cause of the imbalance to prevent further fluid and electrolyte loss. For instance, an antiemetic and an antidiarrheal may be given for vomiting and diarrhea, respectively. GI drainage tubes and the suction applied to them are discontinued as soon as possible.

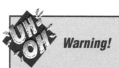

Warning!

Recognizing excessive GI fluid loss

Besides the signs and symptoms related to underlying disorders, the patient with excessive GI fluid loss may show these signs and symptoms of hypovolemia:
• tachycardia
• falling blood pressure
• cool, dry skin
• decreased skin turgor or sunken eyeballs
• decreased urine output
• possible cardiac arrhythmias
• weakness
• confusion or deteriorated mental status
• changes in respirations.

Cheat sheet

Signs and symptoms of GI fluid loss

- Altered respirations
- Altered arterial blood gas and electrolyte levels
- Cardiac arrhythmias
- Cool, dry skin
- Decreased blood pressure
- Decreased skin turgor and sunken eyeballs
- Decreased urine output
- Falsely elevated hematocrit
- Increased heart rate
- Tachycardia
- Weakness and confusion

The patient should also receive I.V. or oral fluid replacement, depending on his tolerance and the cause of the fluid loss. Electrolytes should also be replaced if serum levels are decreased. Long-term parenteral nutrition may be needed. An antibiotic may be administered if infection is the underlying cause of fluid loss.

How you intervene

A patient with a condition that alters fluid and electrolyte balance through GI losses needs to be closely monitored. An increase in the amount of drainage from GI tubes or an increase in the frequency of vomiting or diarrhea should be reported. Follow these recommendations when caring for a patient with GI fluid losses.

Assess

- Measure and record the amount of fluid lost through vomiting, diarrhea, or gastric or intestinal suctioning. Remember to include GI losses as part of the patient's total output. Significant increases in GI loss places the patient at increased risk for fluid and electrolyte imbalances and metabolic alkalosis or acidosis
- Assess the patient's fluid status by monitoring intake and output, daily weight, and skin turgor.
- Assess vital signs and report any changes that may indicate fluid deficits, such as a decreased blood pressure or increased heart rate.

Teaching points

Teaching about GI fluid loss

Make sure you cover these points with your patient, and then evaluate his learning:
• basics of the condition and its treatment
• need to report prolonged vomiting or diarrhea
• importance of avoiding repeated use of enemas and laxatives
• proper technique for irrigating a gastric tube, if appropriate
• proper technique for monitoring I.V. infusion, if appropriate.

• Report vomiting to keep imbalances from becoming severe and to initiate prompt treatment.

Administer and maintain

• Administer oral fluids containing water and electrolytes, such as Gatorade or Pedialyte, if the patient can tolerate fluids. (See *Teaching about GI fluid loss* and *Documenting GI fluid loss*, page 252.)
• Maintain patent I.V. access, as ordered. Administer I.V. replacement fluids as prescribed. Monitor the infusion rate and volume to prevent hypervolemia. (See *Don't go too fast with fluids.*)
• If the patient is undergoing gastric suctioning, check GI tube placement often to prevent fluid aspiration.
• Irrigate the suction tube with isotonic normal saline solution as ordered. *Remember, never use plain water for irrigation. It draws more gastric secretions into the stomach in an attempt to make the fluid isotonic for absorption.* Also,

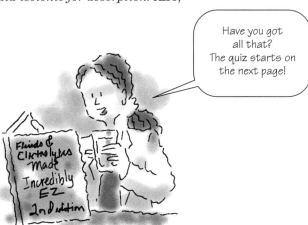

Chart smart

Documenting GI fluid loss

If your patient has the potential for or is experiencing excessive GI fluid loss, here are some things to include in your documentation:

• vital signs
• intake and output
• daily weight
• presence and characteristics of vomitus, diarrhea, or GI fluid drainage
• skin turgor
• correct placement of GI tube, if present, plus care related to the tube
• interventions used to decrease GI fluid loss
• I.V. or oral fluid and electrolyte replacement therapy and the patient's response.

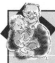

Ages and stages

Don't go too fast with fluids

Elderly patients can develop heart failure if I.V. fluids are infused too rapidly. Therefore, take caution when administering I.V. fluids to replace fluid losses in these patients.

the fluid is suctioned out of the stomach, causing further depletion of fluids and electrolytes.

• When the patient is connected to gastric suction, restrict the amount of ice chips given by mouth and explain the reason for the restriction. Gastric suctioning of ice chips can deplete fluid and electrolytes from the stomach.

• Administer medications, such as an antiemetic or antidiarrheal, as prescribed, to control the patient's underlying condition.

• Evaluate serum electrolyte levels and pH to detect abnormalities and to monitor the effectiveness of therapy.

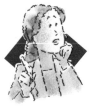

Quick quiz

1. Large amounts of fluid may be lost through the GI system because:

    A.   the intestines normally reabsorb little of the fluids contained in food.

    B.   large amounts of fluid circulate through the GI system each day.

    C.   GI fluids are isotonic.

Answer: B. Because large amounts of fluids circulate through the GI system, anything that disrupts the system can promote excessive fluid loss.

2. The excessive use of Fleet enemas can cause which of the following imbalances?

    A.   Hypophosphatemia

    B.   Hyponatremia

    C.   Hypernatremia

Answer: C. Hypernatremia can result from the excessive use of Fleet enemas because they contain sodium. If the enema is retained for a long time before it's expelled, the bowel absorbs the excess sodium, resulting in hypernatremia.

3. Which of the following fluid and electrolyte imbalances can occur with excessive GI fluid loss?

    A.   Hypomagnesemia, hypermagnesemia, and hyponatremia

    B.   Hypomagnesemia, hypernatremia, and hyperchloremia

    C.   Hypervolemia, hyponatremia, and hypernatremia

Answer: A. Hypomagnesemia, hypermagnesemia, and hyponatremia — and others — may occur with varying types of GI fluid loss.

4. A patient with fluid losses from the upper GI tract is likely to suffer which of the following imbalances?

    A.   Metabolic alkalosis

    B.   Metabolic acidosis

    C.   Respiratory acidosis

Answer: A. GI fluid losses from the upper GI tract can result in metabolic alkalosis; losses from the lower GI tract can result in metabolic acidosis.

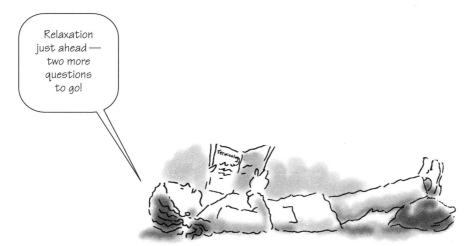

Relaxation just ahead — two more questions to go!

5. Warning signs of hypovolemia associated with GI losses include:
- A. tachycardia, decreased blood pressure, decreased urine output.
- B. tachycardia, increased blood pressure, increased urine output.
- C. decreased blood pressure, increased urine output, and warm, flushed skin.

Answer: A. Tachycardia, decreased blood pressure, and decreased urine output indicate that the patient is experiencing hypovolemia from GI losses.

6. You carefully observe the characteristics of the patient's vomitus. You document your finding as brown with fecal odor. This type of vomitus may indicate:
- A. excessive hydrochloric acid in gastric contents.
- B. intestinal obstruction.
- C. obstruction below the pylorus.

Answer: B. Vomitus that's brown with fecal odor may indicate intestinal obstruction or infarction.

Scoring

☆☆☆ If you answered all six questions correctly, here's a high five! You're a GI genius!

☆☆ If you answered four or five correctly, we want to shake your hand! You're certainly not at a loss for the right answers!

☆ If you answered fewer than four correctly, slap us some skin! With a little (certainly not excessive!) review, you'll get this down just fine.

Renal failure

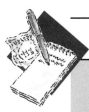

Just the facts

This chapter will help you understand the effects of fluid imbalances associated with renal failure. It will also provide guidelines for treatment and preventive care. In this chapter, you'll learn:

♦ how to tell the difference between acute and chronic renal failure

♦ which fluid, electrolyte, and acid-base imbalances occur with renal failure and why

♦ the signs and symptoms of renal failure

♦ which nursing interventions are appropriate for patients with renal failure.

A look at renal failure

Renal failure involves a disruption of normal kidney function. The kidneys play a major role in regulating fluids, electrolytes, acids, and bases. Acute renal failure occurs suddenly and is usually reversible. In contrast, chronic renal failure occurs slowly and is irreversible.

Both acute and chronic renal failure affect the kidneys' functional unit, the nephron, which forms urine. Imbalances occur as the kidneys lose the ability to excrete water, electrolytes, wastes, and acid-base products through the urine. Patients may also develop hypertension, anemia, uremia, and renal osteodystrophy, the latter of which includes softening of bones and a reduction of bone mass. The following discussion examines how acute and chronic renal failure develop.

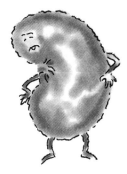

How acute renal failure happens

Acute renal failure can stem from intrarenal conditions, which damage the kidneys themselves; from prerenal conditions such as heart failure, which causes a diminished blood flow to the kidneys; or from obstructive postrenal conditions such as prostatitis, which can cause urine to back up into the kidneys. (See *Causes of acute renal failure.*)

About 5% of hospitalized patients develop acute renal failure at some point during their hospitalizations. Many conditions reduce blood flow or otherwise damage the kidneys' nephrons. Acute renal failure normally passes through three distinct phases: oliguric-anuric, diuretic, and recovery.

Phase 1: A drop-off

A decrease in urine output is the first clinical sign of acute renal failure during the first phase, called the oliguric-anuric phase. Typically, as the glomerular filtration rate (GFR) decreases, the patient's urine output decreases to less than 400 ml during a 24-hour period.

When the kidneys fail, nitrogenous waste products accumulate, which causes an elevation in blood urea nitrogen (BUN) and serum creatinine levels. The result is uremia. Electrolyte imbalances, metabolic acidosis, and other effects follow as the patient becomes increasingly uremic, and renal dysfunction disrupts other body systems. Left untreated, the condition is fatal.

The oliguric-anuric phase generally lasts 1 to 2 weeks but may last for several more. The longer the patient remains in this phase, the poorer the prognosis for a return to normal renal function.

Phase 2: Rebound

The second phase, or diuretic phase, starts with a gradual increase in daily urine output from 400 ml/24 hours to 1 to 2 L/24 hours. The BUN level stops rising. Although urine output begins to increase in this phase, a potential for fluid and electrolyte imbalances still exists as glomerular filtration increases. The diuretic phase lasts about 10 days.

Phase 3: Feeling better

The third phase, the convalescent or recovery phase, begins when fluid and electrolyte values start to stabilize, indicating a return to normal kidney function. The patient may experience a slight reduction in kidney function for the rest of his life, so he'll still be at risk for fluid and electrolyte imbalances. The recovery phase generally lasts a few months.

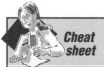

Cheat sheet

Facts about acute renal failure

- Occurs suddenly
- Usually reversible
- May stem from intrarenal conditions, prerenal conditions, or obstructive postrenal conditions
- Divided into three phases: oliguric-anuric, diuretic, and recovery

Causes of acute renal failure

The causes of acute renal failure can be broken down into three categories (illustrated here)—prerenal, intrarenal, and postrenal. Prerenal causes include conditions that diminish blood flow to the kidneys. Intrarenal causes include conditions that damage the kidneys themselves. Postrenal causes include conditions that obstruct urine outflow, which causes urine to back up into the kidneys.

Prerenal causes
- Serious cardiovascular disorders
- Hypovolemia
- Peripheral vasodilation
- Severe vasoconstriction
- Renal vascular obstruction
- Trauma

Intrarenal causes
- Acute tubular necrosis
- Nephrotoxins
- Heavy metals
- Aminoglycosides or non-steroidal anti-inflammatory drugs
- Ischemic damage from poorly treated renal failure
- Eclampsia, postpartum renal failure, or uterine hemorrhage
- Crush injury, myopathy, sepsis, or transfusion reaction
- Trauma

Postrenal causes
- Bladder obstruction
- Ureteral obstruction
- Urethral obstruction
- Trauma

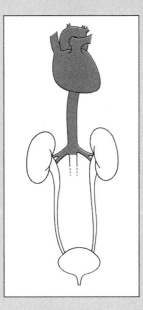
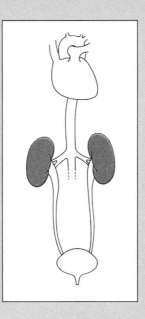
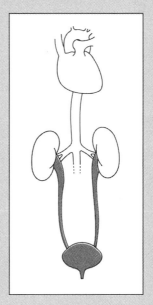

How chronic renal failure happens

Chronic renal failure, which has a more insidious onset than acute renal failure, may result from:
- chronic glomerular disease such as glomerulonephritis
- chronic infections, such as chronic pyelonephritis or tuberculosis
- congenital anomalies such as polycystic kidney disease
- vascular diseases, such as renal nephrosclerosis or hypertension
- obstructions such as those from calculi
- collagen diseases such as systemic lupus erythematosus
- long-term therapy with nephrotoxic drugs such as aminoglycosides
- endocrine diseases such as diabetes mellitus.

Setting the stage

Because chronic renal failure has a slow onset, identifying specific time frames for its stages may be difficult. The rate at which kidney function deteriorates depends as well on the specific disease causing the deterioration. It's possible, however, to stage progression of the disease by the degree of kidney function.

Chronic renal failure can be divided into four basic stages:
- reduced renal reserve (GFR 40 to 70 ml/minute)
- renal insufficiency (GFR 20 to 40 ml/minute)
- renal failure (GFR 10 to 20 ml/minute)
- end-stage renal disease (GFR less than 10 ml/minute).

Depleting the reserve

The kidneys have great functional reserve. Few symptoms develop until more than 75% of glomerular filtration is lost. The remaining functional nephrons then deteriorate progressively; symptoms worsen as renal function diminishes. Failing kidneys can't regulate fluid balance or filter solutes or participate effectively in acid-base balance. If chronic renal failure continues unchecked, uremic toxins accumulate and produce potentially fatal physiologic changes in all major organ systems.

Imbalances caused by renal failure

Renal failure—acute or chronic—can cause a number of fluid, electrolyte, and acid-base imbalances, including hypervolemia, hypovolemia, hyperkalemia, hyperphosphatemia, hypocalcemia, hyponatremia, hypernatremia, hypermagnesemia, metabolic acidosis, and metabolic alkalosis.

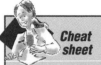

Cheat sheet

Facts about chronic renal failure

- Occurs slowly
- Irreversible
- May stem from chronic glomerular disease, chronic infections, congenital anomalies, vascular disease, long-term therapy with nephrotoxic drugs, and endocrine diseases.
- Divided into four stages: reduced renal reserve, renal insufficiency, renal failure, and end-stage renal disease

Water, water, everywhere...or not

When urine output decreases, especially with the more sudden onset of acute renal failure, the body retains fluid, which can lead to hypervolemia. That condition may also occur if fluid intake exceeds urine output. The resulting fluid retention can lead to hypertension, peripheral edema, heart failure, or pulmonary edema.

Hypovolemic water losses usually occur during the diuretic phase of acute renal failure and can result in hypotension or circulatory collapse.

Potassium to the max

As the kidneys' ability to excrete potassium is impaired, serum potassium levels increase, resulting in hyperkalemia. In chronic renal failure, a patient tends to tolerate high potassium levels more than a patient with acute renal failure, in which the onset is more sudden.

Metabolic acidosis, which occurs with renal failure, causes potassium to move from inside the cells into the extracellular fluid. The release of potassium from any necrotic or injured cells worsens hyperkalemia. Additional stressors — such as infection, GI bleeding, trauma, and surgery — can also lead to high serum potassium levels.

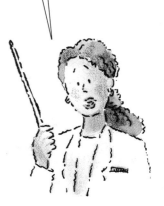

Such stressors as infection, GI bleeding, trauma, and surgery can also lead to high serum potassium levels.

Balancing act

Serum calcium and phosphorus have an inverse relationship, so when one goes out of balance, the other follows suit. Secondary imbalances can occur as a result.

Hyperphosphatemia develops when the kidneys lose the ability to excrete phosphorus. High serum phosphorus levels cause a decrease in calcium levels because calcium and phosphorus have an inverse relationship.

Decreased activation of vitamin D by the kidneys results in decreased GI absorption of calcium — another cause for low serum calcium levels.

Salt shakers

Sodium levels may be either abnormally high or unusually low during renal failure.

Hyponatremia can occur with acute renal failure because a decreased GFR and damaged tubules increase water and sodium retention. This dilutional hyponatremic state can also be caused by the intracellular-extracellular exchange between sodium and potassium during metabolic acidosis.

Hypernatremia can occur with chronic renal failure. A progression in the degree of kidney failure causes less sodium to be excreted and makes hypernatremia worse.

Too much magnesium

The patient with renal failure may retain magnesium as a result of a decreased GFR and destruction of the tubules. However, a high serum magnesium level usually isn't recognized unless the patient receives external sources of magnesium, such as laxatives, antacids, I.V. solutions, or hyperalimentation solutions.

The acid-base seesaw

Metabolic acidosis is the most common acid-base imbalance occurring with renal failure. It develops as the kidneys lose the ability to secrete hydrogen ions—an acid—in the urine. The imbalance is also exacerbated as the kidneys fail to hold onto bicarbonate—a base.

Patients with chronic renal failure have more time to compensate for this acid-base imbalance than patients with acute renal failure. The lungs try to compensate for the excess acid by increasing the depth and rate of respirations in an attempt to blow off carbon dioxide.

Metabolic alkalosis rarely occurs with renal failure. When it does, it usually results from excessive intake of bicarbonate, given in an effort to correct metabolic acidosis.

What to look for

The patient's history may reveal a disorder that can cause renal failure; it may also include a recent episode of fever, chills, GI problems (such as anorexia, nausea, vomiting, diarrhea, or constipation), and central nervous system problems such as headache.

Signs and symptoms vary, depending on the length of time in which renal failure develops. (See *Laboratory results associated with acute renal failure.*) Fewer signs may appear in patients with acute renal failure because of the condition's shorter clinical course. In patients with chronic renal failure, however, almost all body systems are affected. Your assessment findings may involve several body systems. (See *Recognizing renal failure.*)

Salt shortage

In cases of renal failure in which the kidneys are unable to retain salt, hyponatremia may occur. The patient may complain of dry mouth, fatigue, and nausea. You may note hypotension, loss of skin turgor, and listlessness that progresses to somnolence and confusion.

Later, as the number of functioning nephrons decreases, so does the kidney's capacity to excrete sodium and potassium. Urine output decreases. The urine may be dilute, with casts or

---

Laboratory results associated with acute renal failure

Keep alert for these early signs of acute renal failure:
• urine output below 400 ml over 24 hours
• increased blood urea nitrogen level
• increased serum creatinine level.

As the number of functioning nephrons decreases, so does the kidney's capacity to excrete sodium and potassium. Oy.

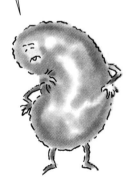

Warning!

Recognizing renal failure

The following signs and symptoms are associated with renal failure. Your patient may develop some or all of them.

Neurologic
- Burning, itching, and pain in the legs and feet
- Coma
- Confusion
- Fatigue
- Hiccups
- Irritability
- Listlessness and somnolence
- Muscle irritability and twitching
- Seizures
- Shortened attention span and memory

Cardiovascular
- Anemia
- Cardiac arrhythmias
- Heart failure
- Hypertension
- Hypotension
- Irregular pulse
- Pericardial rub
- Tachycardia
- Weight gain with fluid retention

Pulmonary
- Crackles
- Decreased breath sounds, if pneumonia is present
- Dyspnea
- Kussmaul's respirations

GI
- Ammonia smell to the breath
- Anorexia
- Bleeding
- Constipation or diarrhea
- Dry mouth
- Inflammation and ulceration of GI mucosa
- Metallic taste in the mouth
- Nausea and vomiting
- Pain on abdominal palpation and percussion

Integumentary
- Dry, brittle hair that may change color or fall out easily
- Dry, scaly skin with ecchymoses, petechiae, and purpura

- Dry mucous membranes
- Loss of skin turgor
- Severe itching
- Thin, brittle fingernails with lines
- Uremic frost (in later stages)
- Yellow-bronze skin color

Genitourinary
- Amenorrhea in women
- Anuria or oliguria
- Changes in urinary appearance or patterns
- Decreased libido
- Dilute urine with casts and crystals
- Impotence in men
- Infertility

Musculoskeletal
- Bone and muscle pain
- Gait abnormalities or loss of ambulation
- Inability to ambulate
- Muscle cramps
- Muscle weakness
- Pathologic fractures

crystals present. Accumulation of potassium causes muscle irritability and then muscle weakness, irregular pulse, and life-threatening cardiac arrhythmias. Sodium retention causes fluid overload, and edema becomes palpable. The patient gains weight from fluid retention. Metabolic acidosis can also occur.

Rubs and crackles

When the cardiovascular system is involved, you'll find hypertension and an irregular pulse. Tachycardia may occur. Signs of a pericardial rub, related to pericarditis, may be heard, especially in patients with chronic renal failure. Crackles at the bases of the lungs may be heard, and peripheral edema may be palpated if heart failure occurs.

The lungs take a plunge

Pulmonary changes include reduced pulmonary macrophage activity with increased susceptibility to infection. If pneumonia is present, breath sounds may decrease over areas of consolidation. Crackles at the lung bases occur with pulmonary edema. Kussmaul's respirations occur with metabolic acidosis.

Down in the mouth

With inflammation and ulceration of GI mucosa, inspection of the mouth may reveal gum ulceration and bleeding. The patient may complain of hiccups, a metallic taste in the mouth, anorexia, nausea, and vomiting (caused by esophageal, stomach, or bowel involvement). You may note an ammonia smell to the breath. Abdominal palpation and percussion may cause pain.

Dry skin

Inspection of the skin typically reveals a yellow-bronze color. The skin is dry and scaly with purpura, ecchymoses, and petechiae that form as a result of thrombocytopenia and platelet dysfunction caused by uremia. In later stages, the patient may experience uremic frost (powdery deposits on the skin as a result of urea and uric acid being excreted in sweat) and thin, brittle fingernails with characteristic lines. Mucous membranes are dry. Hair is dry and brittle and may change color and fall out easily. The patient usually complains of severe itching.

Sexual effects

With chronic renal failure, the patient may have a history of infertility and decreased libido. Women may have amenorrhea, and men may be impotent.

Bone and muscle pain

The patient may have a history of pathologic fractures and complain of bone and muscle pain, which may be caused by an imbalance in calcium and phosphorus or in the amount of parathyroid hormone (PTH) produced. You may note gait abnormalities or, possibly, that the patient is no longer able to ambulate.

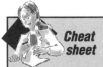

Cheat sheet

Diagnostic tests for renal failure

- Arterial blood gas analysis: reveals metabolic acidosis
- Electrocardiogram: peak T waves; widened QRS
- Hematocrit: low
- Hemoglobin level: low
- Urinalysis: reveals casts; decreased specific gravity, proteinura

More problems

You may note that the patient has changes in his level of consciousness that may progress from mild behavior changes, shortened memory and attention span, apathy, drowsiness, and irritability to confusion, coma, and seizures. The patient may complain of muscle cramps and twitching caused by muscle irritability. The patient may also complain of pain, burning, and itching in the legs and feet that may be relieved by voluntarily shaking, moving, or rocking them. Those symptoms may eventually progress to paresthesia and motor nerve dysfunction.

What tests show

Diagnostic test results typical of patients with renal failure include:
• elevated serum BUN, creatinine, potassium, and phosphorus levels (See *Age-related kidney changes*.)
• arterial blood gas (ABG) results that indicate metabolic acidosis — specifically, a low pH and bicarbonate level
• low hematocrit, low hemoglobin level, and mild thrombocytopenia
• urinalysis showing casts, cellular debris, decreased specific gravity, and proteinuria
• electrocardiogram (ECG) showing tall, peaked T waves; a widened QRS complex; and disappearing P waves if hyperkalemia is present.

Other studies, such as kidney-ureter-bladder radiography and kidney ultrasonography, may also be performed to determine the cause of renal failure.

How renal failure is treated

Treatment of renal failure aims to correct specific symptoms and to alter the disease process.

Go low pro

A patient with renal failure needs to make dietary changes. A low-protein diet will reduce end products of protein metabolism that the kidneys are unable to excrete. The protein a patient needs should be consumed only in foods, such as eggs, milk, poultry, and meat, that contain all essential amino acids to prevent breakdown of body protein.

The patient should also follow a high-calorie diet to meet daily requirements and to prevent breakdown of body protein. The diet also should restrict sodium and potassium.

Ages and stages

Age-related kidney changes

As people age, nephrons are lost and kidneys decrease in size. These changes decrease renal blood flow and may result in doubled blood urea nitrogen levels in older patients.

> A patient with renal failure must make dietary changes. Garcon! I'll have the low protein special!

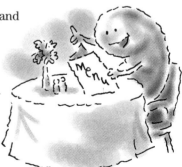

Fine tuning fluids

Maintaining fluid balance requires careful monitoring of vital signs, weight changes, and urine output. Fluid retention can be reduced, if some renal function remains, with the use of a loop diuretic such as furosemide (Lasix) and with restriction of fluid.

Careful monitoring of serum potassium levels is necessary to detect hyperkalemia. If the patient develops this condition, emergency treatment should be initiated. (See *Emergency treatment of hyperkalemia.*) A phosphate-binding antacid may be given to lower serum phosphorus levels.

A kick to the marrow

In patients with chronic renal failure, kidney production of erythropoietin is diminished. This hormone controls the rate of red blood cell (RBC) production in bone marrow and functions as a growth factor and differentiating factor. Treatment includes administration of synthetic erythropoietin to stimulate bone marrow to produce RBCs.

Filling in for the kidneys

Hemodialysis and peritoneal dialysis are used in both acute and chronic renal failure. By assuming the function of the kidneys, these measures help correct fluid and electrolyte disturbances and relieve some of the symptoms of renal failure.

How you intervene

Caring for a patient with renal failure requires careful monitoring, administration of various medicines and therapeutic regimens, and empathic ministering to the patient and family.

Assess and monitor

- Assess the patient carefully to determine the type and severity of fluid, electrolyte, and acid-base imbalances.
- Maintain accurate fluid intake and output records.
- Weigh the patient daily, and compare the results with the 24-hour intake and output record. (See *Teaching about renal failure.*)
- Monitor vital signs, including breath sounds and central venous pressure when available, to detect changes in fluid volume. Report hypertension, which may occur as a result of fluid and sodium retention.
- Observe the patient for signs and symptoms of fluid overload, such as edema, bounding pulse, and shortness of breath.

Emergency treatment of hyperkalemia

Emergency treatment of hyperkalemia includes dialysis and administration of 50% hypertonic glucose I.V., regular insulin, calcium gluconate I.V., and sodium bicarbonate I.V. Kayexalate may also be administered.

> **Teaching points**
>
> ## Teaching about renal failure
>
> Make sure you cover the following points with your patient and his family, and then evaluate his learning:
> - basics of renal failure and its treatment
> - prescribed medications
> - avoidance of high-sodium and high-potassium foods
> - importance of weighing himself daily
> - warning signs and symptoms and when to report them
> - need for frequent rest for the anemic patient
> - referrals to counseling services, if indicated
> - proper methods of caring for shunt, fistula, or vascular access device
> - proper method of performing peritoneal dialysis at home, if appropriate.

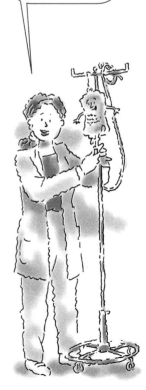

Drugs excreted through the kidney or removed during dialysis will need their dosages adjusted.

- Monitor serum electrolyte and ABG levels for abnormalities. Report significant changes to the doctor.
- Observe the patient for signs and symptoms that may indicate an electrolyte or acid-base imbalance — for example, tetany, paresthesia, muscle weakness, tachypnea, or confusion.
- Monitor ECG readings to detect electrolyte imbalances.
- Monitor hemoglobin levels and hematocrit.
- If the patient requires dialysis, check the vascular access site every 2 hours for patency and signs of clotting, and feel for a bruit. Check the site for bleeding after dialysis.

Administer

- Restrict fluids as prescribed.
- Administer prescribed diuretic to patients whose kidneys can still excrete excess fluid.
- Administer other prescribed medications, such as oral or I.V. electrolyte replacement to correct electrolyte imbalances and vitamin supplements to correct nutritional deficiencies.
- Know the route of excretion for medications being given. Drugs excreted through the kidney or removed during dialysis will need their dosage adjusted.
- Expect to administer sodium bicarbonate I.V. to control acute acidosis and orally to control chronic acidosis. Remember that sodium bicarbonate has a high sodium content. Multiple doses of the drug may result in hypernatremia, which could contribute to the onset of heart failure and pulmonary edema.

• As necessary, restrict electrolyte intake, especially potassium and phosphorus, to prevent imbalances. Monitor and document the patient's response. (See *Documenting renal failure*.)
• Be prepared to initiate dialysis when electrolyte or acid-base imbalances don't respond to drug therapy or when fluid removal isn't possible.

Maintain

• Maintain nutritional status. Provide a diet high in calories and low in protein, sodium, and potassium. Initiate a nutritional consultation as needed.
• If a shunt or fistula for dialysis has been placed in the patient's arm, don't use that extremity for measuring blood pressure, drawing blood, or inserting I.V. catheters.
• Provide emotional support to the patient and his family.
• Teach the patient and his family about renal failure and its treatment.

Chart smart

Documenting renal failure

If your patient is experiencing renal failure, include the following points in your documentation:
• assessment findings, such as those related to fluid, electrolyte, or acid-base imbalances
• vital signs, including breath sounds and central venous pressure readings (if available)
• daily weight
• laboratory test results
• intake and output
• administration of I.V. or oral electrolyte replacement therapy
• dialysis and care of the vascular access site
• patient and family teaching and patient's response
• notification of the doctor.

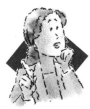

Quick quiz

1. Patients with chronic renal failure may not experience symptoms until later stages of the disease because:
    A.   liver hormones mask the symptoms.
    B.   the kidneys have great functional reserve.
    C.   other body systems take over some renal functions.

Answer: B. Because the kidneys have great functional reserve, chronic renal failure develops more slowly than acute renal failure and without apparent signs and symptoms until later stages of the disease.

2. Metabolic acidosis worsens which of the following electrolyte imbalances?
    A.   Hyperkalemia
    B.   Hypervolemia
    C.   Hypokalemia

Answer: A. Metabolic acidosis causes the movement of potassium from intracellular to extracellular fluid, causing high blood potassium levels.

3. Low serum calcium levels in patients with renal failure may result from:
- A. decreased amounts of PTH.
- B. decreased activation of vitamin D.
- C. demineralization of bone.

Answer: B. Decreased activation of vitamin D in patients with renal failure causes a decreased GI absorption of calcium. Although bone demineralization can occur with renal failure, the condition is caused by repeated episodes of hypocalcemia.

4. In the oliguric phase of acute renal failure, urine output drops to less than:
- A. 800 ml/24 hours.
- B. 400 ml/24 hours.
- C. 100 ml/24 hours.

Answer: B. The oliguric phase involves a urine output below 400 ml/24 hours.

5. A patient with hyperkalemia may experience several ECG changes, including:
- A. flat T waves, a small QRS complex, and normal P waves.
- B. tall, peaked T waves; a widened QRS complex; and disappearing P waves.
- C. no T waves, a normal QRS complex, and flattened or misshaped P waves.

Answer: B. High potassium levels may result in disappearing P waves, a widened QRS complex, and tall, peaked T waves because of the effect on cardiac cells.

6. Which of the following is the optimal diet for a patient with renal failure?
- A. High-calorie, low-protein, low-sodium, low-potassium
- B. High-calorie, high-protein, high-sodium, high-potassium
- C. Low-calorie, high-protein, low-sodium, low-potassium

Answer: A. A high-calorie, low-protein, low-sodium, and low-potassium diet is the optimal diet for meeting the metabolic and nutritional requirements of a patient with renal failure.

7. Laboratory results associated with acute renal failure include:

    A.   increased BUN level and decreased serum creatinine level.

    B.   decreased BUN level and increased urine output.

    C.   increased BUN and serum creatinine levels.

Answer: C. The patient with acute renal failure has increased BUN and serum creatinine levels and decreased urine output.

Scoring

☆☆☆ If you answered all seven items correctly, great job! You're dominant in the renal arena!

☆☆ If you answered five or six correctly, way to go! You're intelligence is still acute and your diagnosis is one of chronic success!

☆ If you answered fewer than five correctly, don't look so glum, it's not like you just took a kidney punch! Shake it off and good luck with the next chapter.

Burns

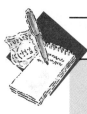

Just the facts

This chapter explains how burn injuries affect the entire body system. In this chapter, you'll learn:

♦ what physiologic changes occur with a severe burn injury

♦ what fluid, electrolyte, and acid-base imbalances occur as a result of a severe burn injury

♦ what signs and symptoms occur with a burn injury

♦ how treatment methods vary for burn injuries

♦ how to provide appropriate nursing care for a burn patient.

A look at burns

A major burn is a horrifying injury, requiring painful treatment and a long period of rehabilitation. The destruction of the epidermis, dermis, or subcutaneous layers of the skin can affect the entire body and commonly is life-threatening. If not fatal, it can be permanently disfiguring and incapacitating, both emotionally and physically.

A burn, like any injury to the skin, interferes with the skin's ability to help keep out infectious organisms, maintain fluid balance, and regulate body temperature. Burn injuries cause major changes in the body's fluid and electrolyte balance. Many of those imbalances change over time as the initial injury progresses.

The extreme heat from a burn can be severe enough to completely destroy cells. Even with a lesser injury, normal cell activity is disrupted. With minimal injury, the cell may recover its function. The burn patient's prognosis depends on the size and severity of the burn.

Several factors determine the severity of a burn, including the cause, degree, and extent of the burn as well as the part of the body involved. The outcome for the burned patient is also affected by the presence of preexisting medical conditions and the patient's age.

Types of burns

Burns can result from thermal, mechanical, or electrical injuries as well as from exposure to chemicals or radiation.

Thermal burns

Thermal burns, the most common type of burn injury, result from exposure to either dry (flames) or moist (steam, hot liquids) heat. They commonly occur with residential fires, motor vehicle accidents, childhood accidents, exposure to improperly stored gasoline, exposure to space heaters, electrical malfunctions, and arson. Other causes may include the improper handling of firecrackers, contact with scalding liquids, and kitchen accidents.

Because its effects are similar to those of thermal burn, frostbite is included in this category.

Mechanical burns

Mechanical burns are caused by the friction or abrasion that occurs when the skin is rubbed harshly against a coarse surface. A motorcycle accident in which a person experiences "road rash" is an example of this type of burn.

Electrical burns

Electrical burns commonly occur after contact with faulty electrical wiring, high-voltage power lines, or immersion in water that has been electrified. Those injuries may also be caused by lightning strikes. *When caring for a patient with an electrical burn, keep in mind that there may be more damage internally than meets the eye.* Check the patient for entrance and exit wounds. Tissue damage from an electrical burn is difficult to assess because internal destruction along the conduction pathway is usually greater than the surface burn indicates.

An electrical burn that ignites the patient's clothing may cause thermal burns as well.

Chemical and radiation burns

Chemical burns result from the direct contact, ingestion, inhalation, or injection of acids, alkali, or vesicants. The chemical destroys protein in tissues, leading to necrosis. The type and extent

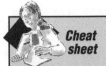

Cheat sheet

Burn basics

• May result from thermal, mechanical, electrical, chemical, or radiation injury
• Classified as partial thickness, deep partial thickness, or full thickness
• Place patient at risk for infection, fluid and electrolyte imbalances, and altered body temperature

of damage caused depends on the properties of the particular chemical.

Radiation burns are typically associated with sunburn or radiation treatment for cancer. These burns tend to be superficial, involving the outer layer of skin.

Classification of burns

Burn thickness affects cell function. Therefore, classifying the degree of burn helps to determine the type of intervention needed.

First-degree

Partial-thickness (first-degree) burns affect the superficial layer of the epidermis. These burns are usually pink or red and dry and painful. No blistering occurs with a partial-thickness burn; however, some edema may be present.

These burns aren't classified as severe because the epidermis remains intact and continues to prevent water loss from the skin, so they don't affect fluid and electrolyte balance. Regrowth of the epidermis occurs, and healing is generally rapid without scarring.

Second-degree

Deep partial-thickness (second-degree) burns affect both the epidermis and dermis. These burns are caused by prolonged exposure — usually longer than 10 seconds — to intense heat or by prolonged contact with hot liquids or objects.

To identify a deep partial-thickness burn, look for the area to be painful, swollen, and red, with blister formation. When pressure is applied to the burn, it blanches and refills.

Regeneration of the epithelial layer may occur. The amount of scarring varies with this type of burn. Fluid and electrolyte imbalances are associated with second-degree burns that cover significant areas of the body.

Third-degree

Full-thickness (third-degree) burns affect the epidermis, the dermis, and tissues below the dermis. These burns look dry and leathery, are painless (because nerve endings are destroyed), and don't blanch when pressure is applied. The color of the burned area varies from white to black or charred.

Third-degree burns require skin grafting. Full-thickness burns carry the greatest risk of fluid and electrolyte imbalance.

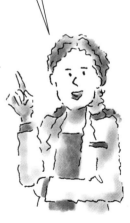

Second-degree burns will be painful, swollen, and red with blister formation.

Extent of a burn

Assessment tools, such as the Rule of Nines or the Lund-Browder chart, are used to estimate the percentage of body surface area involved in a burn. (See *Estimating the extent of a burn.*)

The severity of a burn can be estimated by correlating its depth and size. Burns are categorized as major, moderate, and minor.

Major burn

Major burns include:
• second-degree burns covering more than 25% of an adult's body surface area
• third-degree burns covering more than 10% of the body surface area
• burns of the hands, face, eyes, ears, feet, or genitalia
• all inhalation burns
• all electrical burns
• burns complicated by fractures or other major trauma
• all burns in poor-risk patients, such as children younger than age 2, adults older than age 60, and patients who have preexisting medical conditions such as heart disease.

Moderate burn

Moderate burns include:
• third-degree burns on 2% to 10% of the body surface area, regardless of body size
• second-degree burns on 15% to 25% of an adult's body surface area and 10% to 20% of a child's.

Minor burn

Minor burns include:
• third-degree burns that appear on less than 2% of the body surface area, regardless of body size
• second-degree burns on less than 15% of an adult's body surface area and 10% of a child's.

Phases of a burn

Burn phases describe the physiologic changes that occur after a burn and include the fluid accumulation, fluid remobilization, and convalescent phases. Burns affect many body systems and can

Estimating the extent of a burn

You can quickly estimate the extent of an *adult* patient's burns by using the Rule of Nines (below, left). This method divides an adult's body surface into percentages.

To use this method, match your adult patient's burns to the body chart shown here. Then add up the corresponding percentages for each burned section. The total — a rough estimate of the extent of your patient's burns — enters into the for-mula to determine his initial fluid replacement needs.

An infant or a child's body-section percentages differ from those of an adult. For instance, an infant's head accounts for a greater percentage of his total body surface when compared with an adult's. For an *infant* or *child,* use the Lund-Browder chart (below, right).

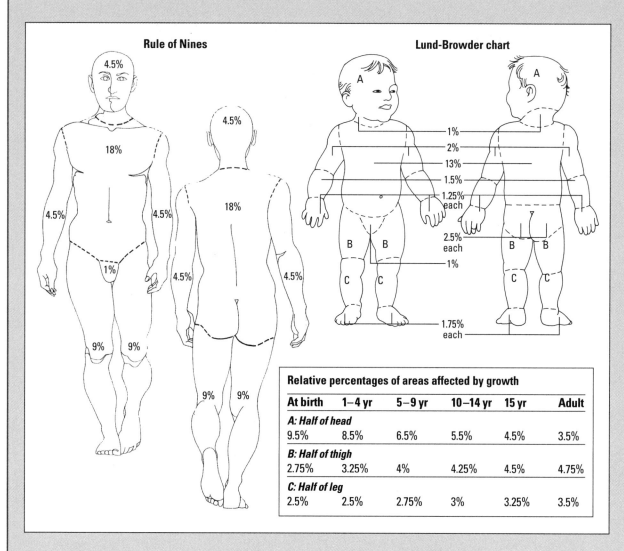

Rule of Nines

Lund-Browder chart

Relative percentages of areas affected by growth					
At birth	1–4 yr	5–9 yr	10–14 yr	15 yr	Adult
A: Half of head					
9.5%	8.5%	6.5%	5.5%	4.5%	3.5%
B: Half of thigh					
2.75%	3.25%	4%	4.25%	4.5%	4.75%
C: Half of leg					
2.5%	2.5%	2.75%	3%	3.25%	3.5%

lead to several serious fluid and electrolyte imbalances, which vary depending on the phase of the burn.

Fluid accumulation phase

The fluid accumulation phase lasts for 36 to 48 hours after a burn injury. During that phase, fluid shifts from the vascular compartment to the interstitial space, a process known as third-space shift. This shift of fluids causes edema. Typically, the edema reaches its maximum extent within 8 hours after the injury. Severe edema may compromise circulation and diminish pulses. Other conditions occur during this phase.

Permeability and plasma

Because of the burn injury, capillary damage alters the permeability of the vessels. Plasma—the liquid and protein part of blood—also escapes from the vascular compartment into the interstitium. Because less fluid is available to dilute the blood, the blood becomes hemoconcentrated and the patient's hemoglobin level and hematocrit rise.

Because of the third-space shift (fluids moving out of the vascular compartment), hypovolemia occurs. Hypovolemia causes decreased cardiac output, tachycardia, and hypotension. The patient may develop shock or cardiac arrhythmias or his mental status may decrease.

With the burn's damage to the skin surface, the skin's ability to prevent water loss is also decreased. As a result, the patient can lose up to 8 L of fluid per day, or 400 ml/hour.

Back in the kidneys...

Diminished kidney perfusion causes decreased urine output. In response to a burn, the body produces and releases stress hormones (aldosterone and antidiuretic hormone) that cause the kidneys to retain sodium and water.

Uneasy breathing

Depending on the type of burn, a patient may have a compromised, edematous airway. Look for burns of the head or neck, singed nasal hairs, soot in the mouth or nose, coughing, voice changes, mucosal burns, and stridor. You may hear crackles or wheezes over the lung fields. The patient may breathe rapidly or pant. Circumferential burns and edema of the neck or chest can restrict respirations and cause shortness of breath.

Acid test

Injured tissue causes the release of acids that can cause a drop in the pH level of the blood and subsequent metabolic acidosis. Dam-

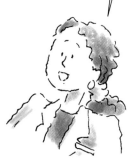

Depending on the type of burn, a patient may have a compromised, edematous airway.

age to muscle tissue in full-thickness burns causes a release of myoglobin, which can cause renal damage and acute tubular necrosis. Myoglobin gives urine a darkened appearance.

The GI takes a hit

Hypovolemia can cause a decrease in circulation to the GI system, resulting in paralytic ileus. The development of gastric ulceration is also common among severe burn patients. Due to tissue destruction, protein loss, and the body's stress response, a negative nitrogen balance can occur after a burn injury. In these instances, protein loss exceeds intake and leads to a negative nitrogen balance.

Also, the body's metabolic needs are increased due to the burn injury. The increase in metabolic need is usually proportional to the size of the burn wound.

Unbalanced!

Many electrolyte imbalances can occur during the fluid accumulation phase because of the hypermetabolic needs and the priority that fluid replacement takes over nutritional needs during the emergent phase.

Potassium and fluid

Hyperkalemia can result from massive cellular trauma, metabolic acidosis, or renal failure. The condition develops as potassium is released into the extracellular fluid in the initial days following the injury.

Hypovolemia can occur as a result of fluid losses and fluids moving from the vascular space to the interstitial space. Lost fluid resembles intravascular fluid in composition and contains proteins and electrolytes.

Sodium

Hyponatremia can result from the increased loss of sodium and water from the cells. Large amounts of sodium become trapped in edematous fluid during the fluid accumulation phase. Aqueous silver nitrate dressings may also contribute to this electrolyte imbalance.

Other imbalances

Hypernatremia can occur as a result of the aggressive use of hypertonic sodium solutions during fluid replacement therapy.

Hypocalcemia can occur because calcium travels to the damaged tissue and becomes immobilized at the burn site. That movement can occur 12 to 24 hours after the burn injury. It may also occur due to an inadequate dietary intake of calcium or inadequate supplementation during treatment.

Metabolic acidosis can develop as a result of the accumulation of acids released from the burned tissue. It can also occur due to decreased tissue perfusion from hypovolemia.

Respiratory acidosis can result from inadequate ventilation, as happens in inhalation burns.

Fluid remobilization phase

The fluid remobilization phase, also known as the diuresis stage, starts about 48 hours after the initial burn. Here, the fluid shifts back to the vascular compartment. Edema at the burn site decreases, and blood flow to the kidneys increases, which increases urine output. Sodium is lost through the increase in diuresis, and potassium either moves back into the cells or is lost through the urine.

A shift in balance

Fluid and electrolyte imbalances present during the initial phase after a burn can change during the fluid remobilization phase. Here's a rundown of these imbalances.

• Hypokalemia can develop as potassium shifts from the extracellular fluid back into the cells. The condition usually occurs 4 to 5 days after a major burn.

• Hypervolemia can occur as fluid shifts back to the vascular compartment. Excessive administration of I.V. fluids may exacerbate the condition.

• Hyponatremia may occur when sodium is lost during diuresis.

Convalescent phase

The convalescent phase begins after the first two phases have been resolved and is characterized by the need to focus on the healing or reconstruction of the burn wound. Although the major fluid shifts have been resolved, further fluid and electrolyte imbalances may continue as a result of inadequate dietary intake. Anemia commonly develops at this time because severe burns typically destroy red blood cells.

What tests show

Diagnostic test results you may see when caring for a burn patient include:
- increased hemoglobin levels and hematocrit
- increased serum potassium levels
- decreased serum sodium levels
- increased blood urea nitrogen and creatinine levels, indicating renal failure
- low pH and bicarbonate levels, indicating metabolic acidosis
- increased carboxyhemoglobin levels, indicating smoke inhalation
- electrocardiogram (ECG) changes reflecting electrolyte imbalances or myocardial damage
- myoglobin in the urine.

Be alert!

Watch for signs and symptoms of pulmonary edema, which can result from fluid replacement therapy and the shift of fluid back to the vascular compartment. Check for decreased hemoglobin levels and hematocrit, due to hemodilution from that shift of fluid.

Skin impairment leads not only to body temperature alterations and chills but also to infection. Blisters, charring, and scarring may appear, depending on the type and age of the burn. With infected wounds, a foul odor and purulent drainage may also be present.

How burns are treated

Priorities in treating a burn patient reflect the ABCs — airway, breathing, and circulation. For a patient with severe facial burns or suspected inhalation injury, treatment to prevent hypoxia includes endotracheal (ET) intubation, administration of high concentrations of oxygen, and positive-pressure ventilation. Be aware that adult respiratory distress syndrome may develop from both the body's immune response to injury and the leakage of fluid across the alveolocapillary membrane.

Rehydrate

Fluid resuscitation is a vital part of treatment. Several formulas have been created to guide initial treatment for the burn victim. The Parkland formula is one of the more commonly used formulas. (See *Fluid replacement formula*, page 278.)

Initial treatment includes administration of lactated Ringer's solution through a large-bore I.V. line to expand vascular volume. This balanced isotonic solution supplies water, sodium, and other

Fluid replacement formula

Here's a commonly used formula, the Parkland formula, for calculating fluid replacement in burn patients. Vary volumes of infusions depending on the patient's response, especially his urine output.

Formula

4 ml of lactated Ringer's solution per kilogram of body weight per percentage of body surface area over 24 hours.

    Example: for a 68 kg person with 27% body surface area burns: 4 ml x 68 kg x 27 = 7,344 ml over 24 hours. Give one-half of the total over the first 8 hours after the burn and the remainder over the next 16 hours.

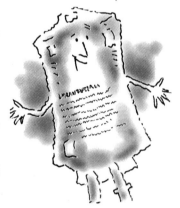

Fluid resuscitation is a vital part of treatment.

electrolytes; it can help correct metabolic acidosis because the lactate in the solution is quickly metabolized into bicarbonate.

Colloid controversy and insensible losses

Hypertonic solutions called colloids may be used to increase blood volume. Colloids draw water from the interstitial space into the vasculature. However, the use of colloids in the immediate postburn period is controversial because they increase colloid osmotic pressure in the interstitial space, which may worsen edema at the burn site. Examples of colloid solutions are plasma, albumin, and dextran.

A solution of dextrose 5% in water may be used to replace normal insensible water loss as well as water loss associated with damage to the skin barrier. Central and peripheral I.V. lines are inserted as necessary. Potassium may be added to I.V. fluids 48 to 72 hours after the burn injury.

More help

An indwelling urinary catheter permits accurate monitoring of urine output. Administration of 2 to 4 mg of morphine I.V. alleviates pain and anxiety. The patient may need a nasogastric (NG) tube to prevent gastric distention from paralytic ileus.

All burn patients need a booster of 0.5 ml of tetanus toxoid given I.M. Most burn centers don't recommend administering a prophylactic antibiotic because overuse of antibiotics fosters the development of resistant bacteria.

Caring for the wound

Treatment of the wound includes:
• initial debridement by washing the surface of the wound area with mild soap

• sharp debridement of loose tissue and blisters because blister fluid contains vasospastic agents that can worsen tissue ischemia
• coverage of the wound with an antibacterial agent, such as silver sulfadiazine, and an occlusive cotton gauze dressing
• removal of eschar (escharotomy) if the patient is at risk for vascular, circulatory, or respiratory compromise — for example, if the patient has a circumferential burn that circles around an extremity, the chest cavity, or the abdomen. Skin grafts may be required.

How you intervene

For a burn patient, good nursing care can mean the difference between life and death. The priority during the emergent phase is to provide immediate, aggressive burn treatment to increase the patient's chance for survival. Later, the priority shifts to providing supportive measures and using strict aseptic technique to minimize the risk of infection. (For tips on how to handle burns outside the health care system, see *Emergency burn care.*)

First steps

• Maintain head and spinal alignment until head and spinal cord injuries have been ruled out.
• Give emergency treatment for electric shock if needed. If an electric shock caused ventricular fibrillation and subsequent cardiac and respiratory arrest, begin cardiopulmonary resuscitation

---

Emergency burn care

Here's what you should do if you come upon a person who has just been burned:
• Extinguish any remaining flames on the patient's clothing.
• Don't directly touch the patient if he's still connected to live electricity. Unplug or disconnect the electrical source if possible.
• Assess the ABCs (airway, breathing, circulation), and initiate cardiopulmonary resuscitation if necessary.
• Assess the scope of the burns and other injuries.
• Remove the patient's clothing, but don't pull at clothing that sticks to the skin.
• Irrigate areas of chemical burns with copious amounts of water.
• Remove from the patient any jewelry or other metal objects that can retain heat and constrict patient movement.
• Cover the patient with a blanket.
• Send for emergency medical assistance.

at once. Try to obtain an estimate of the voltage that caused the injury.

• Make sure the patient has an adequate airway and effective breathing and circulation. If needed, assist with ET intubation. The patient may have a tracheostomy tube inserted if ET intubation isn't possible. Administer 100% oxygen as ordered, and adjust the flow to maintain adequate gas exchange. Draw blood for arterial blood gas (ABG) analyses as ordered.

• Assess vital signs every 15 minutes. Assess breath sounds, and watch for signs of hypoxia and pulmonary edema.

• Take steps to control bleeding, and remove clothing that's still smoldering. If clothing is stuck to the patient's skin, soak it in saline solution. Remove rings and other constricting items.

• Assess the skin for the location, depth, and extent of the burn.

• Assist with the insertion of a central venous line and additional arterial and I.V. lines.

• Start I.V. therapy at once to prevent hypovolemic shock and maintain cardiac output. Follow the Parkland formula or another fluid resuscitation formula, as ordered by the doctor.

• Insert an indwelling urinary catheter as ordered, and monitor intake and output every 15 to 30 minutes.

• Maintain adequate pulmonary hygiene by turning the patient and performing postural drainage regularly.

Assess and monitor

• Watch for signs of decreased tissue perfusion, increased confusion, and agitation. Assess peripheral pulses for adequacy.

• Assess the patient's heart and hemodynamic status for changes that might indicate fluid imbalances, such as hypervolemia or hypovolemia.

• Observe the pattern of third-space shifting (generalized edema, ascites, and pulmonary or intracranial edema), and document your findings.

• Monitor potassium levels, and watch for signs and symptoms of hyperkalemia, such as cardiac rhythm strip changes, weakness, diarrhea, and a slowed, irregular heart rate.

• Monitor sodium levels, and watch for signs and symptoms of hyponatremia, such as increasing confusion, twitching, seizures, abdominal pain, nausea, and vomiting. (See *Teaching about burns.*)

• Watch for signs and symptoms of metabolic acidosis, such as headache, disorientation, drowsiness, nausea, vomiting, and rapid, shallow breathing.

• Monitor ABG results.

• Monitor other laboratory results.

• Monitor ECG results for arrhythmias.

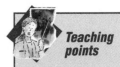

Teaching points

Teaching about burns

Teach the patient and his family about burns and then evaluate their learning. Include:

• what a burn is and how to prevent it

• the patient's particular plan of treatment and wound management

• signs and symptoms to report to the doctor

• long-term care issues, such as home care follow-up and rehabilitation.

Maintain

• Anticipate the need to administer maintenance I.V. replacement fluids, based on daily assessment of fluid, electrolyte, acid-base, and nutritional status.
• Maintain core body temperature by covering the patient with a sterile blanket and exposing only small areas of his body at a time.
• Insert an NG tube, if ordered, to decompress the stomach. Avoid aspiration of stomach contents during the procedure.

Weigh and measure

• Obtain a preburn weight from the patient or from a family member or friend.
• If bowel sounds are present, provide a diet high in potassium, protein, vitamins, fats, nitrogen, and calories to maintain the patient's preburn weight. If necessary, feed the patient enterally until he can tolerate oral feedings. If he can't tolerate oral or enteral feedings, administer hyperalimentation as ordered.
• Weigh the patient every day at the same time with the same amount of linen, clothes, and dressings.

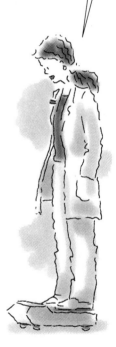

Obtain a preburn weight from the patient.

Care for the wounds

• Use strict aseptic technique for all patient care, including routinely washing your hands and using protective isolation clothing.
• Observe the patient for signs of infection, such as fever, tachycardia, and purulent wound drainage. Burn patients have an increased risk of infection from destruction of the skin barrier and the loss of nutrients.
• Administer an analgesic 30 minutes before wound care.
• Culture wounds before applying a topical antibiotic for the first time.
• Cover burns with a dry, sterile dressing. Never cover large burns with saline-soaked dressings because they can drastically lower body temperature. A topical ointment and an antibiotic may be applied as appropriate. Silver nitrate and mafenide acetate (Sulfamylon) can cause electrolyte imbalances and metabolic alterations.
• Maintain joint function with physical therapy and use of support garments and splints.
• Notify the doctor of significant changes in the patient's condition or pertinent laboratory test results.

Communicate with the patient

• Explain all procedures to the patient before performing them. Speak calmly and clearly to help alleviate anxiety. Encourage the patient to participate in self-care as much as possible.
• Provide opportunities for the patient to voice concerns, especially about altered body image. If appropriate, arrange a meeting

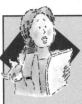

Chart smart

Documenting burn care

Your documentation for a burn victim should include:
- assessment findings
- depth, extent, and severity of burn injury
- extent of edema
- pertinent laboratory results
- I.V. therapy
- patient and family teaching along with the patient's response
- support made available to the patient and family
- other interventions such as wound care.

with another patient with similar injuries. When possible, show the patient how bodily functions are improving. If necessary, refer the patient for mental health counseling.
- Prepare the patient and family to go home.
- Document all care given, all teaching done, and the patient's reaction to each. (See *Documenting burn care.*)

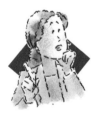

Quick quiz

1. During the fluid accumulation phase of a major burn injury, fluids shift from the:
- A.   intravascular space to the interstitial space.
- B.   interstitial space to the intravascular space.
- C.   intracellular space to the interstitial space.

Answer: A. During the fluid accumulation phase, fluids shift from the intravascular space to the interstitial space.

2. Hypovolemia usually occurs during which major burn phase?
- A.   Fluid remobilization
- B.   Fluid accumulation
- C.   Convalescent

Answer: B. Hypovolemia usually occurs during the fluid accumulation phase as fluid moves from the intravascular space to the interstitial space, a process known as third-space shift.

3. Hypervolemia can occur during the fluid remobilization phase of a major burn as a result of:

    A.   fluids shifting back into the intracellular space.

    B.   fluids shifting back into the interstitial space.

    C.   giving too much I.V. fluids.

Answer: C. Hypervolemia can be exacerbated by administering excessive I.V. fluids.

4. Your patient has second- and third-degree burn injuries to his anterior chest, anterior abdomen, and entire right arm. Using the Rule of Nines, the percentage of total body surface area involved can be estimated at what percent?

    A.   18%

    B.   27%

    C.   45%

Answer: B. The anterior chest and abdomen make up 18% of the body surface area; the entire right arm, 9%. Therefore, the estimated total is 27%.

5. You insert an I.V. line and begin fluid resuscitation. The doctor wants you to use the Parkland formula. The patient is a 155-lb (70-kg) male and is estimated at having 50% of his total body surface area burned. What amount of lactated Ringer's solution should be administered over the first 8 hours?

    A.   700 ml

    B.   7,000 ml

    C.   1,400 ml

Answer: B. The Parkland formula is 4 ml $\times$ the percentage of total body surface area burned $\times$ weight in kg. So, 4 ml $\times$ 50% $\times$ 70 kg = 14,000 ml or 14 L of lactated Ringer's solution in the first 24 hours. Therefore, you would give 7,000 ml (or half) in the first 8 hours.

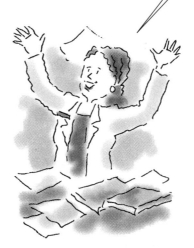

Only one more question to go!

6. During the fluid accumulation phase of a patient with burn injuries, the nurse would expect to see signs of which electrolyte imbalance?

    A.   Hypokalemia

    B.   Hyperkalemia

    C.   Hyponatremia

Answer: A. Hypokalemia occurs in the fluid accumulation phase as potassium shifts from the extracellular fluid back into the cells.

Scoring

☆☆☆ If you answered all six items correctly, outstanding! You're on fire (sorry)!

☆☆ If you answered four or five correctly, way to go! There's not much left to learn when it comes to burns!

☆ If you answered fewer than four correctly, don't feel the heat just yet. There's still a few chapters to go!

Part IV

Treating imbalances

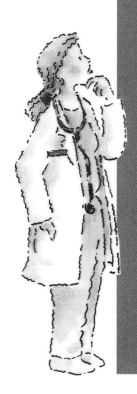

I.V. fluid replacement

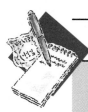

Just the facts

This chapter focuses on I.V. fluid replacement therapy. In this chapter, you'll learn:

♦ what the types of I.V. fluids are and how they're used

♦ what methods are used to administer I.V. fluids

♦ which complications are associated with I.V. therapy

♦ how to provide nursing care for a patient receiving I.V. therapy.

A look at I.V. therapy

To maintain health, the balance of fluids and electrolytes in the intracellular and extracellular spaces needs to remain relatively constant. Whenever a person experiences an illness or a condition that prevents normal fluid intake or causes excessive fluid loss, I.V. fluid replacement may be necessary.

I.V. therapy that provides the patient with life-sustaining fluids, electrolytes, and medications offers the advantages of immediate and predictable therapeutic effects. The I.V. route is, therefore, the preferred route, especially for administering fluids, electrolytes, and drugs in an emergency.

This route also allows for fluid intake when a patient has GI malabsorption. I.V. therapy permits accurate dosage titration for analgesics and other medications. Potential disadvantages associated with I.V. therapy include drug and solution incompatibility, adverse reactions, infection, and other complications.

Types of solutions

Solutions used for I.V. fluid replacement fall into the broad categories of crystalloids (which may be isotonic, hypotonic, or hypertonic) and colloids (which are always hypertonic).

Crystalloids

Crystalloids are solutions with small molecules that flow easily from the bloodstream into cells and tissues. Isotonic crystalloids contain about the same concentration of osmotically active particles as extracellular fluid, so fluid doesn't shift between the extracellular and intracellular areas.

Hypotonic crystalloids are less concentrated than extracellular fluid, so they move from the bloodstream into the cell, causing the cell to swell. In contrast, hypertonic crystalloids are more highly concentrated than extracellular fluid, so fluid is pulled into the bloodstream from the cell, causing the cell to shrink. (See *Comparing fluid tonicity*.)

Isotonic solutions

Isotonic solutions, such as dextrose 5% in water (D_5W), have an osmolality (or concentration) of 275 to 295 mOsm/L. The dextrose metabolizes quickly, however, acting like a hypotonic solution and leaving water behind. Large amounts of the solution may cause hyperglycemia.

More isotonic solutions

Normal saline solution, another isotonic solution, contains only the electrolytes sodium and chloride. Other isotonic fluids are more similar to extracellular fluid. For instance, Ringer's solution contains sodium, potassium, calcium, and chloride. Lactated Ringer's solution contains those electrolytes plus lactate, which the liver converts to bicarbonate.

Hypotonic fluids

Hypotonic fluids are fluids that have an osmolality less than 275 mOsm/L. Examples of hypotonic fluids include:
• half-normal saline solution
• 0.33% sodium chloride solution
• dextrose 2.5% in water.

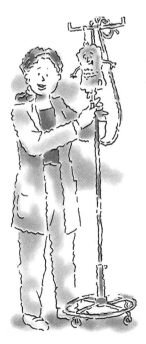

Now I get it!

Comparing fluid tonicity

The illustrations below show the effects of different types of I.V. fluids on fluid movement and cell size.

Isotonic	**Hypertonic**	**Hypotonic**
Isotonic fluids, such as normal saline solution, have a concentration of dissolved particles, or tonicity, equal to that of the intracellular fluid. Osmotic pressure is therefore the same inside and outside the cells, so they neither shrink nor swell with fluid movement.	Hypertonic fluid has a tonicity greater than that of intracellular fluid, so osmotic pressure is unequal inside and outside the cells. Dehydration or rapidly infused hypertonic fluids, such as 3% saline or 50% dextrose, draws water out of the cells into the more highly concentrated extracellular fluid.	Hypotonic fluids, such as half-normal saline solution, have a tonicity less than that of intracellular fluid, so osmotic pressure draws water into the cells from the extracellular fluid. Severe electrolyte losses or inappropriate use of I.V. fluids can make body fluids hypotonic.

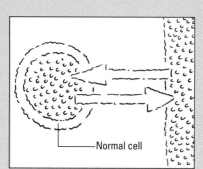

Normal cell

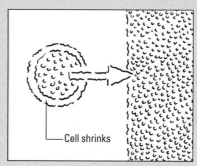

Cell shrinks

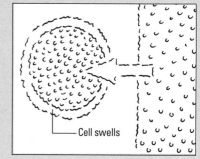

Cell swells

It makes a cell swell

Hypotonic solutions should be given cautiously because fluid then moves from the extracellular space into cells, causing them to swell. That fluid shift can cause cardiovascular collapse from vascular fluid depletion. It can also cause increased intracranial pressure (ICP) from fluid shifting into brain cells.

Hypotonic solutions shouldn't be given to a patient at risk for increased ICP—for example, those who have had a stroke, head trauma, or neurosurgery. Signs of increased ICP include a change in the patient's level of consciousness, motor or sensory deficits, and changes in the size, shape, or response to light in the pupils. Hypotonic solutions also shouldn't be used for patients who suffer from abnormal fluid shifts into the interstitial space or the body cavities—for example, as a result of liver disease, a burn, or trauma.

Hypertonic solutions

Hypertonic solutions are those that have an osmolality greater than 295 mOsm/L. Examples include:
- dextrose 5% in half-normal saline solution
- dextrose 5% in normal saline solution
- dextrose 5% in lactated Ringer's solution
- dextrose 10% in water.

The incredibly shrinking cell

A hypertonic solution draws fluids from the intracellular space, causing cells to shrink and the extracellular space to expand. Patients with cardiac or renal disease may be unable to tolerate extra fluid. Watch for fluid overload and pulmonary edema.

Because hypertonic solutions draw fluids from cells, patients at risk for cellular dehydration (patients with diabetic ketoacidosis [DKA], for example) shouldn't receive them. (See *A look at I.V. solutions.*)

Colloids

The use of colloids over crystalloids is controversial. Still, the doctor may prescribe a colloid—or plasma expander—if your patient's blood volume doesn't improve with crystalloids. Examples of colloids that may be given include:
- albumin (available in 5% solutions, which are osmotically equal to plasma, and 25% solutions, which draw about four times their volume in interstitial fluid into the circulation within 15 minutes of administration)
- plasma protein fraction
- dextran
- hetastarch.

Flowing into the stream

Colloids pull fluid into the bloodstream. The effects of colloids last several days if the lining of the capillaries is normal. The patient needs to be closely monitored during a colloid infusion for increased blood pressure, dyspnea, and bounding pulse, which are all signs of hypervolemia.

If neither crystalloids nor colloids are effective in treating the imbalance, the patient may require a blood transfusion or other treatment.

A look at I.V. solutions

This chart shows examples of some commonly used I.V. fluids and includes some of the clinical uses and special considerations associated with their use.

Solution	Uses	Special considerations
Isotonic Dextrose 5% in water	• Fluid loss and dehydration • Hypernatremia	• Solution is isotonic initially; becomes hypotonic when dextrose is metabolized. • Don't use for resuscitation; can cause hyperglycemia. • Use cautiously in renal or cardiac disease; can cause fluid overload. • Doesn't provide enough daily calories for prolonged use; may cause eventual breakdown of protein.
0.9% sodium chloride (normal saline solution)	• Shock • Hyponatremia • Blood transfusions • Resuscitation • Fluid challenges • Metabolic alkalosis • Hypercalcemia • Fluid replacement in patients with diabetic ketoacidosis (DKA)	• Because this replaces extracellular fluid, don't use in patients with heart failure, edema, or hypernatremia; can lead to overload.
Lactated Ringer's	• Dehydration • Burns • Lower GI tract fluid loss • Acute blood loss • Hypovolemia due to third-space shifting	• Electrolyte content is similar to serum but doesn't contain magnesium. • Contains potassium; don't use with renal failure; can cause hyperkalemia. • Don't use in liver disease because the patient can't metabolize lactate; a functional liver converts it to bicarbonate; don't give if patient's pH > 7.5.
Hypotonic 0.45% sodium chloride (half-normal saline solution)	• Water replacement • DKA after initial normal saline solution and before dextrose infusion • Hypertonic dehydration • Sodium and chloride depletion • Gastric fluid loss from nasogastric suctioning or vomiting	• Use cautiously; may cause cardiovascular collapse or increased intracranial pressure. • Don't use in patients with liver disease, trauma, or burns.

(continued)

A look at I.V. solutions *(continued)*

Solution	Uses	Special considerations
Hypertonic Dextrose 5% in half-normal saline solution	• DKA after initial treatment with normal saline solution and half-normal saline solution — prevents hypoglycemia and cerebral edema (occurs when serum osmolality is reduced too rapidly)	• In DKA, use only when glucose falls < 250 mg/dl.
Dextrose 5% in normal saline solution	• Hypotonic dehydration • Temporary treatment of circulatory insufficiency and shock if plasma expanders aren't available • Syndrome of inappropriate antidiuretic hormone (or use 3% sodium chloride) • Addisonian crisis	• Don't use in cardiac or renal patients because of danger of heart failure and pulmonary edema.
Dextrose 10% in water	• Water replacement • Conditions in which some nutrition with glucose is required	• Monitor serum glucose levels.

Delivery methods

The choice of I.V. delivery is based on the purpose of the therapy and its duration; the patient's diagnosis, age, and health history; and the condition of the patient's veins. I.V. solutions can be delivered through a peripheral or a central vein. Catheters and tubing are chosen based on the therapy and the site to be used. Here's a look at how to choose a site — peripheral or central — and which equipment you'll need for each.

Peripheral lines

Peripheral I.V. therapy is administered for short-term or intermittent therapy through a vein in the arm, hand, leg, or foot. Potential I.V. sites include the metacarpal, cephalic, basilic, median cubital, and greater saphenous veins. Using veins in the leg or foot is unusual because of the risk of thrombophlebitis.

Choose the right site

Choose a site that meets the patient's need for fluids, while keeping the patient as comfortable as possible. Place I.V. catheters in the hand or the lower arm so sites can be moved upward as needed. Use the patient's nondominant hand, if possible. For a patient who has suffered trauma or cardiac arrest, use a large vein in the antecubital area to gain rapid access. Avoid the antecubital site in a mobile patient because the catheter may kink with movement or cause other discomfort. Avoid using veins over joints. Catheters in those veins are uncomfortable and awkward and can be displaced easily.

Pick a cath, not just any cath

Three main types of catheters are used for insertion into a peripheral vein.
• Steel scalp-vein (winged-infusion) needles are inserted easily, but infiltration is common. These catheters are small, nonflexible, and used when access with another device proves unsuccessful. The catheters are also used for short-term therapy in adults, especially for giving medications by I.V. push (through a syringe over a short period of time).
• Indwelling catheters inserted over a steel needle are easy to use and less likely to infiltrate. Once in place, these catheters are more comfortable for the patient. They're also more difficult to insert than a scalp-vein needle.
• Plastic catheters inserted through a hollow needle are longer and are more commonly used for central-vein infusions. The catheter must be threaded through the vein for a greater distance, which makes these catheters more difficult to use.

Needle size

Choosing the right diameter (or gauge) needle or catheter is important for ensuring adequate flow and patient comfort. The higher the gauge, the smaller the diameter of the needle.

If you want to give a lot of fluid over a short period of time, use a catheter with a lower gauge (such as 14G, 16G, or 18G) and a shorter length, which offers less resistance to fluid flow. For routine I.V. fluid administration, use higher-gauge catheters, such as a 20G or a 22G. French catheters are the exception to the needle-gauge rule: The higher the number, the *greater* the diameter.

Central lines

Central venous therapy involves administering solutions through a catheter placed in a central vein, typically the subclavian or inter-

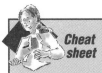

nal jugular vein, less commonly the femoral vein. Central venous therapy is used for patients who have inadequate peripheral veins, need access for blood sampling, require a large volume of fluid, need a hypertonic solution to be diluted by rapid blood flow in a larger vein, or need a high-calorie nutritional supplement.

Pick a cath, part 2

Three main types of catheters are used for short- and long-term central venous therapy.
• The traditional central venous catheter is a multilumen catheter usually used for short-term therapy. Although the lumen size may vary, a multilumen catheter provides multiple I.V. access using one insertion site.
• A peripherally inserted central catheter is now commonly used in hospitals and in home care. A certified nurse can insert this catheter through a vein in the antecubital area, at bedside. Fewer, less-severe adverse effects occur with these catheters than with traditional central venous catheters. Also, the catheters can be left in place for several months, making them ideal for long-term therapy.
• For extended long-term therapy, the patient may receive a vascular access port implanted in a pocket surgically constructed in the subcutaneous tissue or a tunneled catheter, such as a Hickman, Broviac, or Groshong. Some of these catheters have multiple lumens and are used in the health care facility and at home.

Tubing systems

The mechanics of infusing a solution require a tubing system that can deliver a drug at the correct infusion rate. I.V. tubing is available principally in microdrip sets, which are designed so that 60 gtt equal 1 ml. Microdrip sets are useful for infusion rates lower than 100 ml/hour—for instance, when using a solution to keep a vein open.

A macrodrip set, on the other hand, is designed so that 10 to 15 gtt equal 1 ml, depending on the manufacturer. Macrodrip sets are preferred for infusion rates greater than 100 ml/hour—for instance, when treating a patient with shock.

Limiting exposure to needles

The Occupational Safety and Health Administration requires health care organizations to initiate controls to isolate or remove hazardous blood-borne pathogens from the workplace. Several products now available are designed to minimize exposure to contaminated needles. These products include blunt metal cannulas,

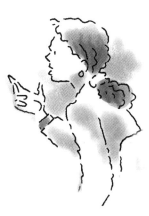

needles that recess into a plastic housing, and blunt plastic cannulas.

Infusion pumps

Electronic infusion pumps deliver fluids at precisely controlled infusion rates. Because each machine requires its own type of tubing, check the directions before use.

Most tubings contain back-check valves to prevent drugs from mixing inside piggyback systems (one I.V. line plugged into another at a piggyback port). Filters on some tubing eliminate particulate matter, bacteria, and air bubbles. Other types of tubing are available specifically for administering individual drugs or for piggybacking multiple drugs.

Complications of I.V. therapy

Caring for a patient with an I.V. line requires careful monitoring as well as a clear understanding of what the possible complications are, what to do if they arise, and how to deal with flow issues.

Infiltration, infection, phlebitis, and thrombophlebitis are the most common complications of I.V. therapy. Other complications include extravasation, a severed catheter, an allergic reaction, an air embolism, speed shock, and fluid overload.

Infiltration

During infiltration, fluid may leak from the vein into surrounding tissue. This occurs when the access device dislodges from the vein. Look for coolness at the site, pain, swelling, leaking, and lack of blood return. Also, look for a sluggish flow that continues even if a tourniquet is applied above the site. If you see infiltration, stop the infusion, elevate the extremity, and apply warm soaks.

Go small

To prevent infiltration, use the smallest catheter that will accomplish the infusion, avoid placement in joint areas, and anchor the catheter in place.

Infection

I.V. therapy involves puncturing the skin, the body's barrier to infection. As a result, the patient may develop an infection. Look for purulent drainage at the site, tenderness, erythema, warmth, or hardness on palpation. Signs and symptoms that the infection has become systemic include fever, chills, and an elevated white blood cell count.

Monitoring vital signs is vital

Nursing actions for an infected I.V. site include monitoring vital signs and notifying the doctor. Swab the site for culture, and remove the catheter as ordered. Always maintain aseptic technique to prevent this complication.

Phlebitis and thrombophlebitis

Phlebitis is inflammation of the vein; thrombophlebitis is an irritation of the vein with the formation of a clot and is usually more painful than phlebitis. Either poor insertion technique or the pH or osmolality of the solution or medication can cause these complications. Look for pain, redness, swelling, or induration at the site; a red line streaking along the vein; fever; or a sluggish flow of the solution.

Prevention begins with big veins

When phlebitis or thrombophlebitis occurs, remove the I.V., monitor the patient's vital signs, notify the doctor, and apply warm soaks to the site. To prevent these complications, choose large-bore veins and change the catheter every 72 hours when infusing a medication or solution with high osmolality.

Extravasation

Extravasation, similar to infiltration, is the leakage of fluid into surrounding tissues. It results when medications — such as dopamine, calcium solutions, and chemotherapeutic agents — seep through veins and produce blistering and, eventually, necrosis. Initially, the patient may experience discomfort, burning, or pain at the site. Look also for skin tightness, blanching, and lack of blood return. Delayed reactions include inflammation and pain within 3 to 5 days and ulcers or necrosis within 2 weeks.

Review policy

When administering medications that may extravasate, know your facility's policy. Nursing actions include stopping the infusion, notifying the doctor, infiltrating the site with an antidote as ordered (this is usually done through the I.V. before removing the catheter), applying ice early and warm soaks later, and elevating the extremity. Assess the circulation and nerve function of the limb.

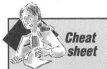

Cheat sheet

Complications of I.V. therapy

Most common
- Infiltration
- Infection
- Phlebitis
- Thrombophlebitis

Others
- Extravasation
- Severed catheter
- Allergic reaction
- Air embolism
- Speed shock
- Fluid overload

Severed catheter

A severed catheter can occur when a piece of catheter becomes dislodged and is set free in the vein. Look for pain at the fragment site, decreased blood pressure, cyanosis, loss of consciousness, and a weak, rapid pulse. If this extremely rare but serious complication occurs, apply a tourniquet above the site of pain, notify the doctor immediately, monitor the patient, and provide support as needed. To simply avoid the problem altogether, avoid reinserting a needle through its plastic catheter once the needle has been withdrawn.

Allergic reaction

A patient may suffer an allergic reaction to the fluid, medication, I.V. catheter, or even the latex port in the I.V. tubing. However, the source of the reaction may not be known. Look for a red streak extending up the arm, rash, itching, watery eyes and nose, and wheezing.

Watch out for anaphylaxis

Left untreated, the condition may progress rapidly to anaphylaxis. Nursing measures for allergic reaction include stopping the I.V. immediately, notifying the doctor, monitoring the patient, and giving oxygen and medications as ordered.

Air embolism

An air embolism occurs when air enters the vein and can cause a decrease in blood pressure, an increase in the pulse rate, respiratory distress, an increase in ICP, and a loss of consciousness.

Clamp the I.V. off

If the patient develops an air embolism, notify the doctor, and clamp off the I.V. Place the patient on his left side, and lower his head to allow the air to enter the right atrium, where it can disperse more safely by way of the pulmonary artery. Monitor him, and administer oxygen. To avoid this serious complication in the future, prime all tubing completely, tighten all connections securely, and use an air detection device on an I.V. pump.

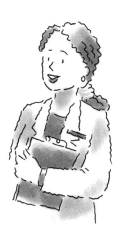

Speed shock

Speed shock occurs when I.V. solutions or medications are given too rapidly. Almost immediately, the patient will have facial flushing, an irregular pulse, a severe headache, and decreased blood pressure. Loss of consciousness and cardiac arrest may also occur.

Clamp off the I.V. here, too

If speed shock occurs, clamp off the I.V., and notify the doctor immediately. Provide oxygen, obtain vital signs frequently, and administer medications as ordered. Also, keep in mind that the use of infusion control devices can prevent this complication.

Fluid overload

Fluid overload can happen gradually or suddenly, depending on how well the patient's circulatory system can accommodate the fluid. Look for neck-vein distention, increased blood pressure, increased respirations, shortness of breath, cough, and crackles in the lungs on auscultation.

Slow it down

If the patient develops fluid overload, slow the I.V. rate, notify the doctor, and monitor vital signs. Keep the patient warm, keep the head of the bed elevated, and give oxygen and other medications (such as a diuretic) as ordered.

How you intervene

Nursing care for the patient with an I.V. includes the following actions.

Check, measure, monitor. . .

• Check the I.V. order for completeness and accuracy. Most I.V. orders expire after 24 hours. A complete order should specify the amount and type of solution, specific additives and their concentrations, and the rate and duration of the infusion. If the order is incomplete or confusing, clarify the order before proceeding.
• Monitor daily weights to document fluid retention or loss. A 2% increase or decrease in body weight is significant. A 2.2-lb (1-kg) change corresponds to 1 qt (1 L) of fluid gained or lost.
• Measure intake and output carefully at scheduled intervals. The kidneys attempt to restore fluid balance during dehydration by reducing urine production. Urine output less than 30 ml/hour signals retention of metabolic wastes. Notify the doctor if your patient's urine output falls below 30 ml/hour.
• Always carefully monitor the infusion of solutions that contain medication because rapid infusion and circulation of the drug can be dangerous.

. . .and all the rest

• Keep in mind the size, age, and history of your patient when giving I.V. fluids to prevent fluid overload. For pediatric patients, use

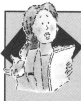

Chart smart

Documenting an I.V. infusion

Your documentation for a patient receiving an I.V. infusion should include:
* patient teaching and the patient's response to it
* the date, time, and type of catheter inserted
* the site of insertion and its appearance
* the type and amount of fluid infused
* the patient's tolerance of, and response to, therapy.

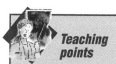

Teaching points

Teaching about I.V. therapy

Make sure you cover the following points with your patient and then evaluate his learning:
* what to expect before, during, and after the I.V. procedure
* signs and symptoms of complications and when to report them
* activity or diet restrictions
* how to care for an I.V. line at home.

a Buretrol or other device to limit the amount of fluid the patient receives hourly and to prevent the accidental administration of excessive amounts of fluid. (See *Teaching about I.V. therapy.*)
* Note the pH of the I.V. solution. The pH can alter the effect and stability of drugs mixed in the I.V. bag. Consult medication literature or the doctor if you have questions.
* Change the site, dressing, and tubing as often as facility policy requires. Solutions should be changed at least every 24 hours. (See *Documenting an I.V. infusion.*)
* When changing I.V. tubing, be sure not to move or dislodge the I.V. device. If you have trouble disconnecting the tubing, use a hemostat to hold the I.V. hub while twisting the tubing. Don't clamp the hemostat shut because doing so may crack the hub.
* Always report needle-stick injuries. Exposure to a patient's blood increases the risk of infection with blood-borne viruses such as human immunodeficiency virus (HIV), hepatitis B virus, hepatitis C virus, and cytomegalovirus. About 1 out of 300 people with occupational needle-stick injuries become HIV-seropositive.

Focus on the patient

* Always listen to your patient carefully. Subtle statements such as, "I just don't feel right" may be your clue to the beginning of an allergic reaction.
* Keep in mind that a candidate for home I.V. therapy must have a family member or friend who can safely and competently administer the I.V. fluids as well as a backup helper, a suitable home environment, a telephone, available transportation, adequate reading skills, and the ability to prepare, handle, store, and dispose of equipment properly. Procedures for caring for the I.V. are the same at home as in a health care facility, except at home the patient uses clean technique instead of sterile technique.

300

I.V. FLUID REPLACEMENT ....

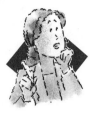

Quick quiz

1. Extravasation of I.V. fluid is associated with administration of which of the following?
- A. Hypertonic fluid
- B. D_5W
- C. An antineoplastic

Answer: C. Antineoplastics are highly irritating to the veins and are typically administered using a steel needle. Extravasation is common in those situations.

2. Hypertonic solutions cause fluids to move from the:
- A. interstitial space to the intracellular space.
- B. intracellular space to the extracellular space.
- C. extracellular space to the intracellular space.

Answer: B. Hypertonic solutions, because of their increased osmolality, draw fluids out of the cells and into the extracellular space.

3. Which of the following is the initial solution to be used in treating patients with DKA?
- A. D_5W
- B. Dextrose 5% in half-normal saline solution
- C. Normal saline solution

Answer: C. Normal saline solution is the optimal choice for patients with DKA because the fluid is isotonic and helps to replenish the intravascular volume.

4. Hypotonic fluids shouldn't be used for a patient with:
- A. increased ICP.
- B. DKA whose blood glucose level is 200 mg/dl or more.
- C. blood loss as a result of trauma.

Answer: A. Hypotonic fluids cause swelling of the cells and can further increase ICP.

5. Which of the following is a sign of an allergy to I.V. tubing?
   A.   Shortness of breath
   B.   Dry throat
   C.   Slow, bounding pulse

Answer: A. Signs and symptoms of an allergic reaction include shortness of breath, rash, and itching.

6. Your patient is a 90-year-old male with a history of heart failure. When you make rounds, you notice that an I.V. of normal saline solution was mistakenly hung an hour before and has infused 600 ml since then. You should observe this patient for signs of:
   A.   septic shock.
   B.   decreased ICP.
   C.   circulatory overload.

Answer: C. Because of his advanced age and cardiac condition, the type of fluid infused, and the infusion rate, the patient is at risk for circulatory overload.

7. When a hypotonic crystalloid solution is infused into the bloodstream, it causes the cells to:
   A.   shrink.
   B.   swell.
   C.   release chloride.

Answer: B. Hypotonic crystalloids are less concentrated than extracellular fluids, so they move from the bloodstream into the cell and cause the cell to expand with fluid.

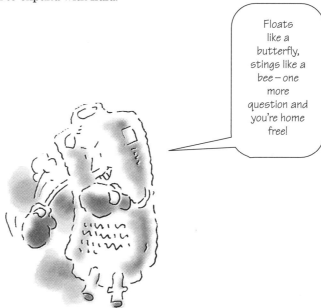

Floats like a butterfly, stings like a bee — one more question and you're home free!

8. Hypertonic solutions should be used cautiously in patients with:

- A. cancer or burns.
- B. cardiac or renal disease.
- C. respiratory or GI disease.

Answer: B. A hypertonic solution draws fluids from the intracellular space into the bloodstream. Patients with cardiac or renal disease may be unable to tolerate that extra fluid volume.

Scoring

☆☆☆ If you answered all eight items correctly, bravo! Here's my arm: plug me in with an I.V., you ace!

☆☆ If you answered five to seven correctly, excellent, you infusion hot shot, you!

☆ If you answered fewer than five correctly, no biggie. With a little more I.V. training you'll be whipping in 18-gaugers in no time!

Total parenteral nutrition

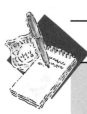

Just the facts

This chapter will help you understand total parenteral nutrition (TPN). In this chapter, you'll learn:

♦ how to identify patients who could benefit from TPN

♦ what each TPN component is and how TPN is delivered

♦ how to recognize complications associated with TPN

♦ how to care for a patient receiving TPN.

A look at TPN

TPN is a highly concentrated, hypertonic nutrient solution administered by way of an infusion pump through a large central vein. For patients with high caloric and nutritional needs due to illness or injury, TPN provides crucial calories, restores nitrogen balance, and replaces essential fluids, vitamins, electrolytes, minerals, and trace elements. (See *Understanding common TPN additives,* page 304.)

TPN also promotes tissue and wound healing and normal metabolic function; gives the bowel a chance to heal; reduces activity in the gallbladder, pancreas, and small intestine; and is used to improve a patient's response to surgery.

Who needs TPN?

Patients who can't meet their nutritional needs by oral or enteral feedings may require I.V. nutritional supplementation or TPN. Generally, this treatment is prescribed for any patient who can't absorb nutrients from the GI tract for more than 10 days. More specific indications include:
• debilitating illnesses lasting longer than 2 weeks
• loss of 10% or more of pre-illness weight

Understanding common TPN additives

Common components of total parenteral nutrition (TPN) solutions—such as dextrose 5% in water (D_5W), amino acids, and other additives—are used for specific purposes. For instance, D_5W provides calories for metabolism. Here's a list of other common additives and the purposes each serves. (Lipids may be infused separately.)

Electrolytes
- *Calcium* promotes development of bones and teeth and aids in blood clotting.
- *Chloride* regulates acid-base balance and maintains osmotic pressure.
- *Magnesium* helps the body absorb carbohydrates and protein.
- *Phosphorus* is essential for cell energy and calcium balance.
- *Potassium* is needed for cellular activity and cardiac function.
- *Sodium* helps control water distribution and maintains normal fluid balance.

Vitamins
- *Folic acid* is needed for DNA formation and promotes growth and development.
- *Vitamin B complex* helps the final absorption of carbohydrates and protein.
- *Vitamin C* helps in wound healing.
- *Vitamin D* is essential for bone metabolism and maintenance of serum calcium levels.
- *Vitamin K* helps prevent bleeding disorders.

Other additives
- *Acetate* prevents metabolic acidosis.
- *Micronutrients* (such as zinc, cobalt, and manganese) help in wound healing and red blood cell synthesis.
- *Amino acids* provide the proteins necessary for tissue repair.

- serum albumin level below 3.5 g/dl
- excessive nitrogen loss from a wound infection, a fistula, or an abscess
- renal or hepatic failure
- nonfunction of the GI tract lasting for 5 to 7 days. (See *PPN*.)

TPN triggers

Common illnesses or treatments that can trigger the need for TPN include inflammatory bowel disease, ulcerative colitis, bowel obstruction or resection, radiation enteritis, severe diarrhea or vomiting, acquired immunodeficiency syndrome, chemotherapy, and severe pancreatitis, all of which hinder a patient's ability to absorb nutrients. Also, patients may benefit from TPN if they've undergone major surgery or if they have a high metabolic rate due to sepsis, trauma, or burns of more than 40% of total body surface area. Infants with congenital or acquired disorders may need TPN to promote proper growth and development.

TPN has limited value for well-nourished patients with GI tracts that are healthy or are likely to resume normal function within 10 days. The treatment also may be inappropriate for a patient with a poor prognosis or when the risks of TPN outweigh its benefits.

Today's TPN trends

The trend of today's nutritional supplementation is to tailor TPN formulas to the patient's specific needs. As a result, standard TPN mixtures are becoming less popular. Nutritional support teams consisting of nurses, doctors, pharmacists, and dietitians assess, prescribe for, and monitor patients receiving TPN. The solutions may consist of:
- protein (amino acids in a 2.5% to 8.5% solution), with varying types available for patients with renal or liver failure
- dextrose (15% to 50% solution)
- fat emulsions (10% to 20% solution)
- electrolytes
- vitamins
- trace element mixtures
- medications.

Lipid emulsions

Lipid emulsions are thick emulsions that supply patients with both essential fatty acids and calories. These emulsions assist in wound healing, red blood cell (RBC) production, and prostaglandin synthesis. Although they're typically given with TPN, they may be given alone through a peripheral or central venous line, or they may be mixed with amino acids and dextrose in one container (providing a three-in-one-system) and infused over 24 hours.

The limits on lipids

Lipid emulsions should be given cautiously to patients with hepatic or pulmonary disease, anemia, or a coagulation disorder and to patients at risk for developing a fat embolism. These emulsions shouldn't be given to patients who have conditions that disrupt

PPN

Peripheral parenteral nutrition (PPN) is prescribed for patients who are able to take oral feedings but not enough to meet nutritional levels. PPN is infused peripherally in various combinations of lipid (fat) emulsions and amino acid-dextrose solutions.

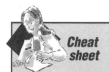

Cheat sheet

Key facts about TPN

- For patients with high caloric and nutritional needs due to injury or illness
- Provides calories, restores nitrogen balance, and replaces fluid, vitamins, electrolytes, minerals, and trace elements
- Infused through a central vein
- For therapy lasting 3 months or more, infused through a peripherally inserted central catheter

Warning!

Adverse reactions to lipid emulsions

Immediate or early adverse reactions to lipid emulsions include:
- back and chest pain
- cyanosis
- diaphoresis or flushing
- dyspnea
- headache
- hypercoagulability
- irritation at the site
- lethargy or syncope
- nausea or vomiting
- slight pressure over the eyes
- thrombocytopenia.

Delayed complications associated with prolonged administration include:
- blood dyscrasias
- fatty liver syndrome
- hepatomegaly
- jaundice
- splenomegaly.

normal fat metabolism, such as pathologic hyperlipidemia, lipid nephrosis, and acute pancreatitis.

Also, make sure you report any adverse reactions to the doctor so the TPN regimen can be changed as needed. (See *Adverse reactions to lipid emulsions.*)

How to infuse TPN

TPN must be infused through a central vein. As a hypertonic solution, it may be up to six times the concentration of blood and, therefore, too irritating for a peripheral vein.

TPN may be infused around the clock or for part of the day — for instance, as the patient sleeps at night. A sterile catheter made of polyurethane, polyvinyl chloride, or silicone rubber (Silastic) is inserted into the subclavian or jugular vein. A polyurethane catheter is for short-term use only because it stiffens within a short period of time and can cause thrombophlebitis. A Silastic catheter is a better alternative for therapy lasting months or years because it's more flexible and durable and it's compatible with many medications and solutions.

Looking to the peripheral

A peripherally inserted central catheter, a variation of central venous therapy, can be used for therapy lasting 3 months or more. The catheter is inserted through the basilic or cephalic vein and threaded so that the tip lies in the superior vena cava.

The patient generally experiences less discomfort with a peripheral catheter, especially if he can move around easily. Movement stimulates blood flow and decreases the risk of phlebitis. Peripherally inserted central catheters are becoming the preferred choice for intermediate-term therapy, at home and in the hospital.

What to look for

Signs and symptoms of electrolyte imbalances caused by TPN administration include abdominal cramps, lethargy, confusion, malaise, muscle weakness, tetany, convulsions, and cardiac arrhythmias. Acid-base imbalances can also occur due to the patient's condition or the TPN content. Look for these other complications:
• heart failure or pulmonary edema from fluid and electrolyte administration, conditions that can lead to tachycardia, lethargy, confusion, weakness, and labored breathing
• hyperglycemia from dextrose infusing too quickly, a condition that may require an adjustment in the patient's insulin dosage
• adverse reactions to medications added to TPN — for example, added insulin can cause hypoglycemia, which can result in confusion, restlessness, lethargy, pallor, and tachycardia
• complications from I.V. cannulas and central venous catheters.

Constant assessment and rapid intervention are critical for patients receiving TPN.

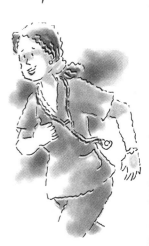

How you intervene

Constant assessment and rapid intervention are critical for patients receiving TPN. When caring for a patient on TPN, you'll want to take these actions.

Assess and monitor

• Carefully monitor patients receiving TPN to detect early signs of complications, such as metabolic problems, heart failure, pulmonary edema, or allergic reactions. Adjust the TPN regimen as needed.

• Assess the patient's nutritional status, and weigh the patient at the same time each morning after he voids, in similar clothing, and on the same scale. Weight is indicative of nutritional progress and also determines fluid overload. Patients ideally should gain 1 to 2 lb (0.5 to 1 kg)/week. Weight gain greater than 1 lb/day indicates fluid retention.

• Assess the patient for peripheral and pulmonary edema. Edema is a sign of fluid overload.

• Monitor serum glucose levels every 6 hours initially, then once a day. Watch for thirst and polyuria, indications that he may have hyperglycemia. Periodically confirm serum glucose meter readings with laboratory test results. Serum glucose levels should be less than 200 mg/dl. This indicates the patient's tolerance of the glucose solution.

• Monitor for signs and symptoms of glucose metabolism disturbance, fluid and electrolyte imbalances, and nutritional problems. Some patients may require insulin added directly to the TPN for the duration of treatment.

• Monitor electrolyte and protein levels daily at first, and then twice a week for serum albumin. Albumin levels may drop initially as treatment restores hydration.

• Check renal function by monitoring blood urea nitrogen (BUN) and creatinine levels; increases may indicate excess amino acid intake.

• Assess nitrogen balance with 24-hour urine collection.

• Assess liver function with liver function tests, bilirubin, triglyceride, and cholesterol levels. Abnormal values may indicate intolerance.

• In most facilities, central lines and peripherally inserted central catheters require an order and a patient-consent form. Only an RN specializing in inserting those lines should obtain the form. (See *Teaching about TPN.*)

• Obtain a chest X-ray to check catheter placement after insertion.

Infuse properly

• Review the patient's serum chemistry and nutritional studies, and alert the doctor of abnormal results, which may indicate that the TPN fluid concentration or ingredients may need to be adjusted to meet the patient's specific needs.

• Avoid an adverse reaction by starting TPN slowly — about 1,000 calories over 24 hours — and increasing gradually. Occasionally, a patient may react adversely to specific ingredients in the TPN solution. Protein may need to be reduced if BUN and creatinine levels are elevated. Continually monitor the patient's cardiac and respiratory status.

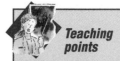

Teaching points

Teaching about TPN

Be sure to cover these topics with your patient, and evaluate his learning:

• basics of total parenteral nutrition (TPN) and its specific use for the patient

• adverse reactions or catheter complications and when to report them

• basic care of a TPN line

• maintenance of equipment

• how to monitor weight, calorie count, intake and output, and glucose levels.

• Because the TPN solution is high in glucose, starting the infusion slowly will also allow the patient's pancreatic beta cells to adapt to the glucose by increasing insulin output. Within the first 3 to 5 days of TPN, the typical adult can tolerate about 3 qt (3 L) of solution a day without experiencing an adverse reaction.
• When a patient is severely malnourished, starting TPN may spark refeeding syndrome, which includes a rapid drop in potassium, magnesium, and phosphorus levels. To avoid compromising cardiac function, initiate feeding slowly and monitor the patient's electrolyte levels closely until they stabilize.

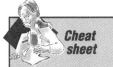

Cheat sheet

TPN complications

• Electrolyte imbalances
• Acid-base imbalances
• Heart failure or pulmonary edema
• Hyperglycemia
• Rebound hypoglycemia

Set up

• Use an infusion pump for rate control.
• Flush central lines according to protocol.
• If using a single-lumen central venous line, don't use the line for blood or blood products, give a bolus injection, administer simultaneous I.V. solutions, measure the central venous pressure, or draw blood for laboratory tests.
• Never add medications to a TPN solution container.
• Don't use a three-way stopcock unless absolutely necessary; add-on devices increase the risk of infection.
• Explain the insertion procedure to the patient.

Monitor during the infusion

• Record vital signs at least every 4 hours. Temperature elevation is one of the earliest signs of catheter-related sepsis.
• Assess the patient daily. Measure arm circumference and skinfold thickness over the triceps, if ordered.
• Perform site care and dressing changes at least three times a week (once a week for transparent semipermeable dressings), or whenever the dressing becomes wet, soiled, or nonocclusive. Use strict aseptic technique.
• Monitor the patient for signs of inflammation and infection, and document any you find. (See *Documenting TPN*, page 310.)
• Change the I.V. administration set according to facility policy, and always use aseptic technique. Changes of I.V. administration sets are usually done every 24 hours for TPN.
• Don't allow TPN solutions to hang for more than 24 hours.
• The TPN solution should be clear or pale yellow if multivitamins are added to the solution. If you see particulate matter, cloudiness, or an oily layer in the bag when preparing to hang a TPN solution, return the bag to the pharmacy.

Don't allow TPN solutions to hang for more than 24 hours.

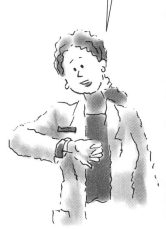

Follow up

• Provide emotional support, especially if eating is restricted due to the patient's condition.
• Provide frequent mouth care.

• While weaning the patient from TPN, document his dietary intake and total calorie and protein intake. Use percentages when recording food intake. For instance, chart that, "The patient ate 50% of a baked potato," rather than "The patient had a good appetite."

• When discontinuing TPN, decrease the infusion slowly, depending on current glucose intake. Slowly decreasing the infusion minimizes the risk of hyperinsulinemia and resulting hypoglycemia. Weaning usually takes place over 24 to 48 hours but can be completed in 4 to 6 hours if the patient receives sufficient oral or I.V. carbohydrates.

• Promptly report any adverse reactions to the doctor.

• Prepare your patient for home care.

• Accurately document all aspects of care, according to facility policy.

Chart smart

Documenting TPN

When documenting total parenteral nutrition, you'll want to include these points:

• adverse reactions or catheter complications

• signs of inflammation or infection at the I.V. site

• nursing interventions (including infusion rate) and the patient's response

• time and date of administration set changes

• specific dietary intake.

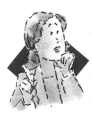

Quick quiz

1. The patient most likely to benefit from TPN is:
    A.   a well-nourished patient whose GI tract will resume normal function within 10 days.
    B.   a patient with a chronic, intractable condition.
    C.   a patient with a nonfunctioning GI tract lasting 5 to 7 days.

Answer: C. A patient whose GI tract is nonfunctioning for 5 to 7 days is a good candidate for TPN; however, TPN has only limited value if the patient is well nourished and normal function is expected to resume within 10 days of function loss. TPN may be inappropriate for a patient with a poor prognosis.

2.   When a severely malnourished patient starts receiving TPN, his laboratory tests show a rapid drop in potassium, magnesium, and phosphorus levels. The findings indicate which of the following conditions?
    A.   Fluid shock
    B.   Refeeding syndrome
    C.   Hypovolemia

Answer: B. These findings are signs of refeeding syndrome.

3. Which of the following types of I.V. catheter is recommended for TPN expected to last months or years?
  A. Silastic catheter
  B. Polyvinyl chloride catheter
  C. Metal-winged catheter

Answer: A. The Silastic catheter is a hardy catheter and may be used for months or years.

4. When preparing to hang a TPN solution, you see an oily layer in the bag. You should:
  A. gently agitate the solution to disperse the contents.
  B. hang the solution; the oily layer will disperse in time.
  C. return the solution to the pharmacy.

Answer: C. The solution should be clear. An oily layer indicates that the fluid may be contaminated or may have been improperly prepared.

5. Site care and dressing changes for a patient with TPN should be performed at least:
  A. once a week.
  B. three times a week.
  C. every day.

Answer: B. It's recommended that site care and dressing changes be performed three times a week; however, the patient's condition or facility policy may dictate the need for more frequent care.

6. Infusions of lipid emulsions are useful for promoting:
  A. wound healing.
  B. coagulation in bleeding disorders.
  C. a reduction in inflammation from pancreatitis.

Answer: A. Lipid emulsions assist in wound healing, in the production of RBCs, and in prostaglandin synthesis. Their use should be avoided in patients with acute pancreatitis or a coagulation disorder.

I see one more question in your future.

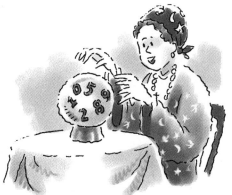

7.   Where is the tip of a peripherally inserted central catheter usually placed?

A.   Right atrium

B.   Internal jugular vein

C.   Superior vena cava

Answer: C. Peripherally inserted central catheters are generally inserted through the basilic or cephalic vein and threaded so that the tip lies in the superior vena cava.

Scoring

☆☆☆   If you answered all seven items correctly, totally cool! Your daily nutritional intake must include plenty of brain food!

☆☆   If you answered four to six correctly, you should still be pumped up! Your TPN knowledge is top 10!

☆   If you answered fewer than four correctly, let me give you some "parenteral" advice: Get your energy up and review the chapter!

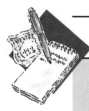

Blood products

Just the facts

This chapter discusses blood products and their uses. In this chapter, you'll learn:

♦ how blood is typed

♦ what types of blood products are available and when each is used

♦ which complications can occur with a transfusion

♦ how to care for a patient receiving a transfusion.

A look at blood transfusions

Transfusion therapy can restore blood volume as well as correct deficiencies in the blood's oxygen-carrying capacity and its coagulation components. Nursing responsibilities in blood transfusion include administering blood products and monitoring patients receiving the therapy. Nurses need to be knowledgeable about the various blood products available to safely transfuse blood to their patients.

Compatibility

Blood contains various antigens that affect how compatible one person's blood is with another's. The antigens include the ABO blood group, the rhesus (Rh) factor, and the human leukocyte antigen (HLA) blood group. Laboratory technologists crossmatch these characteristics — especially the Rh factor and the ABO blood type — to ensure compatibility between the donor's and recipient's blood before transfusion.

Identifying compatible blood types

A transfusion most likely will be safe if the donor and recipient have compatible blood types. The illustration here provides a guide to blood-type compatibility.

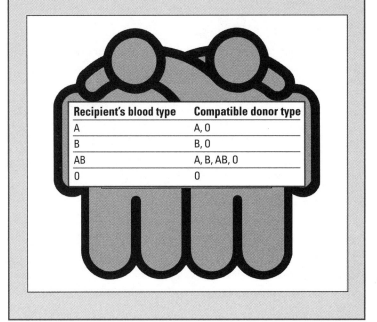

Recipient's blood type	Compatible donor type
A	A, O
B	B, O
AB	A, B, AB, O
O	O

The ABOs of typing blood

The ABO method of typing blood identifies two antigens on red blood cells (RBCs) — A and B. A person has both A and B antigens (type AB), only one antigen (type A or type B), or neither (type O). In the United States, 85% of the population has either type A or type O (with type O being the most common), 10% has type B, and 5% has type AB.

If a patient has A antigens, he has anti-B antibodies floating freely in his plasma. If a patient has B antigens, he has anti-A antibodies in his plasma. A patient may suffer a transfusion reaction if he receives a blood type for which he has antibodies.

Patients who have type AB blood are called universal recipients. They don't have antibodies and, therefore, can receive blood type O, A, B, or AB without having an ABO reaction. Patients with type O blood, by contrast, are universal donors. Their blood may be transfused into a person with any blood type, but because type

Transfusing in a crisis

In a crisis situation, during which it may not be possible to wait for blood crossmatching, the following can be given until tested blood is available:
• type O Rh-negative blood (blood from a universal donor)
• plasma protein solution (albumin)
• artificial plasma substitute (dextran, heta-starch)
• artificial blood substitutes.

O patients have both anti-A and anti-B antibodies, they may receive only type O blood safely.

Ideally, transfusions should be done using the same type of blood as the patient's. If that isn't possible, patients should receive blood that's compatible with their own blood type to keep transfusion reactions to a minimum. (See *Identifying compatible blood types.*)

In an emergency, when waiting for a crossmatch would be inadvisable, blood from a universal donor or plasma volume expanders may be given. (See *Transfusing in a crisis.*)

Perflurocarbons — milky, white emulsions that act like plasma but carry oxygen like RBCs — may provide an alternative in some hospitals.

The positives and negatives of Rh

About 85% of the U.S. population is Rh-positive, which means possessing the Rh antigen, an antigen found on the membrane of RBCs. People who don't have the Rh antigen are said to be Rh-negative.

No natural antibodies to Rh exist. However, Rh-negative people may develop an Rh antibody if exposed to Rh-positive blood. The first exposure usually causes sensitization, but the second exposure may result in a fatal hemolytic reaction. These reactions can occur during transfusions or pregnancy. (See *Fixing an Rh problem.*)

HLA story

HLA is located on the surface of circulating platelets, white blood cells (WBCs), and most tissue cells. HLA is responsible for febrile reactions in patients receiving a transfusion that contains platelets from several donors.

In that instance, an antigen-antibody reaction causes platelet destruction. As a result, the patient becomes less responsive to platelet transfusions. Giving HLA-matched platelets greatly decreases the risk of such antigen-antibody reactions. Generally, HLA tests benefit patients who receive multiple transfusions over a long period of time or frequent transfusions during a short-term illness.

Types of blood products

Many blood products are available for transfusion, including whole blood, RBCs, packed RBCs, granulocytes, fresh frozen plasma, cryoprecipitate, albumin, and platelets. What's more, patients

Fixing an Rh problem

If an Rh-negative patient is exposed to Rh-positive blood, an injection of $Rh_0(D)$ immune globulin can be given within 72 hours of exposure. $Rh_0(D)$ immune globulin inhibits antibody formation. Names of common preparations include Gamulin Rh, HypRho-D, and RhoGAM.

may also receive transfusions of their own blood through a process called autologous transfusion.

The whole story

Whole blood is rarely used unless the patient has lost more than 25% of total blood volume. It's generally available in bags of 500 ml and may be used to treat hemorrhage, trauma, or major burns.

Whole blood should be avoided if fluid overload is a concern. Stored whole blood is also high in potassium. After 24 hours, the viability and function of RBCs decreases. ABO compatibility and Rh matching are required before administration.

Packed and preserved

Packed RBCs are prepared by removing about 90% of the plasma surrounding the cells and adding an anticoagulant preservative. A 250-ml bag of packed RBCs can help restore or maintain the oxygen-carrying capacity of the blood in patients with anemic conditions or can correct blood losses during or after surgery. About 70% of the leukocytes in packed cells have been removed, which reduces the risk of febrile, nonhemolytic reactions. ABO compatibility and Rh matching are still required, however, for these transfusions.

Grand ol' granulocytes

Granulocyte, or WBC, transfusions are rarely indicated; however, they may be used to treat gram-negative sepsis or progressive soft-tissue infection that's unresponsive to an antimicrobial. HLA compatibility tests are preferable, and Rh matching is required. Daily granulocyte transfusions should be given until the infection resolves or the neutrophil count exceeds 50 mg/ml.

The big thaw

Fresh frozen plasma is prepared by separating the plasma from the RBCs and freezing it within 6 hours of collection. The resulting solution contains plasma proteins, water, fibrinogen, some clotting factors, electrolytes, sugar, vitamins, minerals, hormones, and antibodies.

Fresh frozen plasma is used to treat hemorrhage, expand plasma volume, correct undetermined coagulation factor deficiencies, replace specific clotting factors, and correct factor deficiencies resulting from liver disease. ABO compatibility testing is unnecessary; Rh matching is preferred. Large-volume transfusions of fresh frozen plasma may require correction for hypocalcemia because citric acid in the transfusion binds with and depletes the patient's own serum calcium.

VIII is enough

Cryoprecipitate (also called factor VIII) is the insoluble portion of plasma recovered from fresh frozen plasma. It's used to treat von Willebrand's disease, hypofibrinogenemia, factor VIII deficiency (antihemophilic factor), hemophilia A, and disseminated intravascular coagulation. ABO compatibility testing is unnecessary.

What an extract!

Albumin, which comes in an isotonic 5% solution or in a hypertonic 25% solution, is extracted from plasma and contains globulin and other proteins. It's used for patients who have acute liver failure, burns, or trauma or who have had surgery as well as for neonates with hemolytic disease when crystalloids prove ineffective.

As a colloidal solution, albumin's large molecules increase plasma oncotic pressure, coaxing fluid from the interstitial space across normal capillary membranes and into the intravascular space. Albumin may actually do more harm than good in shock patients by leaking through damaged capillary membranes and dragging intravascular fluid along to worsen interstitial edema. It's also used to treat hypoproteinemia with or without edema. ABO matching is unnecessary.

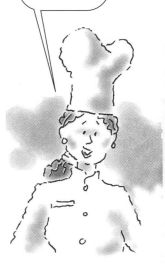

You've got your vanilla extract, your anise extract, and your albumin extract...

People, people who need platelets

Platelets are used for patients who have platelet dysfunctions or thrombocytopenia. They're also used for patients who have had multiple transfusions of stored blood, acute leukemia, or bone marrow abnormalities. Patients may have febrile or mild allergic reactions to platelet transfusions. Rh matching is preferred.

Banking on your own blood

The term *autologous transfusion*, also called autotransfusion, refers to the reinfusion of a patient's own blood or blood components. Indications for autologous transfusion include:
• elective surgery in which blood has been donated during a period of time leading up to the procedure
• elective or nonelective surgery in which anticoagulated blood is withdrawn immediately before the procedure and replaced with colloid or crystalloid volume. In open-heart surgery, the resultant hemodilution helps reduce RBC sludging during periods of induced hypothermia, low flow, and circulatory arrest. Whole blood sequestered outside the cardiopulmonary bypass circuit also escapes the ravages the heart-lung machine can wreak. Such blood is simply reinfused into the patient after bypass.
• preoperative hemorrhage or as a continuous intraoperative procedure when considerable blood loss is anticipated. Heparinized

Cheat sheet

Key facts about blood products

Whole blood
- Rarely used unless more than 25% of total blood volume is lost
- Available in 500-ml bags
- Used to treat hemorrhage, trauma, and major burns
- Avoid if fluid overload is a concern

Packed red blood cells
- Prepared by removing 90% of plasma around cells and adding anticoagulant preservative
- Available in 250-ml bags

Granulocytes, or white blood cells
- Rarely used except in cases of sepsis (gram-negative) or progressive soft-tissue infection that's unresponsive

Fresh frozen plasma
- Prepared by separating plasma from the red blood cells and freezing it within 6 hours of collection
- Used to treat hemorrhage, expand plasma volume, correct undetermined coagulation factor deficiencies, replace specific clotting factors, and correct factor deficiencies resulting from liver disease

Cryoprecipitate, or factor VIII
- Insoluble portion of plasma recovered from fresh frozen plasma
- For von Willebrand's disease, hypofibrinogenemia, factor VIII deficiency (antihemophilic

factor), hemophilia A, and disseminated intravascular coagulation
- ABO compatibility testing unnecessary

Albumin
- Extracted from plasma
- Contains albumin, globulin, and other proteins
- For acute liver failure, burns, trauma, and hemolytic disease of neonates

Platelets
- For platelet dysfunction and thrombocytopenia
- For patients who have had multiple transfusions of stored blood, acute leukemia, or bone marrow abnormalities

Patient's own blood or blood components
- Autologous transfusion, or autotransfusion
- Donated for a period of time before elective surgery
- Withdrawn immediately before procedure and replaced with I.V. fluid for nonelective surgery and some elective surgery; then reinfused after procedure
- Used with preoperative hemorrhage or intraoperative procedure with considerable blood loss (shed blood is collected, then reinfused)

shed blood is aspirated into a filtered reservoir, centrifuged, and saline-washed. RBCs are reinfused. Examples of operations using autologous transfusions include cardiovascular surgery, hip and knee operations, liver resection, ruptured ectopic pregnancy, and hemothorax.

Possible complications of autologous transfusions include hemolysis, embolus, coagulation disorders, and thrombocytopenia. Autologous transfusions are advantageous, however, because they avoid the risk of transfusion reaction, prevent the transmission of disease-causing organisms such as human immunodeficiency virus (HIV), and avoid depleting the local blood supply.

Win, lose, or drawbacks

Drawbacks to autologous transfusions include the following: Autologous blood donors need more counseling than patients who aren't donating their own blood, blood is commonly wasted, and storage, preparation, and testing are expensive. Furthermore, some patients — such as those with malignant neoplasms, coagulopathies, excessive hemolysis, or active infections — simply aren't candidates for these transfusions.

What to look for

Transfusions of blood and blood products aren't without risk. Concerns have surfaced over the years about the risk of transmitting disease-causing organisms — particularly HIV — through transfusions. With HIV-antibody testing being done on all donated blood and stringent criteria being used to exclude high-risk blood donors, studies now show that HIV transmission through infusion is rare. Testing for hepatitis B and hepatitis C viruses has become more specific, which also has helped to make the blood supply safer.

No matter how safe the blood supply is, however, transfusion reactions can still occur. (See *Guide to transfusion reactions*, pages 320 and 321.) Watch for signs of transfusion complications, including endogenous reactions caused by antigen-antibody reaction in the recipient and exogenous reactions caused by external factors related to blood administration. If a transfusion reaction occurs, the transfusion should be discontinued immediately and appropriate therapy initiated.

How blood transfusions are administered

Administering a blood transfusion of any kind requires cooperation and vigilance on the part of various personnel, from the blood bank technologist to the nurse at the bedside to the support personnel throughout the facility. Follow these steps when caring for a patient having a blood transfusion.

(Text continues on page 322.)

Guide to transfusion reactions

This chart describes endogenous reactions (those caused by antigen-antibody reactions) and exogenous reactions (those caused by external factors in administered blood).

	What causes it	What to look for	What to do
E N D O G E N O U S	**Allergic reaction** • Allergen in donated blood • Donor blood hypersensitive to certain drugs	Anaphylaxis (chills, facial swelling, laryngeal edema, pruritus, urticaria, wheezing), fever, nausea, vomiting	• Stop the infusion. • Give antihistamines as ordered. • Monitor vital signs and continue to assess the patient. • Give epinephrine and a corticosteroids as ordered.
	Bacterial contamination • Organisms that survive the cold, such as *Pseudomonas* and *Staphylococcus*	Abdominal cramping, chills, diarrhea, fever, shock, signs of renal failure, vomiting	• Stop the infusion. • Give antibiotics, corticosteroids, and epinephrine as prescribed. • Maintain strict blood storage control. • Change the administration set and filter every 4 hours or every 2 units. • Infuse each unit of blood over 2 to 4 hours; stop the infusion if it lasts more than 4 hours. • Maintain sterile technique.
	Febrile • Bacterial lipopolysaccharides • Antileukocyte recipient antibodies directed against donor white blood cells	Chest tightness, chills, cough, facial flushing, fever up to 104° F (40 ° C), flank pain, headache, increased pulse rate, palpitations	• Stop the infusion. • Administer antipyretics and antihistamines as ordered. • If the patient needs further transfusions, use frozen red blood cells (RBCs) and a leukocyte filter, and give acetaminophen as ordered.
	Hemolytic • ABO or Rh incompatibility • Intradonor incompatibility • Improper crossmatching • Improperly stored blood	Bloody oozing at infusion site, burning along the vein receiving blood, chest pain, chills, dyspnea, facial flushing, fever, flank pain, hypotension, hemoglobinuria, oliguria, shock, signs of renal failure	• Stop the infusion. • Monitor vital signs, including pulse oximetry. • Manage shock with I.V .fluids, oxygen, epinephrine, and vasopressors as ordered. • Obtain a posttransfusion reaction blood sample and urine sample for analysis. • Observe for signs of hemorrhage from disseminated intravascular coagulation.
	Plasma protein incompatibility • Immunoglobulin A incompatibility	Abdominal pain, chills, diarrhea, dyspnea, fever, flushing, hypotension	• Stop the infusion. • Administer oxygen, fluids, epinephrine, and corticosteroids as ordered. *(continued)*

Guide to transfusion reactions *(continued)*

	What causes it	What to look for	What to do
E X O G E N O U S	**Bleeding tendencies** • Low platelet count in stored blood, causing thrombocytopenia	Abnormal bleeding and oozing from cuts or breaks in the skin or the gums, abnormal bruising and petechiae	• Give platelets, fresh frozen plasma, or cryoprecipitate as ordered. • Monitor platelet count.
	Circulatory overload • Possibly from infusing whole blood too rapidly	Back pain, chest pain or tightness, chills, distended neck veins, dyspnea, fever, flushed feeling, headache, hypertension, increased central venous pressure, increased plasma volume	• Slow or stop the infusion. • Monitor vital signs. • Use packed RBCs instead of whole blood. • Give diuretics as ordered.
	Hypocalcemia • Citrate toxicity, which occurs when citrate-treated blood is infused too rapidly and binds with calcium, causing a calcium deficiency	Arrhythmias, hypotension, muscle cramps, nausea, seizures, tingling in fingers, vomiting	• Slow or stop the transfusion if ordered. Expect a more severe reaction in hypothermic patients or patients with elevated potassium levels. • Give calcium gluconate I.V. slowly if ordered.
	Hypothermia • Rapid infusion of large amounts of cold blood, which decreases body temperature	Arrhythmias (especially bradycardia), cardiac arrest if core temperature falls below 86° F (30° C), chills, hypotension, shaking	• Stop the transfusion. • Warm the patient. • Obtain an electrocardiogram (ECG). • Warm the blood if the transfusion is resumed.
	Potassium intoxication • An abnormally high level of potassium in stored plasma caused by hemolysis of RBCs	Bradycardia, cardiac arrest, diarrhea, ECG changes (such as tall, peaked T waves), flaccidity, intestinal colic, muscle twitching, oliguria, signs of renal failure	• Stop the infusion. • Obtain an ECG and serum electrolyte levels, such as potassium and glucose levels. • Give Kayexalate as ordered. • Give glucose 50% and insulin, bicarbonate, or calcium, as ordered, to force potassium into cells. • Give mannitol, and maintain vigorous hydration to force diuresis and prevent renal damage.

In the beginning

Before starting a blood transfusion, take the following steps:
• Make sure the patient or his next of kin has signed an informed consent form. Explain the procedure to the patient. Many people are still afraid of receiving a blood transfusion because of the fear of contracting HIV. Educate the patient as indicated about the extremely low risk of infection due to highly effective screening procedures.
• The religious beliefs of Jehovah's Witnesses preclude the use of blood products. Therefore, when treating patients who follow this faith, make sure that refusal of blood reflects the patient's own decision and not coercion by family members or clergy. Consider consulting your facility's legal counsel on behalf of minors and adults incapable of giving their own consent.
• Review facility policy for administering blood.
• Assess your patient, documenting vital signs and other pertinent information. Notify the doctor if the patient has a fever of 100° F (37.8° C) or higher before the transfusion.
• Keep in mind your patient's other treatment needs. If he's receiving an I.V. medication that can't be mixed with blood products, for example, another I.V. line may need to be inserted.
• Check the orders for the type of transfusion to be given. (See *How to avoid transfusion errors.*)
• Triple-check your patient's identity to ensure that the right patient receives the right transfusion at the right time.
• Ask the patient if he has ever had a transfusion reaction and, if so, under what conditions the transfusion was given and how it was resolved.

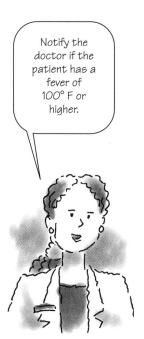

Notify the doctor if the patient has a fever of 100° F or higher.

Ready, get set, transfuse

When preparing for the transfusion — and while it's in progress — take these actions:
• Maintain sterile technique to protect the patient.
• Observe standard precautions to protect yourself. Wear a gown, gloves, and a face shield.
• Infuse blood products through at least an 18G or 20G I.V. catheter. Never use a smaller-gauge catheter or needle.
• Transfuse blood using a Y-type I.V. administration set (with filter), and infuse the blood over 2 to 4 hours.
• When you start the transfusion, remain with the patient and observe him carefully for the first 15 minutes. (See *Teaching about blood transfusions*, page 324.) Most acute adverse reactions occur within that time period, although delayed reactions can occur up to 2 weeks later. Recheck vital signs 15 minutes after hanging the blood, and again every hour.

How to avoid transfusion errors

Proper identification of the patient and the blood product he's to be given is essential, as is following your facility's policy and taking these precautions:

• Match the patient's name, medical record number, ABO and Rh status, and blood bank identification numbers with the label on the blood bag.

• Check the expiration date.

• Have another nurse verify the information.

• Sign the blood slip, filling in the required data. The blood slip will prove useful if the patient develops an adverse reaction.

• Double-check the doctor's order to make sure you're transfusing the correct product.

• Be sure that the blood was typed and crossmatched within the last 48 hours—a Food and Drug Administration requirement for transfusions.

• Use a pressure bag or a specialized infusion pump to administer blood more rapidly, if needed.

Flushing and filters

• Flush with normal saline solution before and after infusing blood products. You may need to flush the I.V. line during the transfusion if the blood is dripping too slowly. Don't use a dextrose solution, which can cause hemolysis, or lactated Ringer's solution, which contains calcium and can clog the tubing.

• Filters work best when completely filled with blood. Special filters are available to trap leukocytes (leukocyte-depleting filters) or tiny clots and debris that can get through standard filters (microaggregate filters).

• If you're transfusing whole blood, you can reduce the risk of an adverse reaction by adding a microfilter to trap platelets.

Getting blood ready

• Obtain blood from the laboratory *when you're ready to hang it.* Check the bag for leaks, discoloration, bubbles, and clots. Return questionable products to the blood bank.

• Don't store blood in a nursing-unit refrigerator because the temperature may be inaccurate, and the blood could be damaged. Blood that isn't refrigerated for 4 hours or more carries a high risk of bacterial contamination.

• If the order calls for blood to be warmed before administration, use a blood-warming device and special tubing. The temperature should be maintained between 89.6° and 98.6° F (32° and 37° C). Blood-warming devices are useful when transfusing large quantities of blood.

Giving platelets

- Transfuse platelets over 15 minutes. If the patient history includes a platelet transfusion reaction, premedicate with an antipyretic or an antihistamine as ordered.
- Avoid giving platelets when a patient is febrile.
- Check the platelet count 1 hour after the transfusion ends.

Giving albumin and other fluids

- Don't mix albumin with other solutions.
- Be aware that albumin may be given as a volume expander until crossmatching for a whole blood transfusion is completed.
- Don't use albumin for patients with severe anemia, and give cautiously to patients with a cardiac or pulmonary disorder because heart failure may occur.
- Because factor VIII's half-life is 8 to 10 hours, give repeated transfusions at those intervals to maintain normal factor VIII levels.
- If a patient will receive WBCs, premedicate him with diphenhydramine hydrochloride (Benadryl), if prescribed, and give an antipyretic for fever. Agitate the blood container to prevent cells from settling and unintentional delivery of a bolus infusion. WBC transfusions may be given along with an antibiotic to treat infection, but they shouldn't given with amphotericin B.

After the transfusion

- Continue to assess the patient as you remove the blood and tubing, and hang an infusion of normal saline solution to keep the vein open.
- Watch for signs of circulatory overload, especially in elderly patients. Carefully monitor the rate of infusion and the I.V. site.
- Obtain laboratory tests as ordered to determine the effectiveness of the treatment. The hemoglobin level of an adult patient receiving 1 unit of packed RBCs should increase by 1 g/dl. The hematocrit should increase by 3%. You should see a rise in platelets of 5,000 to 10,000/mm^3 with each unit of platelets infused, and an improvement in prothrombin time and partial thromboplastin time after giving clotting factors.
- Document your administration of blood products according to facility policy. (See *Documenting transfusions*.)

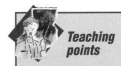

Teaching points

Teaching about blood transfusions

Be sure to cover the following topics with your patient, and then evaluate his learning:
- need for transfusion
- reason for informed consent, if required
- risks
- length of time required
- related procedures, such as vital signs checks and follow-up blood tests
- adverse reactions and when to report them
- activity restrictions during the transfusion.

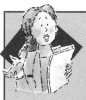

Chart smart

Documenting transfusions

When administering blood products to your patient, make sure you record:
• patient teaching
• patient identification
• identification of blood products, including date of expiration
• vital signs before, during, and after the transfusion
• date, time, type, amount, and duration of the transfusion
• adverse reactions and actions taken
• patient response, including relevant laboratory test results
• patient assessment after the transfusion.

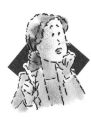

Quick quiz

1. If a hematologically stable patient receives 1 unit of RBCs, you can expect an increase in:
    A.   hematocrit by 3% and hemoglobin level by 1 g/dl.
    B.   hematocrit by 5% and hemoglobin level by 2 g/dl.
    C.   platelet count by 5,000/mm^3.

Answer: A. The hematocrit should rise by 3%, and the hemoglobin level by 1 g/dl.

2. Which of the following blood types is considered the universal recipient?
    A.   Type A
    B.   Type AB
    C.   Type O.

Answer: B. Type AB blood is considered the universal recipient and can receive type A, B, AB, or O transfusions.

3. Whole blood is rarely used unless the patient has lost more than:

   A.   10% of the total blood volume.
   B.   25% of the total blood volume.
   C.   50% of the total blood volume.

Answer: B. The cutoff for using whole blood is generally 25%.

4. An Rh-negative mother would be most likely to have a serious hemolytic reaction when:

   A.   she's first exposed to Rh-positive blood.
   B.   she delivers her first child.
   C.   she has a second exposure to Rh-positive blood.

Answer: C. A mother initiates antibody formation after the first exposure. By the second exposure, the antibodies already present react and cause a hemolytic reaction to the infused Rh-positive blood.

5. To expand plasma volume or to replace clotting factors, you would expect to give which of the following blood products?

   A.   Albumin
   B.   Fresh frozen plasma
   C.   Whole blood

Answer: B. Fresh frozen plasma would be the product of choice.

6. About 10 minutes after you start an infusion of packed RBCs, your patient complains of chills, chest and back pain, and nausea. His face is flushed, and he's anxious. His blood pressure is 90/60 mm Hg; temperature, 101.5° F (38.6° C); heart rate, 120 beats/minute; and respiratory rate, 24 breaths/minute. Your assessment indicates that the patient is experiencing:

   A.   an HLA antibody-antigen reaction.
   B.   a hemolytic reaction.
   C.   circulatory overload.

Answer: B. The signs and symptoms indicate a hemolytic reaction.

Scoring

☆☆☆   If you answered all six items correctly, you've done a great job! You could even say you're compatible with greatness.

☆☆   If you answered four or five correctly, super! You're a platelet-giving powerhouse.

☆   If you answered fewer than four correctly, no problem. Review your ABOs and you'll be transfused with new confidence.

Appendices and index

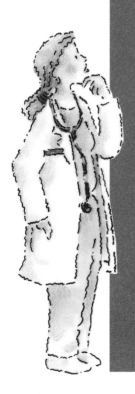

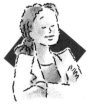

Practice makes perfect

1. A construction worker labors outside in 90° F (32.2° C) temperatures. What hormone will his body release in larger quantities to help him retain water?
    A.   Insulin
    B.   Antidiuretic hormone
    C.   Renin

2. A postoperative patient is ordered an I.V. solution of dextrose 5% in normal saline solution. What type of fluid is this solution?
    A.   Hypertonic
    B.   Hypotonic
    C.   Isotonic

3. You're teaching a group of athletes how to prevent excessive fluid loss. You should tell them to consume fluids when they:
    A.   experience dry mouth.
    B.   feel light-headed or dizzy.
    C.   are thirsty.

4. A patient with hyponatremia caused by diabetes insipidus requires I.V. fluid replacement. Which I.V. fluid would provide the greatest concentration of sodium replacement if the patient were to develop a subnormal serum sodium level?
    A.   Dextrose 5% in water
    B.   Half-normal saline solution
    C.   Ringer's solution

5. A 29-year-old patient comes to the ED after being involved in a motor vehicle crash. Chest radiography reveals a right pneumothorax. You interpret his ABG results as respiratory acidosis. Why?
    A.   His pH is low; $Paco_2$ is high, and HCO_3^- is normal.
    B.   His pH is low, $Paco_2$ is low, and HCO_3^- is low.
    C.   His pH is low, $Paco_2$ is high, and HCO_3^- is low.

6. A patient is transferred to the ICU in septic shock. ABG results show that the patient is acidotic. You expect the anion gap to be:
    A.   0 to 8 mEq/L.
    B.   8 to 14 mEq/L.
    C.   greater than 14 mEq/L.

7. A patient who sustained multiple abdominal injuries in a motor vehicle crash 2 days ago becomes hypotensive. His urine output for the past 4 hours totals 45 ml. The doctor decides to insert a pulmonary artery catheter. During measurement of pulmonary artery pressures, what specific information is being obtained when the balloon is wedged in a branch of the pulmonary artery?

A. Left-sided heart function
B. CVP
C. Cardiac output

8. A patient with Alzheimer's disease is admitted with suspected dehydration after her daughter reports that the patient has refused to drink anything for the past 3 days. The doctor orders several laboratory tests. Which laboratory result is most expected with dehydration?
A. Urine specific gravity of 1.005
B. Serum sodium level of 150 mEq/L
C. Hematocrit of 38%

9. A 53-year-old homeless person is admitted with dehydration. Which type of I.V. fluid should be avoided when treating this patient?
A. Isotonic fluid
B. Hypertonic fluid
C. Hypotonic fluid

10. A 78-year-old patient is admitted with pulmonary edema. The patient is given I.V. morphine sulfate. Why?
A. To lower his blood pressure
B. To promote diuresis
C. To slow his breathing

11. A patient diagnosed with lung cancer develops SIADH, which puts him at risk for hyponatremia. Which serum sodium level indicates hyponatremia?
A. 128 mEq/L
B. 135 mEq/L
C. 142 mEq/L

12. While being treated for hyponatremia, a patient develops iatrogenic hypernatremia. Which treatment is appropriate for resolving this problem?
A. Fluid restriction
B. Diuretic therapy
C. Hypertonic fluid administration

13. A 35-year-old man with a history of food poisoning and subsequent vomiting complains of weakness, palpitations, abdominal pain, and cramping. His body temperature is 99.6° F (37.6° C). ECG results show irregularities. Which imbalance is he most likely to have?
A. Hypervolemia
B. Hypokalemia
C. Acidosis

14. A 65-year-old patient receives daily doses of furosemide (Lasix) and digoxin (Lanoxin) for treatment of heart failure. His serum potassium level is 3.1 mEq/L. Which associated ECG changes would you expect?

    A.   Peaked T wave
    B.   Depressed ST segment
    C.   Narrow QRS complexes

15. As part of a patient's treatment for hypokalemia, the doctor prescribes I.V. potassium supplementation. At which rate should it be administered?

    A.   5 mEq/hour
    B.   10 mEq/hour
    C.   20 mEq/hour

16. A patient with a history of systemic lupus erythematosus develops hyperkalemia. The doctor prescribes sodium polystyrene sulfonate (Kaexylate) to reduce the patient's serum potassium level. This drug works by:

    A.   forcing potassium into the cells.
    B.   promoting renal excretion of potassium.
    C.   pulling potassium into the bowel for excretion.

17. A 28-year-old patient is seen in the obstetrics clinic with a blood pressure of 220/130 mm Hg and abnormal reflexes. The nurse-midwife caring for her suspects pre-eclampsia. A urinalysis for protein is ordered immediately, and proteinuria is detected. The patient is transported to the obstetric unit in the medical center. On admission, the nurse assesses her deep tendon reflexes as 4+. This value means the reflexes are:

    A.   present but diminished.
    B.   slow to respond.
    C.   hyperactive.

18. Which intervention is most appropriate for the patient receiving a continuous magnesium sulfate infusion?

    A.   Insert an indwelling urinary catheter.
    B.   Attach the patient to a continuous cardiac monitor.
    C.   Administer calcium gluconate every 4 hours.

19. Which finding suggests that a patient has received too much magnesium sulfate?

    A.   Muscle weakness
    B.   Tetany
    C.   Tachycardia

20. A patient develops hypermagnesemia. Which intervention is most effective in reducing serum magnesium levels?

    A.   Administer a cation-exchange resin.
    B.   Infuse a bolus of calcium gluconate.
    C.   Increase the volume of I.V. and oral fluids.

21. A 36-year-old woman with a history of hyperthyroidism has undergone a total thyroidectomy. After surgery, she experiences hypotension, irritability, and circumoral paresthesia. Her surgical wound has well-approximated borders, no bleeding, and minimal swelling. Her speech and breathing are unimpaired. Based on the patient's signs and symptoms, her serum calcium level is likely to be:
    A.   10 mg/dl.
    B.   9 mg/dl.
    C.   8 mg/dl.

22. A 35-year-old patient with a history of alcohol abuse is admitted with acute pancreatitis. His calcium level on admission is 7.6 mg/dl. Which finding also suggests hypocalcemia?
    A.   Prolonged ST segment on ECG
    B.   Constipation
    C.   Flaccid reflexes

23. A patient with acute hypocalcemia develops torsades de pointe. Which drug is most commonly given to treat acute hypocalcemia?
    A.   Calcium carbonate
    B.   Calcium gluconate
    C.   Calcium chloride

24. You need to prepare a calcium infusion for a patient with hypocalcemia. You should mix the drug in which solution?
    A.   Normal saline solution
    B.   Dextrose 5% in water
    C.   Half-normal saline solution

25. A public health nurse in a homeless shelter assesses a 57-year-old man with chronic alcoholism. He has a productive cough and a low-grade fever. He's 5'10" (1.8 m) and weighs 135 lb (61.2 kg). The nurse's nutritional assessment reveals he's malnourished. The patient is admitted to a respiratory isolation room in a community hospital because tuberculosis is suspected. Based on his history of alcohol abuse, you expect his serum phosphorous level to be:
    A.   below normal.
    B.   above normal.
    C.   in the normal range.

26. A patient's phosphorous level is elevated. Which of the following electrolytes should you expect to be decreased?
    A.   Calcium
    B.   Potassium
    C.   Sodium

27. You're teaching a patient with hypophosphatemia about the importance of consuming phosphorus-rich foods. You should recommend:
    A.   pumpkin.
    B.   cranberries.
    C.   trout.

28. A 10-year-old girl who recently returned from traveling abroad complains that she's experienced frequent episodes of diarrhea and weakness for the last 3 days. She's diagnosed with gastroenteritis. Her temperature is 102.4° F (39.1° C), her pulses are weak, and her blood pressure is 76/40 mm Hg. She has poor skin turgor, low urine output, and dry mucous membranes. Serum laboratory studies reveal the child's chloride level to be 88 mEq/L. The direct cause of the child's hypochloremia is most likely:

    A.   fever.

    B.   low urine output.

    C.   diarrhea.

29. A 39-year-old patient is admitted with severe vomiting and abdominal pain. His admission laboratory findings reveal hypochloremia. Which other electrolyte would you expect to be deficient?

    A.   Calcium

    B.   Sodium

    C.   Magnesium

30. A 62-year-old patient who underwent a partial gastrectomy 2 days ago develops hypochloremia. This places the patient at risk for:

    A.   respiratory alkalosis.

    B.   metabolic acidosis.

    C.   metabolic alkalosis.

31. A 16-year-old male with a recent history of weight loss, increased appetite, and urinary frequency is seen in the clinic. He complains of weakness and syncope. On initial observation, the nurse notes that his skin and mucous membranes are dry and that his eyeballs appear sunken. The teen's mother reports that he gets up a lot at night to go to the bathroom. His capillary blood glucose measurement is 480 mg/dl. Which acid-base imbalance should you suspect?

    A.   Metabolic acidosis

    B.   Metabolic alkalosis

    C.   Respiratory acidosis

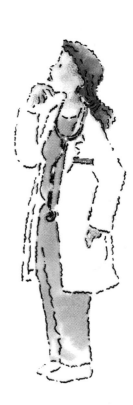

32. A 23-year-old patient is admitted with diabetic ketoacidosis. Which value from the ABG analysis supports the diagnosis?

    A.   pH: 7.48

    B. HCO_3^-: 28 mEq/L

    C.   Anion gap: 17 mEq/L

33. You're caring for a 33-year-old patient who developed Guillain-Barré syndrome 1 week after contracting an upper respiratory infection. This places the patient at risk for which acid-base imbalance?

    A.   Metabolic acidosis

    B.   Respiratory acidosis

    C.   Respiratory alkalosis

34. A 27-year-old woman in her 38th week of pregnancy is admitted to the obstetric unit after her water broke at home. You perform a vaginal examination and note that her cervix is 6 cm dilated. You attach the fetal monitor and find that the fetal heart rate is normal. As her labor progresses, she hyperventilates. Which acid-base imbalance is she most likely to experience if she continues to hyperventilate?

    A.   Metabolic alkalosis

    B.   Respiratory acidosis

    C.   Respiratory alkalosis

35. A 58-year-old man calls for emergency medical services from his home after he experiences excruciating substernal chest pain. He's rushed to the ED where he's given nitroglycerin and morphine for the pain. ECG results show changes consistent with an acute anterior-wall MI. A main complication of an anterior-wall MI is heart failure. Which chamber of the heart is most likely to fail in this patient?

    A.   Right ventricle

    B.   Left atrium

    C.   Left ventricle

36. A patient with a history of heart failure calls you to her room because she's short of breath. You assess her and find that her heart failure is worsening. Which type of fluid volume excess is the patient experiencing because of her heart failure?

    A.   Intravascular volume excess

    B.   Extracellular volume excess

    C.   Intracellular volume excess

37. A 74-year-old man with a 3-day history of worsening COPD is hospitalized. His breathing is labored, breath sounds are congested with rhonchi throughout, and his SaO_2 (as measured by pulse oximetry) is 89%. He's placed on a 35% aerosol mask, and blood is drawn for ABG analysis. The results are pH, 7.33; PaO_2, 68 mm Hg; $PaCO_2$, 53 mm Hg; and HCO_3^-, 18 mEq/L. He's diagnosed with acute respiratory failure. Which acid-base imbalance does the patient most likely have?

    A.   Metabolic alkalosis

    B.   Respiratory acidosis

    C.   Respiratory alkalosis

38. You're caring for a 54-year-old patient who has smoked two packs of cigarettes per day for the past 35 years. He's been admitted with worsening COPD. Why is it important for supplemental oxygen to be carefully monitored in this patient?

    A.   Increasing the PaO_2 beyond what's needed will lead to oxygen toxicity.

    B.   High oxygen levels will promote microbial growth in the patient's lungs.

    C.   Increased PaO_2 levels can depress the drive to breathe in patients with COPD.

39. A patient returned from the postanesthesia care unit with a nasogastric tube in place. The doctor's order states *irrigate NG tube q 4 hours.* Which solution is the best irrigant?

    A.   Saline solution
    B.   Distilled water
    C.   Tap water

40. A 66-year-old woman who survived a cardiac arrest was admitted to the ICU. She experienced a prolonged episode of hypotension and is now in acute renal failure. Frequent electrolyte levels are ordered. Hemodialysis is scheduled to begin within 24 hours. Which type of renal failure did the patient experience?

    A.   Intrarenal
    B.   Prerenal
    C.   Postrenal

41. A patient with a history of hypertension develops chronic renal failure. What should you expect the GFR to be?

    A.   40 to 70 ml/minute
    B.   10 to 20 ml/minute
    C.   20 to 40 ml/minute

42. A patient who sustained massive internal injuries in a motor vehicle crash becomes hypotensive and develops acute renal failure. Which acid-base imbalance is this patient most likely to experience?

    A.   Respiratory acidosis
    B.   Respiratory alkalosis
    C.   Metabolic acidosis

43. A patient received burn injuries 48 hours ago. He's entering the second phase of burn injury, what physiologic changes can be expected?

    A.   Edema development
    B.   Profuse urination
    C.   Decrease in hemoglobin level

44. A fireman sustains burns while fighting an apartment fire. He receives fluid resuscitation using the Parkland formula. Which type of fluid is used?

    A.   Normal saline solution
    B.   Half-normal saline solution
    C.   Lactated Ringer's solution

45. A 42-year-old man with end-stage AIDS has frequent episodes of watery stool. He's nauseated and refuses to drink fluids. His body temperature is 102° F (38.9° C), his blood pressure is 88/52 mm Hg, and his pulse is 112 beats/minute. Normal saline solution is infusing at 150 ml/hour through a large bore I.V. catheter. Which type of fluid is normal saline solution?

    A.   Isotonic
    B.   Hypotonic
    C.   Hypertonic

46. A patient's blood volume doesn't improve after the administration of crystalloids. The doctor prescribes a colloid for this patient. Which of the following solutions is a colloid?

    A.   Dextrose 5% in half-normal saline solution

    B.   Hetastarch

    C.   Dextrose 10% in water

47. An 18-year-old patient sustained a head injury 5 days ago. His ICP has been unstable and attempts at GI feeding have been unsuccessful. TPN is indicated when the patient's serum albumin is less than:

    A.   4.5 g/dl.

    B.   4.0 g/dl.

    C.   3.5 g/dl.

48. A patient receiving TPN requires a transfusion of packed red blood cells. Before you begin the transfusion, you should:

    A.   infuse the blood directly into the TPN line.

    B.   start a separate I.V. line for the blood transfusion.

    C.   stop the TPN, infuse the blood at the TPN site, and then restart the TPN.

49. A patient's postoperative hemoglobin level is 7.9 g/dl. The doctor orders 2 U of packed RBCs for the patient. By what percentage should this increase the patient's hematocrit?

    A.   3%

    B.   6%

    C.   9%

50. A patient experiences a transfusion reaction 15 minutes after you begin a blood transfusion. You collect the appropriate laboratory specimens. Laboratory results reveal hemoglobinuria. Which type of reaction has the patient most likely experienced?

    A.   Hemolytic

    B.   Febrile

    C.   Allergic

Answers

1. B. One way the body conserves water is to release more antidiuretic hormone, which reduces diuresis.

2. A. A solution of dextrose 5% in normal saline is considered hypertonic because the concentration of solutes in the solution is greater than the concentration of solutes in the patient's blood.

3. C. The simplest mechanism for maintaining fluid balance is the thirst mechanism. When an individual senses thirst, he should drink to replace lost fluid.

4. C. Ringer's solution contains 147 mEq of sodium per liter. Half-normal saline solution contains 77 mEq/L. Dextrose 5% in water contains no sodium.

5. A. In patients with respiratory acidosis, pH is low, Pa_{CO_2} is high, and HCO_3^- is normal.

6. C. Patients who are in an acidotic state typically have higher-than-normal amounts of organic acids, which leads to an elevated anion gap (greater than 14 mEq/L).

7. A. When the tip of the pulmonary artery catheter is wedged in a branch of the pulmonary artery, it measures pressures that reflect left-sided heart function.

8. B. Because some of the water present in the serum is lost, causing dehydration, the serum sodium level becomes elevated.

9. B. Dehydration is a hypertonic state; therefore, hypertonic fluid should be avoided because it would worsen the patient's condition. Free water or isotonic or hypotonic fluid would be a safer choice.

10. C. Morphine sulfate is given to the patient with pulmonary edema because it relieves air hunger and dilates blood vessels, which in turn reduces pulmonary congestion and the amount of blood that returns to the heart.

11. A. Normal serum sodium level is 135 to 145 mEq/L. A serum sodium level less than 135 mEq/L indicates hyponatremia.

12. B. Diuretics increase sodium loss in the urine, thereby lowering the serum sodium level.

13. B. Conditions such as vomiting that lead to loss of gastric acids can cause hypokalemia and alkalosis.

14. B. Hypokalemia causes various ECG changes, including a flattened T wave, a depressed ST segment, and a characteristic U wave.

15. B. When supplemental potassium is given by I.V. infusion, it should be administered at a rate of 10 mEq/hour.

16. C. Sodium polystyrene sulfonate is a cation-exchange resin that causes potassium to move out of the blood into the intestines. It's then excreted in the stool.

17. C. Deep tendon reflexes are graded on a 0 to 4+ scale. 0 is absent, 1+ is present but diminished, 2+ is normal, 3+ is increased but not necessarily abnormal, and 4+ is hyperactive.

18. B. Magnesium affects cardiac function and can cause arrhythmias. Therefore, any patient receiving a magnesium sulfate infusion should be on continuous cardiac monitoring.

19. A. Hypermagnesemia causes muscle weakness. Therefore, if a patient develops muscle weakness while receiving magnesium, most likely the dose is too great.

20. C. The best method of reducing serum magnesium levels is to increase urinary excretion of magnesium by increasing the patient's fluid intake.

21. C. Hypotension, irritability, and circumoral paresthesia are signs and symptoms of hypocalcemia. Because 8.9 to 10.1 mg/dl is the normal range for total serum calcium levels, 8 mg/dl is the only value here that indicates hypocalcemia.

22. A. The patient with hypocalcemia may experience diarrhea, hyperactive deep tendon reflexes, a diminished response to digoxin (Lanoxin), decreased cardiac output, prolonged ST segment on ECG, and a lengthened QT interval, which places the patient at risk for torsades de pointe.

23. B. With acute cases of hypocalcemia, I.V. calcium gluconate is usually given. Calcium chloride is a less-common alternative.

24. B. When preparing a calcium infusion, add calcium to a solution containing dextrose 5% in water. Solutions containing normal saline cause renal calcium loss.

25. A. Patients who abuse alcohol typically have serum phosphorous levels that fall below normal.

26. A. Phosphorus and calcium have an inverse relationship: When the levels of one are increased, the levels of the other are decreased. No such relationship exists between phosphorus and potassium, sodium, or magnesium.

27. C. Fish is a food source that's rich in phosphorus, so trout would be helpful to a patient with hypophosphatemia.

28. C. The child's low serum chloride level is probably caused by her diarrhea.

29. B. Chloride is a negatively charged ion that has an electrical attraction to sodium. Therefore, if chloride levels become low, so do serum sodium levels.

30. C. To compensate for a chloride loss (hypochloremia), the kidneys retain bicarbonate. The accumulation of excess bicarbonate in extracellular fluid can raise the arterial pH above 7.45, causing metabolic alkalosis.

31. A. The patient has signs and symptoms of type 1 diabetes mellitus. Because of the accumulation of metabolic wastes (for example, ketones), type 1 diabetes mellitus is most commonly associated with metabolic acidosis.

32. C. Metabolic acidosis causes the anion gap to be greater than 14 mEq/L. With metabolic acidosis, pH will be less than 7.35, HCO_3^- will be less than 22 mEq/L, and $Paco_2$ will typically be unaffected.

33. B. In certain neuromuscular diseases, such as Guillain-Barré syndrome, the respiratory muscles fail to respond properly to the respiratory drive, leading to respiratory acidosis.

34. C. When a patient hyperventilates, excess carbon dioxide is blown off. This raises the arterial pH above 7.45 causing respiratory alkalosis.

35. C. With an anterior-wall MI, the left ventricle usually fails, causing heart failure.

36. B. Because the heart doesn't pump effectively in a patient with heart failure, fluid imbalances develop. The most common fluid imbalance associated with heart failure is extracellular volume excess. This results from the heart's failure to propel blood forward, consequent vascular pooling, and the sodium and water reabsorption triggered by the renin-angiotensin-aldosterone system.

37. B. When a patient's $Paco_2$ is elevated, carbonic acid is retained, leading to acidosis. Because the acidosis is respiratory in origin, the patient most likely has respiratory acidosis.

38. C. Increased Pao_2 can depress the patient's drive to breathe, which is largely driven by hypoxemia.

39. A. The best solution for gastric irrigation is an isotonic solution such as saline solution.

40. B. The patient's renal failure was due to hypotension, which is a prerenal cause. Prerenal causes are those conditions that diminish blood flow to the kidneys.

41. B. Renal failure occurs when the GFR is 10 to 20 ml/minute. A rate of 40 to 70 ml/minute indicates renal reserve; 20 to 40 ml/minute, renal insufficiency; and less than 10 ml/minute, end-stage renal disease.

42. C. As the kidneys lose their ability to excrete hydrogen ions, there's a buildup of hydrogen, which leads to metabolic acidosis.

43. B. The second phase of the burn injury, known as the remobilization phase, starts about 48 hours after the initial injury. During this phase, fluid shifts back to the vascular compartment. Edema at the burn site decreases and blood flow to kidneys increases, which increases diuresis.

44. C. The Parkland formula, which is widely used for burn resuscitation, uses lactated Ringer's solution.

45. A. Normal saline solution is an isotonic crystalloid fluid.

46. B. Examples of colloids include albumin, hetastarch, dextran, and plasma protein fraction.

47. C. TPN is typically indicated when the serum albumin level is less than 3.5 g/dl.

48. B. Blood transfusions shouldn't be infused with TPN; therefore, a separate I.V. line should be secured for the blood transfusion.

49. B. One unit of packed RBCs will increase hematocrit by 3%; 2 U, by 6%.

50. A. Hemoglobinuria is a sign of a hemolytic reaction to a blood transfusion and isn't representative of other reaction types.

Glossary

absorption: taking up of a substance by cells or tissues

acid: substance that donates hydrogen ions

acid-base balance: mechanism by which the body's acids and bases are kept in balance

acidosis: condition resulting from the accumulation of acid or the loss of base

adenosine triphosphate (ATP): vital phosphorus-containing compound that represents stored energy in the cells; needed to carry out the body's functions

afterload: pressure exerted by blood in the large arteries leaving the heart

air embolism: air bubble in the vascular system

aldosterone: adrenocortical hormone that regulates sodium, potassium, and fluid balance

alkalosis: condition resulting from the accumulation of base or the loss of acid

angiotensin: potent vasoconstrictor that increase systemic blood pressure

anion: negatively charged ion, of which proteins, chloride, bicarbonate, and phosphorus are among the body's most plentiful

anion gap: measurement of the difference between the amount of sodium and the amount of bicarbonate and chloride in the blood

antibody: substance produced by the body that reacts with an antigen and causes outward signs or symptoms of that reaction

antidiuretic hormone (ADH): hormone made by the hypothalamus and released by the pituitary gland that decreases the production of urine by increasing the reabsorption of water by the renal tubules

antigen: substance that causes the body to form antibodies against it

anuria: absence of urine formation or output of less than 100 ml of urine in 24 hours

arterial blood gas (ABG) analysis: measurement of arterial pH, partial pressures of oxygen and carbon dioxide, and other levels used to evaluate acid-base balance and pulmonary function

autologous transfusion (autotransfusion): reinfusion of the patient's own blood or blood components

base: substance that accepts hydrogen ions

2,3-biphosphoglycerate (2,3-BPG): compound in red blood cells that contains phosphorus and facilitates the transfer of oxygen from hemoglobin to the tissues

buffer: substance that, when combined with acids or bases, minimizes changes in pH

calcification: deposit of calcium phosphate in soft tissues that can occur with prolonged high serum phosphorus levels; can lead to organ dysfunction

calcium: positively charged ion involved in the structure and function of bones, impulse transmission, the blood-clotting process, and the normal function of heart and skeletal muscles

carboxyhemoglobin: molecule of carbon monoxide and hemoglobin that prevents the normal transfer of oxygen and carbon dioxide; can result in asphyxiation or death

cation: positively charged ion, of which sodium, potassium, calcium, magnesium, and hydrogen are the body's most plentiful

cation-exchange resin: medication used to lower serum potassium levels by exchanging sodium ions for potassium ions in the GI tract

cerebral edema: increase in the brain's fluid content; may result from correcting hypernatremia too rapidly

chemoreceptor: special cell that senses the presence of specific chemicals in the bloodstream

chloride: most abundant anion in extracellular fluid; maintains serum osmolality and fluid, electrolyte, and acid-base balance

Chvostek's sign: abnormal spasm of facial muscles that may indicate hypocalcemia or tetany; tested by lightly tapping the facial nerve (upper cheek, below the zygomatic bone)

colloid: large molecule, such as albumin, that normally doesn't cross the capillary membrane

colloid osmotic pressure: pressure exerted by colloids in the vasculature

compensation: process by which one system (renal or respiratory) attempts to correct an acid-base disturbance in the other system

crystalloid: solute, such as sodium or glucose, that crosses the capillary membrane in solution

deep tendon reflex: involuntary muscle contraction in response to a sudden stretch that can be elicited by a hammer or finger tap on a tendon at its insertion

dehydration: condition in which the loss of water from cells causes them to shrink

diabetes insipidus: condition in which the brain fails to secrete enough antidiuretic hormone causing greater than normal diuresis

diuretics: class of medications acting at various points along the nephron to increase urine output, resulting in the loss of water and electrolytes

electrolyte: solute that separates in a solvent into electrically charged particles called ions

extravasation: leakage of intravascular fluid into surrounding tissue; can be caused by such medications as chemotherapeutic drugs, dopamine, and calcium solutions that produce blistering and, eventually, tissue necrosis

factor VIII (cryoprecipitate): antihemophilic factor recovered from fresh frozen plasma; instrumental in blood clotting

glomerular filtration rate (GFR): rate at which the glomeruli in the kidneys filter blood; normally occurs at a rate of 125 ml/minute

granulocytopenia: fewer than normal number of granular leukocytes in the blood

hydrostatic pressure: pressure exerted by fluid in the blood vessels

hypercalcemia: excess of calcium in extracellular fluid; when the total serum calcium level is above 10.1 mg/dl or the ionized calcium level is above 5.1 mg/dl

hypercapnia: partial pressure of carbon dioxide in arterial blood that's greater than 45 mm Hg

hyperchloremia: excess of chloride in the extracellular fluid; occurs when the serum chloride level is above 106 mEq/L

hyperchloremic metabolic acidosis: condition resulting from a deficit in bicarbonate ions and an increase in chloride ions, which causes a decrease in pH

hyperkalemia: excess potassium in the extracellular fluid; occurs when the serum potassium level is greater than 5 mEq/L

hypermagnesemia: excess magnesium in the extracellular fluid; occurs when the serum magnesium level is above 2.5 mEq/L

hypernatremia: excess sodium in the extracellular fluid; occurs when the serum sodium level is above 145 mEq/L

hyperphosphatemia: excess phosphorus in the extracellular fluid; occurs when the serum phosphorus level is above 2.6 mEq/L

hypervolemia: excess of fluid and solutes in extracellular fluid; can be caused by increased fluid intake, fluid shifts in the body, or renal failure

hypocalcemia: deficit of calcium in extracellular fluid; occurs when the total calcium level is below 8.9 mg/dl or the ionized calcium level is below 4.5 mg/dl

hypocapnia: partial pressure of carbon dioxide in arterial blood that's less than 35 mm Hg

hypochloremia: deficit of chloride in extracellular fluid; occurs when the serum chloride level is below 96 mEq/L

hypochloremic metabolic alkalosis: condition caused by a deficit in chloride and a subsequent increase in bicarbonate that ultimately causes an increase in pH

hypokalemia: deficit in potassium in extracellular fluid; occurs when the serum potassium level is below 3.5 mEq/L

hypomagnesemia: deficit in magnesium in extracellular fluid; occurs when the serum magnesium level is below 1.5 mEq/L

hyponatremia: deficit of sodium in extracellular fluid; occurs when the serum sodium level is below 135 mEq/L

hypophosphatemia: deficit of phosphorus in extracellular fluid; occurs when the serum phosphorus level is below 1.8 mEq/L

hypotonic: solution that has fewer solutes than another solution

hypovolemia: condition marked by the loss of fluid and solutes from extracellular fluid that, if left untreated, can progress to hypovolemic shock

hypovolemic shock: potentially life-threatening condition in which a decreased blood volume leads to low cardiac output and poor tissue perfusion

hypoxemia: oxygen deficit in arterial blood (lower than 80 mm Hg)

hypoxia: oxygen deficit in the tissues

infiltration: leakage of fluid from a blood vessel into surrounding tissue

interstitial fluid: fluid surrounding cells that, with plasma, makes up extracellular fluid

isotonic solution: solution that has the same concentration of solutes as another solution

magnesium: cation located primarily in intracellular fluid that promotes efficient energy use, aids protein synthesis, regulates nerve and muscle impulses, and promotes cardiovascular function

metabolic acidosis: condition in which excess acid or reduced bicarbonate in the blood drops the arterial blood pH below 7.35

metabolic alkalosis: condition in which excess bicarbonate or reduced acid in the blood increases the arterial blood pH above 7.45

oliguria: low urine output; less than 400 ml/24 hours

orthostatic hypotension: drop in blood pressure and increase in heart rate that occur when the body changes position; can be caused by a loss of circulating blood volume

osmolality: concentration of a solution; expressed in milliosmols per kilogram of solution

osmolarity: concentration of a solution; expressed in milliosmols per liter of solution

osmotic pressure: pressure exerted by a solute in solution on a semipermeable membrane

osmoreceptors: special sensing cells in the hypothalamus that respond to changes in the osmolality of blood

osteodystrophy: defective bone development; can occur within the face of prolonged elevated serum phosphorus levels

osteomalacia: softening of bone tissues due to demineralization; often accompanies chronic hypocalcemia

paralytic ileus: obstruction of the bowel due to paralysis of the bowel wall

paresthesia: numbness, tingling, or other abnormal sensations that occur with no apparent cause; possible symptom of electrolyte imbalance

peripherally inserted central catheter (PICC): catheter inserted through a vein above the antecubital area that causes fewer and less severe adverse reactions than a traditional central venous catheter; can be left in place for several months

petechiae: minute hemorrhagic spots in the skin

pH: measurement of the percentage of hydrogen ions in a solution; normal pH is 7.35 to 7.45 of arterial blood

phosphorus: anion located primarily in intracellular fluid; involved in maintaining bone and cell structure, maintaining storage of energy in cells, and aiding oxygen delivery to tissue

pneumothorax: presence of air or gas in the pleural cavity

potassium: major intracellular cation involved in skeletal muscle contraction, fluid distribution, osmotic pressure, and acid-base balance as well as heartbeat regulation

preload: the amount the ventricles are stretched by contained blood

pulmonary edema: abnormal fluid accumulation in the lungs; life-threatening condition

pyelonephritis: inflammation of the renal parenchyma, calyces, and pelvis

reabsorption: taking in, or absorbing, a substance again

renin: enzyme that's released by the kidneys into the blood; it triggers a series of reactions that produce angiotensin, a potent vasoconstrictor

renin-angiotensin-aldosterone system: renal mechanism in which renin, angiotensin, and aldosterone regulate blood pressure and water and sodium levels

resorption: loss of a substance through physiologic or pathologic means such as loss of calcium from bone

respiratory acidosis: acid-base disturbance caused by failure of the lungs to eliminate sufficient carbon dioxide; partial pressure of arterial carbon dioxide above 45 mm Hg and pH below 7.35

respiratory alkalosis: acid-base imbalance that occurs when the lungs eliminate more carbon dioxide than normal; partial pressure of arterial carbon dioxide below 35 mm Hg and pH above 7.45

respiratory failure: condition that occurs when the lungs can't sufficiently maintain arterial oxygenation or eliminate carbon dioxide

rhabdomyolysis: disorder in which skeletal muscle is destroyed; causes intracellular contents to spill into extracellular fluid

Silastic: silicone rubber, the preferred material for sterile catheters intended for long-term total parenteral nutrition because it's more flexible, durable, and biocompatible than plastic

sodium: major cation of extracellular fluid involved in regulating extracellular fluid volume, transmitting nerve impulses, and maintaining acid-base balance

solute: molecules or ions dissolved in a solution

solvent: fluid in which a solute is dissolved

syndrome of inappropriate antidiuretic hormone (SIADH): condition that causes excessive release of antidiuretic hormone, resulting in water retention and sodium excretion

tetany: condition caused by abnormal calcium metabolism; characterized by painful muscle spasms, cramps, and sharp flexion of the wrist and ankle joints

third-space fluid shift: movement of fluid out of the intravascular space into another body space such as the abdominal cavity

Trousseau's sign: carpal (wrist) spasm elicited by applying a blood pressure cuff to the upper arm and inflating it to a pressure 20 mm Hg above the patient's systolic blood pressure; indicates the presence of hypocalcemia

uremia: excess of urea and other nitrogenous wastes in the blood

uremic frost: powdery deposits of urea and uric acid salts on the skin, especially the face; caused by the excretion of nitrogenous compounds in sweat

von Willebrand's disease: syndrome characterized in part by a tendency to bleed and a prolonged bleeding time

water intoxication: condition in which excess water in the cells results in cellular swelling

Index

i refers to an illustration; t refers to a table.

i refers to an illustration; t refers to a table.

i refers to an illustration; t refers to a table.

Notes

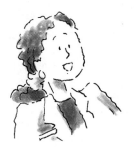

Notes

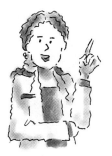

Notes

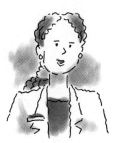